MANUAL OF
SMALL ANIMAL
ANESTHESIA

D1709271

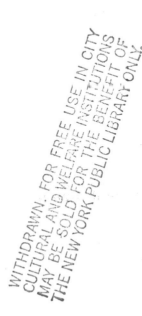

WITHDRAWN. FOR FREE USE IN CITY
CULTURAL AND WELFARE INSTITUTIONS
MAY BE SOLD FOR THE BENEFIT OF
THE NEW YORK PUBLIC LIBRARY ONLY.

THE NEW YORK PUBLIC LIBRARY MM
MID-MANHATTAN LIBRARY HIC
455 FIFTH AVENUE
NEW YORK, NEW YORK 10016

MANUAL OF
SMALL ANIMAL
ANESTHESIA

Second Edition

Robert R. Paddleford, D.V.M.
Diplomate American College of
Veterinary Anesthesiologists
Diplomate American College of
Veterinary Emergency and Critical Care
Associate Professor of Anesthesiology
Director of Anesthesia and
Intensive Care
College of Veterinary Medicine
University of Tennessee
Knoxville, Tennessee

HIC REFERENCE

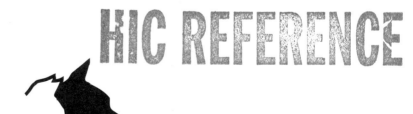

W.B. SAUNDERS COMPANY
A Harcourt Health Sciences Company
Philadelphia   London   Toronto   Montreal   Sydney   Tokyo

W.B. SAUNDERS COMPANY
A *Harcourt Health Sciences Company*

The Curtis Center
Independence Square West
Philadelphia, Pennsylvania 19106

Library of Congress Cataloging-in-Publication Data

Manual of small animal anesthesia / [edited by] Robert R. Paddleford.

p.   cm.

Originally published: New York: Churchill Livingstone, 1988.

Includes bibliographical references and index.

ISBN 0–7216–4060–5

1. Veterinary anesthesia—Handbooks, manuals, etc.   I. Paddleford, Robert R.

SF914.M36 1999   636.089′796—dc21   98–15368

MANUAL OF SMALL ANIMAL ANESTHESIA   ISBN 0–7216–4060–5

Copyright © 1999, 1988 by W.B. Saunders Company.

All rights reserved. No part of this publication may be reproduced or transmitted in any form or by any means, electronic or mechanical, including photocopy, recording, or any information storage and retrieval system, without permission in writing from the publisher.

Printed in the United States of America.

Last digit is the print number: 9   8   7   6   5   4   3

       c. Omni Medical, 7070-C Commerce Circle, Pleasanton, CA 94588; 800-4-Omni-Med

       d. Tri-Anim Health Services, 13170 Telfair Ave., Silmar, CA 91342; 800-874-2646

III. Many varieties of ventilators are available on the new and used markets.

    A. When purchasing a ventilator, it is important to be clear about its intended use.

       1. In general, ventilators are intended for the primary purpose of being used (a) short-term in anesthetized patients in the operating room or (b) long-term in intensive care patients with variable pulmonary complications and weaning difficulties.

       2. Considerable functional overlap exists in that almost any ventilator could be adapted for use in either situation (although if it is used for a purpose different than the one it was designed for, it might be far from ideal.

    B. Ventilators intended for use in the operating room are generally simpler machines than those intended for use in intensive care.

       1. Anesthesia ventilators require a concertina bag (bellows) for the rebreathing of anesthetic gases.

       2. During anesthesia the inspired gas is usually 100% oxygen, and oxygen blenders to regulate the inspired oxygen concentration are unnecessary.

       3. These ventilators generally do not need to have a wide variety of controllable options as ventilatory management is short-term and lungs are usually relatively normal.

       4. Fancy weaning-mode options are usually unnecessary as these patients usually have little trouble regaining adequate spontaneous ventilation.

       5. Numerous alarm and warning functions are less necessary if an anesthetist is sitting right there monitoring the situation.

    C. Ventilators intended for use in intensive care generally have more control options, are more complicated to use, and are more expensive to buy.

       1. A concertina bag is unnecessary, but finite control over inspired oxygen concentrations is essential.

       2. Patients commonly have marginal lung function and neuromuscular debilitation, so the transition from full ventilatory support to spontaneous breathing is often difficult and time-consuming. Multiple weaning-mode options are therefore useful.

       3. Caregivers often have many responsibilities that distract their attention from the ventilator. Numerous alarms and warning functions are therefore necessary.

IV. An automatic ventilator must have some way to initiate an inspiration (after a certain duration of time or in response to the patient's inspiratory effort) and some way to terminate it (at a certain pressure, after a certain volume has been expelled from the ventilator, or after a certain duration of time).

V. The power necessary to operate the ventilator may be provided by compressed gases, electricity, or both.

    A. Compressed-gas ventilators are subject to depleted gas supplies.

    B. Electrically powered ventilators are subject to power outages.

    C. A backup manual means of providing positive pressure ventilation (PPV) must always be available.

VI. Control mechanisms responsible for initiating and terminating the inspiratory phase may be pneumatic-mechanical, pneumatic-fluidic (no moving parts), or electric.

VII. Drive mechanisms (providing the force that causes gas to flow toward the patient) may be pneumatic (gas flows from a high-pressure source to the patient) or piston-driven (usually electrically controlled).

    A. Flow rate is regulated by a variably sized orifice between the high-pressure gas source and the patient or by the rate of movement of the piston.

VENTILATOR TERMINOLOGY

I. *Spontaneous ventilation*—the patient determines both the rate and the volume of each breath.

    A. Most, but not all, normally breathing animals continue to breathe quite satisfactorily while under the influence of a properly administered anesthetic.

II. *Manual ventilation*—a human presence is necessary to make the inspiration happen.

    A. Manual ventilation is necessary to squeeze the rebreathing bag or AMBU bag and to close the thumb-hole on the T-port.

    B. Manual ventilation is necessary to time the breaths with chest compressions during CPR or to gain control over the patient's ventilatory efforts.

III. *Automatic ventilation*—a machine makes the inspiration happen.

    A. The human component of automatic ventilation involves attaching the ventilator to the patient, turning it on, and then evaluating its effectiveness.

IV. *Controlled ventilation*—the ventilator controls both the rate and the volume of each breath.

    A. Controlled ventilation is indicated primarily when an animal is apneic or has medullary disease such that it cannot regulate its carbon dioxide.

    B. It is also indicated when it is desirable to hyperventilate the patient.

V. *Assisted ventilation*—the patient determines the breathing rate, and the ventilator determines the tidal volume.

    A. Assisted ventilation is indicated primarily for animals with normal neuronal responsiveness (they will breath when they need to) but diminished capability to take a deep breath.

    B. If the patient is trying to breathe, but cannot initiate the ventilator, the sensitivity-control knob needs to be adjusted.

VI. *Inspiratory time*—the length of time from the beginning of an inspiration to the end of that inspiration.

VII. *Expiratory time*—the length of time from the end of an inspiration to the beginning of the next inspiration.

    A. Expiratory time includes the exhalation phase and the pause phase.

VIII. *Peak airway pressure*—the highest airway pressure (measured usually at the ventilator) at the end of an inspiration.

    A. Distal airway pressure during a given inspiratory cycle is not as high as proximal airway pressure owing to airway resistance to air flow.

        1. Prolonged inspiratory times close this gap, and vice versa.

        2. Airway diseases that increase resistance to air flow expand this gap.

IX. *Pressure-cycled ventilators*—inspiration will be terminated at a preset pressure.

    A. Tidal volume is determined by the combination of pressure and gas flow rate.

X. *Volume-cycled ventilators*—inspiration will be terminated after a preset volume has been expelled from the ventilator.

    A. High airway pressures may accrue in patients with decreased lung capacity.

XI. *Time-cycled ventilators*—inspiration will be terminated after a preset time.

    A. Tidal volume is determined by the combination of time and gas flow rate.

XII. *Air trapping*—consists of the following:

    A. Lung inflation is active and deflation is passive.

    B. With narrowed lower airways or higher frequency settings, some alveolar units may not empty completely before the next inflation.

    C. These alveolar units become hyperinflated.

        1. The hyperinflation can cause barotrauma.

XIII. *PEEP (positive end-expiratory pressure)*—when the airway pressure is purposely or inadvertently maintained at a level above atmospheric between cycles of the ventilator.

    A. PEEP increases airway (and transpulmonary) pressure and functional residual capacity to help keep small airways open between breaths.

        1. Accumulation of airway fluids increases airway surface tension and the tendency for small-airway and alveolar collapse.

        2. Excessive PEEP can cause thoracic blood flow impairment and barotrauma.

XIV. *Lung (and chest wall) compliance*—consists of the following:

    A. Compliance equals a change in volume per change in pressure.

        1. Virtually all diseases cause the compliance to decrease.

            a. That is, the lung is stiffer and more difficult to ventilate.

            b. That is, a lower volume will be generated from a given change in pressure.

        2. Normal dynamic compliance is about 1 milliliter per centimeter of H_2O of applied airway pressure per kilogram of body weight.

            a. Dynamic lung and chest wall compliance is measured during a normal tidal breath and therefore has a component of airway resistance in it.

            b. Static compliance is measured with an inspiratory hold to allow for redistribution and equilibration of gases throughout the lower airways and air sacs.

                (1) Static compliance is a more accurate measure of lung and chest wall compliance.

                (2) The normal value is somewhat higher than that for dynamic compliance (about 25%).

    B. More important than the actual calculated compliance number are the changes in that number that occur over the course of time.

        1. A progressive decrease in compliance may be due to the following:

            a. Pulmonary parenchymal disease

            b. Pneumothorax

INDICATIONS FOR POSITIVE PRESSURE VENTILATION (PPV)

I. PPV is indicated whenever an animal cannot ventilate adequately on its own.

    A. This indication is usually defined as one of the following:

        1. A Pa_{CO_2} of >60 mm Hg

        2. A low measured/observed minute ventilation (breathing rate or tidal volumes)

    B. PPV is indicated when the hypoventilation is due to neuromuscular disease,

chest wall problems, abdominal enlargements causing anterior displacement of the diaphragm, or pulmonary parenchymal disease.
  1. Treatment should be directed toward the underlying cause when the
     impaired ventilation is due to organic diseases such as airway obstruction
     or pleural space–filling disorders.
  2. *A closed pneumothorax is always an absolute contraindication to PPV.*
  C. PPV is indicated by the following operative procedures:
    1. Those associated with anesthetic-induced respiratory depression in ani-
       mals debilitated by their underlying disease process
    2. Thoracotomies
    3. Prolonged surgical/diagnostic procedures
 II. PPV is indicated whenever an animal cannot oxygenate adequately despite
     oxygen therapy.
  A. This indication is usually defined as one of the following:
    1. A Pa_{O_2} of <60 mm Hg (or Sa_{O_2} is <90%)
    2. Cyanosis
  B. Increased airway pressure opens small airways and alveoli, reestablishing
     their gas-exchange capabilities.
III. PPV is indicated when the animal is having to work excessively hard, irrespec-
     tive of the actual blood gas measurements.
  A. These animals often become exhausted and succumb to hypoxemia.

GOALS OF PPV

  I. The main goal of PPV is to restore oxygenation and ventilation to accept-
     able levels.
  A. This goal is to be attained while minimizing the deleterious effects of PPV.
 II. Short-term 100% oxygen poses no problems.
  A. Inspired oxygen concentrations greater than 60% for longer than 24 hours
     may induce pulmonary oxygen toxicity.
  B. The oxygen-hemoglobin dissociation curve, however, is fairly flat over a
     Pa_{O_2} of 120 mm Hg, and there is little physiologic reason to maintain it
     above this value.
III. The Pa_{CO_2} should be maintained at 30–45 mm Hg.

GENERAL GUIDELINES FOR VENTILATOR SETTINGS
FOR PPV

  I. The general guidelines for PPV of animals with relatively normal lungs apply
     to all methods of mechanical inflation of the lungs, be they manual or
     mechanical.
  A. Proximal airway pressure
    1. 10–20 cm H_2O is enough pressure to inflate a normal lung.
      a. Larger patients need a higher pressure range (15–20 cm H_2O) to lift
         their heavier chest wall.
    2. Some situations are associated with decreased lung or chest wall compli-
       ance, and in these patients higher pressures will be required to inflate
       the lungs.
      a. Patients with pulmonary parenchymal transudative or exudative dis-
         eases may require higher pressures.

     b. Patients with restrictive diseases such as abdominal or pleural space–consuming disorders may require higher pressures.

     c. Pressures may be increased to whatever it takes to ventilate the lung or to the limit of the ventilator, whichever comes first.

     d. Higher pressures may cause thoracic blood flow impairment or barotrauma.

B. Tidal volume

    1. Normal lungs will be well ventilated with a tidal volume of 10–20 ml/kg.

    2. This volume may need to be increased in patients with pulmonary parenchymal disease.

C. Inspiratory time

    1. About 1 second is long enough to achieve a full tidal volume.

     a. Small lungs require less time to fill at the flow rates involved with most cases of PPV.

      (1) In a cat, an inspiratory time of 0.5 second is usually long enough.

     b. Large lungs either require a longer time to fill (at the same gas flow rate) or (as is usual) require higher flow rates to fill them within 1 second.

     c. Long inspiratory times do the following:

      (1) They generate larger tidal volumes at the same airway pressure because the lungs have more time to expand.

      (2) Within reason, long inspiratory times constitute one of the maneuvers used to improve oxygenation in patients with pulmonary parenchymal disease.

      (3) They also predispose the patient to impaired thoracic blood flow and barotrauma.

     d. Very short inspiratory times may not allow time for the distribution of volume to the lower airways.

D. Ventilatory rate

    1. At reasonable tidal volumes, a cycle rate of 10–12 times per minute will generate an adequate minute ventilation in an animal with normal lungs.

    2. The breathing rate may need to be increased in animals with abnormal lung function.

     a. Breathing rate may be increased to whatever it takes to provide acceptable ventilation or to the limit of the ventilator, whichever comes first.

E. Minute ventilation

    1. For a patient with normal lungs, 150–250 ml/kg per minute is an adequate minute ventilation.

    2. The adequacy of the minute ventilation is better defined by the Pa_{CO2}.

     a. The Pa_{CO2} should be maintained at 30–45 mm Hg.

    3. When smaller than normal tidal volumes are applied, the breathing rate may need to be increased to assure adequate minute alveolar ventilation.

    4. When there is an increase in anatomic or physiologic dead space, total minute ventilation may need to be increased to assure adequate minute alveolar ventilation.

F. End-expiratory pressure

    1. Normal lungs ventilate and oxygenate quite well with an end-expiratory pressure of zero (atmospheric).

2. A very small amount of end-expiratory pressure (2 cm H_2O) could be applied to the normal lung to help minimize atelectasis during prolonged positional stasis.
   a. An occasional deep breath (a sigh) to an airway pressure of 30 cm H_2O at regular intervals (30 minutes) will also help prevent intraoperative small-airway and alveolar collapse.
3. An increase in airway fluid (transudate or exudate) increases surface tension and increases the tendency for small-airway and alveolar collapse.
   a. The application of higher airway pressure, higher tidal volumes, longer inspiratory times, and faster breathing rates will improve blood oxygenation in this situation but will also predispose the patient to impaired thoracic blood flow and barotrauma.
   b. The application of higher end-expiratory pressure will maintain higher transmural pressure and higher functional residual capacity and help prevent small-airway and alveolar collapse.
      (1) The pressure should be applied during the expiratory phase of the ventilatory cycle when atelectasis is prominent.
      (2) It should be no higher than necessary so that it will not predispose the patient so much to impaired thoracic blood flow or barotrauma.
4. Positive end-expiratory pressure (PEEP) is available on most ventilators as an adjustable knob.
   a. PEEP can also be achieved by attaching a corrugated breathing tube to the exhalation port of the ventilator or anesthetic machine and then placing the other end underwater.
      (1) The depth to which the end of the tube is submerged determines the airway pressure at the end of exhalation.
   b. PEEP can also be applied by other commercial apparati.
5. Expiratory resistance, achieved by prolonging the duration of time that positive pressure is applied to the airways, functions somewhat like PEEP to improve oxygenation.
   a. Expiratory resistance can be applied by attaching a narrow-aperture device to the exhalation port of the ventilator or patient circuit.
6. Continuous positive airway pressure (CPAP) is an adjustment knob on some ventilators. In this mode the patient breathes spontaneously around a preset airway pressure.

II. Whenever ventilator settings do not seem to meet the needs of the patient or the aforementioned goals, take the following steps:
   A. Make sure that the ventilator settings are indeed what you had planned (including the oxygen supply).
   B. Make sure that there is patient synchrony (that the patient is allowing the ventilator to do its job and is not fighting it).
      1. The level of anesthesia may need to be deepened.
   C. Make sure that other untoward respiratory stimulants are not present (hyperthermia, light level of anesthesia).
   D. Make sure that other organic diseases are not present or worsened (pneumothorax).
   E. Adjust ventilator settings.
III. Optimal ventilator settings
   A. The optimal ventilator settings are the least aggressive ones that provide acceptable ventilation (Pa_{CO_2} of 30–60 mm Hg) and oxygenation (Pa_{O_2} of

at least 60 mm Hg) with the lowest inspired oxygen concentration (only applies when the ventilation procedure exceeds 12–24 hours) (<60%, or Pa_{O_2} of <250 mm Hg) and without thoracic blood flow impairment.

B. The optimal ventilator settings also do the following:
1. Generate the highest oxygen delivery
2. Generate the highest mixed-venous oxygen
3. Are associated with the highest lung-compliance calculation

PROBLEMS WITH AND PRECAUTIONS FOR PPV

I. Thoracic blood flow impairment
   A. Positive pressure inflation of the lungs causes a proportional increase in pleural pressure.
      1. This increase in pleural pressure compresses the vena cavae and pulmonary veins and decreases venous return to both the right and the left side of the heart.
      2. The effect is to decrease stroke volume, cardiac output, and arterial blood pressure.
      3. The degree of impairment of intrathoracic blood flow depends on the following:
         a. Magnitude of increase in pleural pressure
         b. Length of time pressure is applied (inspiratory time)
         c. Ventilatory rate; the faster the rate, the less time the cardiovascular system has to recuperate between inspirations
         d. Baseline central intravenous pressure (the blood volume); the lower the CVP, the greater the impairment
   B. Circulatory impairment is considered excessive if inspiration is associated with a moderate to severe diminution of pulse quality, arterial blood pressure, or cardiac output.
      1. This effect can be checked on a breath-to-breath basis.
   C. If excessive circulatory impairment exists, take the following steps:
      1. Adjust ventilator settings downward if possible.
      2. Increase blood volume (central venous pressure).
   D. Diseased lungs are often poorly compliant, and although higher airway pressures may be required to ventilate them, less of the pressure is transmitted to the pleural space and there is less tendency to impair circulation.

II. Barotrauma
   A. Aggressive ventilator settings may be associated with alveolar septal rupture, pneumomediastinum, pneumothorax, pulmonary hemorrhage, and air embolism.
      1. Preexisting parenchymal bullae, recent parenchymal rupture, and pneumonia lower the threshold to physical lung damage.
   B. Barotrauma can occur even at normal ventilator settings.
   C. All ventilated animals should be monitored continuously for the development of a pneumothorax.
      1. If a pneumothorax develops, a chest drain must be inserted and continuous chest drainage provided.

III. Mechanical problems
   A. The endotracheal tube may become kinked, occluded, or dislodged.

   B. The breathing circuit may become disconnected or filled with condensed water.
   C. The ventilator may malfunction, or its oxygen supply may become depleted.
IV. Iatrogenic hyperventilation
   A. Hypocapnia decreases cerebral blood flow; if flow decreases below 20 mm Hg, some degree of cerebral hypoxia may occur.
   B. Hypocapnia is respiratory alkalosis and, if severe, may be associated with hypokalemia, hypocalcemia (ionized), and ventricular arrhythmias.
V. PPV generally improves alveolar minute ventilation and may be associated with a deepening of the level of anesthesia if the vaporizer is not adjusted.
VI. As with all mechanical equipment, an infection hazard exists with PPV equipment. Precautions follow:
   A. The patient circuit should be regularly washed with soap and water, thoroughly rinsed, and completely dried.
   B. Bacterial filters should be used if the animal has a known respiratory tract infection.
   C. Cold sterilization may be accomplished with 0.25% acetic acid, alkaline glutaraldehyde, or 70% alcohol. Equipment must then be thoroughly washed, rinsed, and dried.
   D. Polypropylene, polycarbonate, FEP-Teflon, and polymethylpentane products are steam-sterilizable.

TROUBLESHOOTING GENERAL VENTILATOR AND PATIENT PROBLEMS

I. Patient-ventilator asynchrony (patient bucking or fighting the ventilator)
   A. Inadequate patient sedation
   B. Hypoxemia (see section II that follows)
   C. Hypercapnia (see section III that follows)
   D. Hyperthermia
   E. Inappropriate ventilator settings
II. Hypoxemia
   A. Low inspired oxygen concentration
      1. Oxygen supply depleted
      2. Oxygen not attached to ventilator
      3. Blender problem
   B. Pneumothorax
   C. Pulmonary parenchymal disease (pneumonia)
   D. Disconnected or loose ventilator tubing
   E. Patient-ventilator asynchrony
III. Hypercapnia (Pa_{CO2} of >45 is the official definition of hypercapnia and hypoventilation; in the interest of minimizing lung barotrauma, it is permissible to allow a Pa_{CO2} of up to 60 mm Hg)
   A. Pneumothorax
   B. Patient-ventilator asynchrony
   C. Endotracheal tube obstruction or malfunction
   D. Disconnected or loose ventilator circuit
   E. Inappropriate ventilator settings

      F. Dead-space rebreathing (if there is a lot of mechanical dead space added to the upper airway for measuring apparati, such as the end-tidal carbon dioxide)

IV. Air-leak sounds during inspiration
      A. Cuff not adequately inflated
      B. Tube that has slipped partially out of the trachea

V. Fluid ("bubbly") sounds
      A. During inspiration only
         1. Leak around the tube
           a. Cuff not properly inflated (maybe the inflation valve or the cuff has a leak)
           b. Tube that has partially pulled out of the trachea
         2. Mucus accumulation in the tracheal tube or trachea
         3. Fluid accumulation in the corrugated ventilator tubing
      B. Both during inspiration and expiration
         1. Mucus accumulation in the tracheal tube or trachea
         2. Fluid accumulation in the lower airways
         3. Fluid accumulation in the corrugated ventilator tubing

VI. Miscellaneous ventilator problems
      A. Ventilator does not cycle.
         1. For an electrically powered ventilator, check whether it is plugged into the power source and is turned on.
         2. For a pneumatically powered ventilator, check whether it is plugged into the oxygen source and whether the tank is turned on, oxygen is in the tank, and the ventilator is turned on.
      B. Ventilator cycles but does not seem to be generating a tidal volume in the patient.
         1. Tidal volume or inspiratory pressure not set high enough
         2. Disconnection between ventilator and patient
         3. Cuff not inflated
         4. Endotracheal tube or airway obstruction
         5. Pressure limit set too low
         6. Low compliance (pneumothorax, respiratory distress syndrome)
      C. Inspiratory times are very long.
         1. Flow rate set too low
         2. Inspiratory time set too long
         3. Peak pressure set too high
         4. Leak in the patient circuit
         5. Driving pressure too low—depleted oxygen supply
      D. Inspiratory times are very short.
         1. Flow rate set too high
         2. Pressure limit set too low
         3. Inspiratory time set too short
         4. Obstruction

WEANING A PATIENT OFF VENTILATORY SUPPORT

I. Weaning an animal off ventilatory support (partially assisting its breathing effort until it gains the capability to ventilate and oxygenate totally on its

own), requires special attention because the animal may be slow to develop
the ability to maintain its own ventilation and oxygenation requirements.

A. For animals that were normal prior to anesthesia induction and have not
   suffered intraoperative complications, weaning is simply a matter of
   allowing carbon dioxide to accumulate to the level that it will stimulate the
   respiratory centers.

   1. Animals should be in a light stage of anesthesia before weaning is
      attempted.
      a. Opioid agents may need to be reversed.
      b. Neuromuscular blocking agents need to be reversed.

   2. Blood oxygen levels will decrease much faster than carbon dioxide levels
      will increase; therefore, the following will apply:
      a. Weaning to spontaneous ventilation should be done while the animal
         is breathing an enriched oxygen mixture (as opposed to room air).
      b. The animal needs to be hypoventilated (as opposed to just letting it
         be apneic until it starts breathing again).
      c. The general rule of thumb is to give the animal one deep breath
         every 30 seconds until it starts breathing again.

B. Weaning should be done more carefully when there is some reason to
   believe that the patient will have trouble reestablishing adequate ventilation
   and oxygenation.

   1. Many ways are available to wean a patient off PPV.
      a. There is no one magic way that always works.

   2. Two types of assisted ventilation follow:
      a. In one type of assisted ventilation, the patient has only to initiate
         each breath.
         (1) You can gradually decrease the automatic frequency of the venti-
             lator, forcing the patient to trigger the ventilator more fre-
             quently.
      b. In another type of assisted ventilation, the ventilator provides every
         breath, so the work demanded of the patient is minimal.
         (1) You can make it progressively harder for the patient to trigger
             the ventilator.

   3. Pressure support
      a. Pressure support is a spontaneous breathing mode.
         (1) It can be used only if the patient is making some effort to breath.
      b. The amount of effort required of the patient depends on the level
         of pressure support.

   4. Intermittent mandatory ventilation (IMV or SIMV)
      a. IMV may or may not be synchronized with the breathing effort of
         the patient.
      b. In IMV, the patient breathes spontaneously and intermittently (at a
         preestablished rate), and the ventilator is triggered to deliver a (pre-
         set) tidal volume.
      c. IMV requires the patient to do some work—it has to breath entirely
         on its own between tidal volumes generated by the ventilator.

   5. Manual technique
      a. The patient is intermittently removed from the ventilator for gradu-
         ally increasing periods of time.

   6. Continuous positive airway pressure (CPAP)

a. In CPAP, spontaneous breathing occurs at an elevated airway pressure.

b. CPAP is primarily intended for patients that can ventilate but cannot oxygenate adequately.

HIGH-FREQUENCY VENTILATION (HFV)

I. High-frequency ventilation (HFV) techniques can be broadly divided into three categories:

  A. High-frequency positive pressure ventilation (HFPPV)

    1. HFPPV is provided by a conventional ventilator with low internal compliance and ventilation rates of about 60–120 per minute.

  B. High-frequency jet ventilation (HFJV)

    1. HFJV utilizes a jet nozzle or a catheter through which gas is forced under high pressure.

    2. Tidal volume depends partly on the jet stream flow and partly on an entrained gas flow.

    3. Cycle rates generally are between 100 and 400 per minute.

  C. High-frequency oscillation (HFO)

    1. HFO utilizes an oscillating diaphragm or piston and a bias flow of fresh gas.

    2. In contrast to other forms of PPV, both inspiration and exhalation are active in HFO.

    3. Cycle rates are generally between 400 and 3000 per minute.

II. Each technique of HFV utilizes progressively smaller tidal volumes.

  A. Tidal volumes as low as about 50% of physiologic dead space are compatible with effective ventilation and oxygenation.

  B. Mechanisms of alveolar ventilation

    1. Bulk convective gas flow

    2. Asymmetric inspiratory and expiratory gas flow profiles

    3. Redistribution of gas volume between alveolar units with unequal inflation time constants

    4. Radial molecular dispersion

    5. Molecular diffusion

    6. Cardiogenic mixing

III. Potential advantages and uses of HFV compared against conventional ventilation techniques

  A. Provides effective ventilation at lower airway pressures that might be associated with less cardiovascular impairment.

    1. The result is to minimize changes in intracranial pressure.

  B. Useful during bronchoscopy

  C. Useful in patients with syndromes associated with airway leakage (bronchopleural fistula, airway surgery)

  D. Provides a quieter operating field during thoracic surgery

  E. Provides access to a small airway via catheter (HFJV) (in newborns and patients undergoing lower airway resections)

  F. Provides emergency ventilatory support via a transtracheal catheter (HFJV)

  G. Minimizes airway trauma (HFO)

  H. Provides ventilatory management during CPR

       I. Provides ventilatory support during weaning procedures

     J. May be more effective than conventional ventilation techniques in the management of pulmonary edema (however, evidence from studies in humans and animals suggests that HFV techniques may also be less, or of equal, efficacy)

IV. Potential disadvantages and precautions for HFV

    A. Requires high fresh gas utilization

    B. Causes tracheal damage (HFJV)

    C. Produces alveolar overinflation caused by inadequate exhalation times (gas trapping)

    D. Is prone to catheter misplacement (HFJV)

       1. Jetting of gases against one spot on the tracheal epithelium—excessive epithelial drying and shear damage

       2. Displacement into the subcutaneous tissues—rapid, severe subcutaneous emphysema

V. Although HFJV can very effectively ventilate even large dogs for short periods of time, results of long-term (>12 hours) HFJV procedures have not been impressive owing to the large amount of mucus accumulation in the trachea.

Perioperative Monitoring

Chapter

7

Steve C. Haskins

WHY MONITOR?

I. The purpose of anesthesia is to provide reversible unconsciousness, amnesia, analgesia, and immobility, with minimal risk to the patient.
   A. Anesthetic drugs and adjuvants may compromise patient homeostasis at unpredictable times and in unpredictable ways.
   B. Anesthetic crises tend to be rapid in onset and devastating in nature.
   C. The purpose of monitoring is to maximize the beneficial aspects of the anesthetic experience while minimizing the decrement of organ function, thereby maximizing the opportunity for a full and uneventful recovery.

WHAT TO MONITOR?

I. Perioperative monitoring begins in the preoperative period when the patient is assessed to determine the existence of any abnormal processes. The monitoring continues for several hours (as many as necessary to ensure an uneventful recovery) into the postoperative period.
   A. Preoperatively, the magnitude of any abnormal disease processes that may compromise the patient's response to anesthesia and the operative procedure is estimated.
      1. This preoperative evaluation provides the basis for tailoring drug selection and intraoperative and postoperative monitoring and support to the specific needs of the patient.
   B. Intraoperative monitoring covers the following:
      1. Adequate depth of anesthesia
      2. Adequate muscular relaxation
      3. Appropriate physiologic response to the anesthetic drugs and the state of general anesthesia
   C. Postoperative monitoring covers the following:
      1. Adequate analgesia
      2. Physiologic recovery from the effects of anesthesia

IS THE ANIMAL ADEQUATELY ANESTHETIZED?

I. Is the animal unconscious, unaware, analgesic, and amnesic, with adequate muscular relaxation?
II. With most anesthetics (barbiturates, etomidate, propofol, and the inhalationals), unconsciousness, unawareness, analgesia, and amnesia are achieved prior to cessation of spontaneous muscular movement.
   A. The lack of spontaneous muscular movement implies unconsciousness and amnesia.

B. This principle applies also to anesthetics that have no inherent analgesic properties (barbiturates, etomidate, propofol, halothane).

C. Muscular movement or an autonomic response to surgical stimulation does not imply conscious perception of the stimulus.
1. Deeper levels of anesthesia may be required if these responses are considered undesirable, per se.

D. The same can probably be said of ketamine even though its pattern of inducing unconsciousness is somewhat different from that of the traditional anesthetics.
1. Hallucinations are not the same as recall or conscious awareness.
2. Ketamine is never used by itself, for reasons of muscle hypertonus, and the adjunctive drugs that must be used produce additive CNS depressant effects.
3. Ketamine is considered to be a good analgesic in human beings.
   a. Electroencephalographic evidence shows that ketamine has antinociceptive qualities in animals as well as humans.
   b. Ketamine appears to be a good analgesic for animals.

E. Opioid-based anesthetic protocols are not potent unconsciousness-producing, nor muscle-relaxing, agents in comparison with other anesthetics.
1. Opioids are considered to produce profound analgesia but not necessarily loss of awareness.

DETERMINING DEPTH OF ANESTHESIA

I. Anesthetic depth is determined by evaluating muscular tone and muscular reflexes.
A. The signs vary from individual to individual, and from moment to moment, depending on the balance between the following:
1. Amount of anesthetic "on board"
2. Amount of surgical stimulation
3. Presence of adjunctive events such as hypotension or hypothermia
B. When the signs are unclear and contradictory, anesthetic administration should be slightly reduced until the signs of light anesthetic depth become clear.

II. All signs should be evaluated. Then a composite estimate of anesthetic depth can be made.
A. The patient's recent history of anesthetic dosages (i.e., the vaporizer settings) is a relatively important index.
1. Larger dosages than those normally recommended should produce a deep level of anesthesia. Smaller dosages should produce a light level.
   a. The anesthetic dosage must also be evaluated in the light of adjunctive diseases.
      (1) Hypothermic animals require smaller than normal dosages; they would be overanesthetized with the usual dosages.
2. The minimum alveolar anesthetic concentration (MAC) of an inhalational anesthetic indicates the amount that will prevent muscular movement in response to a strong surgical stimulus in 50% (MAC_{50}) or 95% (MAC_{95}) of an average patient population.
   a. MAC is not the *definition* of anesthetic depth in an individual patient.
B. Gross, purposeful, spontaneous, muscular movement is a reliable sign of a light level of anesthesia.

    1. The anesthetic level may need to be deepened if surgical stimulation is to be continued.

    2. Muscular twitching may be associated with etomidate, propofol, enflurane, and methoxyflurane even at adequate levels of anesthesia.

    3. Muscle hypertonus may be associated with ketamine anesthesia even at otherwise adequate levels of anesthesia.

    4. Opioids are not particularly good CNS depressants and, unless complemented by other adjuvants, are associated with spontaneous movement.

    5. Shivering may occur at lighter levels of anesthesia but is not, per se, an indication that the anesthetic level is too light.

C. Reflex muscular movement in response to surgical stimulation is a reliable sign of a light level of anesthesia.

    1. It is unlikely that these patients are consciously aware of anything, including discomfort from the surgical stimulation.

    2. Anesthetic level need not be deepened unless the movement interferes with the surgical procedure.

D. Reflex hemodynamic response to surgical stimulation is a reliable sign of a light level of anesthesia.

    1. It is unlikely that these patients are consciously aware of any discomfort.

    2. Anesthetic level need not be deepened unless the hemodynamic response is likely to be harmful to the patient, as in the case of the following:

        a. Excessive tachycardia or hypertension

        b. Ventricular arrhythmias

E. Mandibular and orbicularis oculi muscle tone should be high in light levels of anesthesia, fair in medium levels of anesthesia, and absent in deep levels of anesthesia.

    1. Muscle tone is herein defined as the resistance to being manually opened.

    2. The species and size of the patient must be factored into the evaluation.

    3. Wide individual variation in this sign exists; some animals, and all puppies and kittens, have very little muscle tone even in light anesthesia.

    4. Ketamine enhances muscle tone, so this sign cannot be used to assess depth of anesthesia when ketamine is used.

F. The presence of a palpebral reflex suggests a light level of anesthesia.

    1. The absence of it suggests a medium or deep level of anesthesia.

    2. There is wide individual variation in this sign.

    3. This sign cannot be used with ketamine anesthesia because it is always present with that kind of anesthesia.

G. Ventromedial rotation of the eyeball suggests a medium level of anesthesia.

    1. The eyeball will be central if the animal is in a light or deep level of anesthesia rather than a medium level.

    2. There is wide individual variation in this sign; in some animals, the eyeballs never rotate.

    3. This sign cannot be used with ketamine anesthesia because the eyeballs never rotate with that kind of anesthesia.

H. Pupil size is highly variable but is usually neither constricted nor dilated in a medium level of anesthesia.

    1. Dilated pupils may be caused by the following:

        a. Deep levels of anesthesia

        b. Topical anticholinergic medication
        c. Ketamine
        d. Brain stem disease
        e. Death

I. The pupil should constrict or the eyelid blink when a bright light is shined on the retina while the patient is in light and medium levels of anesthesia.
    1. Lack of this reflex may be caused by the following:
        a. Deep levels of anesthesia
        b. Topical anticholinergic medication (systemic anticholinergics may blunt the response)
        c. Intracranial disease

J. The cornea should be moist.
    1. Dry corneas may be caused by the following:
        a. Deep levels of anesthesia
        b. Open eyelids (including ketamine anesthesia)

K. Heart rate, breathing rate, and arterial blood pressure are unreliable premonitory indicators of the depth of anesthesia.
    1. Physiologic values commonly do not change until after the crisis.
    2. One of the causes of decreasing values is a deep level of anesthesia, but there are many other causes.
    3. Bradycardia and bradypnea are common consequences of opioid-based anesthetic protocols.
    4. Any anesthetic protocol can cause hypotension even at light levels of anesthesia.

L. A positive sign is more reliable than a negative sign.
    1. Strong mandibular muscle tone is a reliable sign of a light level of anesthesia; but the lack of it is not necessarily a sign of a deep level.

HAVING TROUBLE KEEPING THE PATIENT ANESTHETIZED?

I. Inappropriate flowmeter settings
    A. Low flows with VOC vaporizers add little anesthetic to the breathing circuit.
        1. Fresh gas flows should be 20–50 ml/kg per minute for the first 15–30 minutes and then decreased to 10–20 ml/kg per minute.
        2. Tec-type vaporizers reportedly require a flow rate of at least 200 ml/min to output indicated anesthetic concentrations.
    B. High flows with VIC vaporizers cause dilution of the in-circuit anesthetic concentrations.

II. Vaporizer problems
    A. Is the vaporizer turned on, or is it set at a very low setting?
    B. Is dysfunction caused by water or preservative accumulation in the vaporization chamber?
        1. If so, send the machine to the factory for cleaning and recalibration.
    C. Is there anesthetic in the vaporizer?
    D. Is it the correct anesthetic?
        1. Low-vapor-pressure anesthetics placed into vaporizers designed for an-

esthetics with high vapor pressure will result in very low anesthetic vapor output.

   E. Is the vaporizer disconnected from the fresh gas flow? Or are there leaks between the flowmeter and the vaporizer?

   F. Is the vaporizer disconnected from the breathing circuit? Or are there leaks between the vaporizer and the circuit?

III. Endoesophageal or endobronchial intubation

   A. Check the position of the endotracheal tube, and reposition it if necessary.

IV. Uninflated cuff

   A. In this case, the patient is breathing in room air from around the tube.

 V. Anesthetic circuit problems

   A. Are any connections open to room air?

VI. Frequent use of the oxygen flush dilutes in-circuit anesthetic concentrations.

VII. Early redistribution of the injectable induction agent prior to adequate loading with the inhalational agent.

   A. If a patient hypoventilates after induction, give one deep breath per 30 seconds to make sure that the alveoli are exposed to the inhalational agent.

   B. Maybe the vaporizer setting was decreased too rapidly.

VIII. Individual variation in anesthetic requirements.

 IX. Variations in surgical stimulation.

   A. Variations are more likely when the primary anesthetic has no inherent analgesic qualities.

  X. Look-alike problems

   A. Tachypnea, for instance, can be caused by many problems other than a light level of anesthesia, including the following:

      1. Hypercapnia from dead-space rebreathing
      2. Hypoxemia
      3. Hyperthermia
      4. Hypotension

   B. Not all spontaneous movement is due to a light level of anesthesia.

   C. Carefully recheck the patient and the signs of anesthetic depth to avoid misdiagnosing a problem.

WHY IS THIS ANIMAL SO DEEPLY ANESTHETIZED?

 I. An animal that is excited (outwardly or inwardly) prior to induction will require a heavy dose of anesthetic for induction.

   A. In this case, once the emotional stimulus has subsided, the animal will be too deeply anesthetized.

   B. Use sedative premedication to quell preinduction stress and thus avoid using a too-heavy dose of anesthesia for induction.

   C. Handle the animal in a calm, reassuring manner before induction of anesthesia.

 II. Individual variation exists regarding anesthetic requirements.

III. Synergistic diseases

   A. Hypothermia
   B. Hypotension
   C. Systemic debilitation by any preexisting disease
   D. Hypoalbuminemia

1. Most anesthetic agents are highly protein bound.
   a. The lack of binding sites increases the proportion of free drug available for distribution into the brain.
IV. Low flows with VIC vaporizers
V. Non-rebreathing circuits are more efficient than circle systems.
   A. Inspired anesthetic concentration responds rapidly to changes in vaporizer or flowmeter settings.
VI. Positive pressure ventilation increases alveolar ventilation and the respiratory membrane surface area.
   A. Alveolar anesthetic concentration equilibrates more rapidly with that of the circuit.
VII. Improper vaporizer function
   A. When a vaporizer malfunctions, anesthetic output usually, but not always, decreases.
   B. Low fresh gas flow with older (pre–Tec 3) vaporizers are associated with higher anesthetic output.
   C. High-vapor-pressure anesthetics placed into vaporizers designed for anesthetics with low vapor pressure will result in very high anesthetic vapor output.

WHY IS THIS ANIMAL HAVING SUCH A PROLONGED RECOVERY FROM ANESTHESIA?

I. Excessive doses of anesthetic, causing the following:
   A. Too deep a level of anesthesia
   B. Saturation of redistribution sites
      1. The recovery effect from most anesthetics is heavily dependent on the redistribution of anesthetic away from the brain to other tissues.
      2. The animal was not too deeply anesthetized, but muscle and third-space anesthetic accumulations provided a reservoir for significant "reverse" redistribution of anesthetic.
   C. Incomplete reversal of reversible anesthetics
II. Intramuscular administration of an intravenous anesthetic
   A. Because of slower absorption than with intravenous dosages, intramuscular dosages must be higher to achieve the same anesthetic effect.
      1. The animal was not too deeply anesthetized, but the muscle reservoir provided for prolonged and significant anesthetic uptake.
   B. The subcutaneous route (including intramuscular-intended injections that ended up in an intrafascicular fat plane) are associated with slow absorption.
III. Delayed metabolism and elimination of the anesthetic agent, caused by the following:
   A. Severe diffuse liver disease
   B. Portocaval shunts
   C. Oliguria (produced by ketamine in cats)
   D. Slow thiobarbiturate metabolism (in sight hounds)
IV. Postoperative hypoventilation, delaying the elimination of inhalational anesthetics
V. Postoperative administration of sedative analgesics, tranquilizers, or anticonvulsants
VI. Synergistic diseases

WHAT ARE THE PHYSIOLOGIC CONSEQUENCES OF THE ANESTHETIZED STATE?

I. Animals can experience adverse physiologic responses to anesthetic drugs at any anesthetic depth.

II. Although the pharmacodynamic effects of the various anesthetic drugs vary, the mechanisms by which they cause anesthetic emergencies are the same: excessive hypotension, excessive bradycardia, excessive arrhythmias, excessive myocardial depression, excessive vasodilation or vasoconstriction, excessive hypoventilation, excessive hypoxemia, and so on.

III. It is the purpose of the preanesthetic examination to determine to what extent the preexisting underlying disease processes predispose the patient to the preceding problems.

IV. It is the purpose of anesthetic drug planning to select those agents that best complement the underlying disease processes so as to minimize the development of the preceding problems.

V. It is the purpose of the monitoring procedures to watch for these problems in the perioperative period.

PULMONARY

Terminology

I. *Respiratory inadequacy* is the inability of the respiratory system to normally oxygenate the blood or to adequately eliminate carbon dioxide from the blood.

II. *Respiratory failure* is the point at which the patient will succumb to the consequences of the respiratory inadequacy if effective corrective measures are not taken.

III. *Hypoventilation* is a below normal alveolar minute ventilation or an above normal arterial partial pressure of carbon dioxide (Pa_{CO_2}).

IV. *Hyperventilation* is an above normal alveolar minute ventilation or a below normal Pa_{CO_2}.

V. *Tachypnea* is a fast breathing rate.
   A. It does not equate with hyperventilation and is often associated with hypoventilation.

VI. *Bradypnea* is a slow breathing rate.

Breathing Rate and Effort

I. Breathing rates in normal dogs and cats vary between 10 and 50 breaths per minute, preoperatively or intraoperatively.

II. A change in breathing rate is a sensitive indicator of an underlying change in the status of the patient. A single value for breathing rate is, however, of limited diagnostic value for the following reasons:
   A. It defines only itself without reference to the adequacy of overall pulmonary function.
   B. Normal animals can exhibit widely variable breathing rates.
   C. The combination of breathing rate and tidal volume may have diagnostic significance.

III. Bradypnea and decreased breathing effort may be due to the following:
   A. Excessive anesthetic depth
      1. Most anesthetics are potent respiratory depressants.

B. Hypocapnia in an anesthetized patient
C. Medullary depression by severe metabolic disturbances
D. Organic lesions such as cerebral edema
E. Individual variation
1. Some animals are very sensitive to the respiratory depressant effects of anesthetics.
F. Neuromuscular interference
1. Spinal cord edema secondary to needle tap or surgical trauma
2. Neuromuscular blocking agents
3. Aminoglycoside antibiotics (large doses)
IV. Tachypnea and increased breathing effort may be due to the following:
A. Too light a level of anesthesia
B. Too deep a level of anesthesia
1. In patients with anesthetic-induced muscular weakness, the inability to take deep breaths is compensated by taking many small breaths.
2. Positive pressure ventilation should be instituted until the patient is in a light enough stage of anesthesia to maintain a coordinated and adequate minute ventilation.
C. Hypercapnia or hypoxemia
D. Hypotension
E. Hyperthermia
F. Airway obstructions (upper or lower)
G. Pleural space–filling diseases such as pneumothorax
H. Pulmonary parenchymal disease such as pulmonary edema
I. Atelectasis
J. Drug-induced panting
1. Opioids (fentanyl/droperidol, oxymorphone)
K. The normal breathing pattern of some patients during anesthesia is rapid and shallow in nature.

Nature and Rhythm of Breathing Effort

I. Arrhythmic breathing patterns are indicative of a medullary respiratory control problem.
A. Cheyne-Stokes breathing (cycling between hyperventilation and hypoventilation) may be seen in deeply anesthetized animals.
B. Apneustic breathing (inspiratory hold) may be seen in dogs and cats anesthetized with ketamine or tiletamine.
1. Otherwise, apneustic breathing represents *serious* midbrain disease.
C. Marked variations in either rate or volume, cyclic hyperventilation and hypoventilation, cyclic hypoventilation and apnea, rapid breathing interspersed with periods of apnea, and central neurogenic tachypnea are all indicative of central respiratory control disease.
D. Agonal gasps, characterized by a gaping of the mouth and sometimes by spasmodic contraction of the diaphragm, do not constitute real breathing even if there is movement of some air. Such gasps usually occur sometime after the animal has suffered cardiac arrest and are truly a terminal medullary sign.

E. Diaphragmatic breathing with little or no thoracic component may be due to the following:
  1. Deep levels of anesthesia
  2. Upper thoracic spinal cord dysfunction with an intact phrenic nerve
F. Hiccoughs
  1. Diaphragmatic "twitching" associated with each heartbeat
    a. Phrenic nerve "irritability" of unknown cause
G. Apnea may be caused by the following:
  1. In the early postinduction period, a combination of anesthetic-induced respiratory depression and excitement/hyperventilation-induced hypocapnia
    a. Administer one breath every 30 seconds until spontaneous ventilation resumes.
  2. Severe medullary disease: herniation or thromboembolism
  3. Severe cervical spinal cord disease

Mucous Membrane Color

I. Mucous membranes should be evaluated for ashen or cyanotic discoloration.
  A. Cyanosis is a late sign of hypoxemia.
  B. An absolute amount of unoxygenated hemoglobin (usually about 5 gm/dl) in the tissue bed is necessary to show cyanosis.
    1. Anemic animals may not exhibit cyanosis, even in severe hypoxemia.
  C. Other causes of cyanotic discoloration follow:
    1. Sluggish capillary blood flow (caused by the end stage of shock or cardiac arrest)
    2. Methemoglobinemia.

Auscultation

I. Tracheobronchial breath sounds
  A. Loud, high pitched, harsh sounds heard over the trachea or anteroventral quadrant of the thorax
    1. A distinct pause is heard between inspiration and exhalation.
    2. The expiratory phase is slightly longer than the inspiratory phase.
II. Bronchovesicular breath sounds
  A. Subtle, soft, low-pitched, gentle rustling sounds heard over the lung fields away from the anteroventral quadrant of the thorax
    1. The inspiratory phase is longer than the expiratory phase.
    2. No pause is heard between inspiration and exhalation.
III. Abnormal sounds
  A. Low-pitched snoring sounds
    1. Upper airway obstruction
  B. High-pitched squeeking sounds
    1. Severe upper airway obstruction
  C. Mid-pitched "wheezing" sounds
    1. Lower airway narrowing (e.g., bronchoconstriction)
    2. Wheezes have a musical quality and may be high-pitched or low-pitched and either loud and polyphonic or subtle and monophonic.

D. Crackles
   1. Primarily occurring early in the inspiratory phase and late in the expiratory phase
   2. Caused by the sudden opening (inspiratory) or closing (expiratory) of small airways
   3. Could be confused with some pleural friction rubs
E. Fluid "bubbling" sounds
   1. Moderate amount of fluid in the medium-sized to larger airways
   2. Could represent fluid in the endotracheal tube or in the pharynx of an unintubated patient.

Ventilometry

I. Ventilation volume can be estimated by visual observation of chest or rebreathing bag excursions, or it can be measured by ventilometry.
A. Normal tidal volume is 10–20 ml/kg.
B. Normal total minute ventilation is 150–250 ml/kg per minute.
C. Alveolar minute ventilation is normally about one third of total minute ventilation.
   1. It may be as low as 20% of the total minute ventilation in tachypneic animals or those with added upper airway dead space.
   2. It may be as high as 70% of the total if an animal is breathing slowly and deeply and is endotracheally intubated.

Partial Pressure of Carbon Dioxide in Arterial Blood (Pa_{CO_2})

I. The Pa_{CO_2} is the usual working definition of alveolar minute ventilation.
A. Normal values range between 35 mm Hg and 45 mm Hg.
   1. A Pa_{CO_2} of less than 35 mm Hg indicates hyperventilation.
   2. A Pa_{CO_2} of more than 45 mm Hg indicates hypoventilation.
B. Pa_{CO_2} may be estimated by measuring the P_{CO_2} in a sample of gas taken at the end of an exhalation.
   1. The presumption is that alveolar and capillary P_{CO_2} are equilibrated.
   2. End-tidal P_{CO_2} is usually somewhat lower than Pa_{CO_2} (1–5 mm Hg).
II. Hypercapnia is caused by the following:
A. Hypoventilation
   1. Excessive depths of anesthesia
   2. Neuromuscular disorders
   3. Airway obstruction
   4. Thoracic or abdominal restrictive disease
   5. Pleural space–filling disorder
   6. Pulmonary parenchymal disease (late)
   7. Inappropriate ventilator settings
B. Dead-space rebreathing
C. Recent bicarbonate therapy

Arterial Blood Oxygenation

I. The ability of the lungs to oxygenate the blood can be measured by either the partial pressure of oxygen in the arterial blood (Pa_{O_2}) or by the degree of hemoglobin saturation in the arterial blood (Sa_{O_2}).

II. Pa_{O_2}

    A. The Pa_{O_2} measures the tension (the vapor pressure) of oxygen dissolved in physical solution in the plasma.

        1. This measurement is irrespective of the hemoglobin concentration.

    B. Normal Pa_{O_2} is considered to range between 80 mm Hg and 110 mm Hg.

        1. A Pa_{O_2} of less than 80 mm Hg is the common definition of hypoxemia.

        2. A Pa_{O_2} of 50–60 mm Hg represents serious hypoxemia and warrants treatment.

III. Sa_{O_2}

    A. The Sa_{O_2} measures the percent saturation of the hemoglobin.

    B. Pulse oximetry is an indirect, noninvasive method of measuring Sa_{O_2}.

        1. It is usually designated as Sp_{O_2}.

    C. The relationship between Pa_{O_2} and Sa_{O_2} is expressed by the sigmoid oxygen-hemoglobin dissociation curve.

Pa_{O_2}	Sa_{O_2}	Importance
100	98	Normal
< 80	< 95	Hypoxemia
< 60	< 90	Serious hypoxemia
< 40	< 75	Very serious hypoxemia

IV. Oxygen content

    A. Oxygen content depends on both hemoglobin concentration and Pa_{O_2}

        1. Oxygen Content = ([Hemoglobin $\times$ 1.34] $\times$ Percent Saturation) + (0.003 $\times$ P_{O_2})

    B. Hemoglobin concentration is the most important.

    C. The product of oxygen content and cardiac output is oxygen delivery.

Hypoxemia

I. Only three categorical causes of hypoxemia exist:

    A. Low inspired oxygen concentration

        1. Consider this the possible cause of hypoxemia any time an animal is attached to a mechanical apparatus.

    B. Hypoventilation

        1. Hypoventilation can occur when the animal is breathing room air.

        2. But hypoventilation cannot occur when the animal is breathing an enriched oxygen mixture.

    C. Venous admixture

WHAT IS VENOUS ADMIXTURE?

I. Venous admixture is the collective term for all of the ways in which blood can pass from the right chamber of the heart to the left without being properly oxygenated.

    A. The blood is not properly, fully, nor normally oxygenated.

    B. The presence of a venous admixture implies that the animal has either lung disease or an anatomic arteriovenous shunt.

II. How can venous admixture be identified in a patient?

    A. The difference between alveolar and arterial P_{O_2} (A-a P_{O_2}) can reveal the presence of venous admixture.

       1. Alveolar P_{O_2} = Inspired P_{O_2} − Pa_{CO_2} (1.1).

          a. Inspired P_{O_2} = Barometric Pressure × 21%

          b. 1.1 = 1/RQ assuming RQ = 0.9.

       2. The normal A-a PO_2 is about 10 mm Hg when the animal is breathing 21% oxygen and about 100 mm Hg when the animal is breathing 100% oxygen.

          a. An A-a P_{O_2} of more than 20 (21%) or more than 200 (100%) is indicative of a reduced ability of the lung to oxygenate blood.

    B. If a dog or cat is breathing 21% oxygen at sea level and has an approximately normal body temperature, a simplified version of the alveolar air equation is to add the measured Pa_{O_2} and Pa_{CO_2} values.

       1. If the added value is less than 120 mm Hg, there is venous admixture.

       2. The lower the added value is, the greater the magnitude of the venous admixture.

    C. Patients breathing an enriched oxygen mixture should have an elevated Pa_{O_2}.

       1. A rough estimate of the expected Pa_{O_2} at any particular inspired oxygen concentration can be obtained by multiplying the inspired oxygen concentration by 5.

          a. A Pa_{O_2} measurement below this value indicates venous admixture.

    D. A formula that is relatively independent of inspired oxygen concentration is the a/A ratio (Pa_{O_2} / PA_{O_2}).

       1. An a/A ratio of less than 0.85 is indicative of venous admixture.

    E. The "shunt formula" is the most accurate way to quantitate venous admixture as it is less susceptible to errors in assumptions, transitional disequilibrium, and variations in venous oxygen content.

       1. Venous Admixture = $(Cc_{O_2} - Ca_{O_2})/(Cc_{O_2} - Cv_{O_2})$

          a. C = content of oxygen in capillary (c), arterial (a), and pulmonary artery (mixed venous) (v) blood.

          b. Capillary P_{O_2} is assumed to equal alveolar P_{O_2} for the purposes of this calculation.

       2. This calculation represents the percent of cardiac output that would have to bypass the lung (and be totally unoxygenated, assuming that the remainder was perfectly arterialized) in order to account for the observed blood gas measurements.

          a. This is a contrived number, because much of the blood is, in reality, partially arterialized.

       3. Venous admixture assessed by this calculation is normally less than 10%.

    F. When mixed venous blood is not available, the *estimated shunt equation* will provide a close approximation of the venous admixture.

       1. Venous Admixture = $(Cc_{O_2} - Ca_{O_2})/$ 3.5 + $(Cc_{O_2} - Ca_{O_2})$.

III. Animals with venous admixture commonly are hypoxemic and hypocapneic.

    A. The patient compensates for the hypoxemia by hyperventilating.

   B. The more normal units operate on the steep part of the P_{CO_2}-content CO_2 dissociation curve but on the flat part of the P_{O_2}-content O_2 dissociation curve.

   C. Therefore, hyperventilation of these more normal regions has substantive impact on carbon dioxide content but not oxygen content.

   D. Alveolar-capillary units that are functioning more normally can compensate for the effects of venous admixture with respect to carbon dioxide but not oxygen.

WHAT ARE THE MECHANISMS OF VENOUS ADMIXTURE?

I. Lung regions with low ventilation-to-perfusion relationships.
   A. This is a common cause of hypoxemia in patients with pulmonary parenchymal disease.
   B. Diseases associated with diminished ventilation of lung regions
     1. Shallow tidal volumes
     2. Small-airway narrowing
       a. Bronchoconstriction
       b. Accumulation of viscous secretions
       c. Epithelial edema
   C. Diseases associated with enhanced ventral distribution of blood flow
     1. Anesthetic drugs
     2. Bronchodilator interference with pulmonary autoregulation of blood flow
   D. Blood passing through these areas is not normally arterialized, and blood gases are representative of the hypoventilated status of these regions.
   E. This mechanism of hypoxemia is responsive to oxygen therapy.

II. Lung regions that are not being ventilated but that are being perfused.
   A. This is a common cause of hypoxemia in patients with pulmonary parenchymal disease.
   B. It occurs when the small airways or alveoli collapse as a result of the following:
     1. Atelectasis for any reason
     2. Any transudative or exudative pulmonary parenchymal disease associated with the accumulation of airway fluids and airway collapse.
   C. Venous blood flowing through these areas is not arterialized at all.
   D. This mechanism is not particularly responsive to oxygen therapy but is very responsive to PPV.

III. Pathologic arteriovenous shunts (intrapulmonary or extrapulmonary).
   A. Right-to-left shunting patent ductus arteriosus, ventricular septal defect, or atrial septal defect
   B. Anatomic shunts are not responsive to either oxygen or PPV therapy.

IV. Diffusion impairment resulting from a thickened respiratory membrane.
   A. This mechanism is not a common cause of hypoxemia.
   B. It is responsive to oxygen therapy.

CARDIOVASCULAR

Bradycardia

I. Bradycardia is considered to require definitive therapy when it causes an excessive decrease in cardiac output.

    A. That is, when heart rate decreases below 50–60 beats per minute in an animal that has an adequate circulating volume

    B. Also, when mean blood pressure decreases below 60 mm Hg

II. Causes of bradycardia

    A. Excessive anesthetic depth

    B. Excessive vagal tone

       1. Endotracheal intubation, traction or pressure on the eyeball and ocular muscles, visceral traction, and periosteal stimulation

       2. Drug-induced by opioids, atropine (especially low-dose), or anticholinesterase agents

    C. Anesthetic agents that may decrease sympathetic tone (xylazine, beta-receptor blocking agents) or directly depress spontaneously depolarizing cells (halothane, methoxyflurane, barbiturates, lidocaine)

    D. Hypothermia that decreases tissue oxygen demands, resulting in a proportionate decrease in heart rate, cardiac output, and blood pressure

       1. Direct cold-induced myocardial depression may occur at very low core temperatures (<26°C).

    E. Exogenous toxemias and endogenous metabolic disturbances such as hypoxia, acidosis, digitalis intoxication, hypothyroidism, visceral organ failure, hyperkalemia, hypocalcemia, and end-stage shock

III. Prevention and treatment of bradycardia

    A. Atropine or glycopyrrolate is often administered prior to induction to prevent vagal-mediated bradycardia

       1. The duration of vagal blockade is variable.

       2. Although these drugs are not routinely redosed during the operative period, repeat doses can be administered if bradycardia develops.

       3. Large doses of atropine should be avoided because they may predispose the patient to tachycardia and ventricular arrhythmias.

       4. Atropine causes a centrally mediated increase in vagal tone prior to peripheral vagal blockade, and bradyarrhythmias are occasionally seen prior to the peripheral cholinergic blockade.

    B. If the specific cause of the bradycardia cannot be determined, and if it is judged to have deleterious effects on blood pressure and has not responded to atropine, the administration of a beta-receptor stimulant may be indicated.

       1. Dopamine, dobutamine, and ephedrine are the sympathomimetics of choice for this purpose because they support blood pressure without causing excessive peripheral vasodilation or vasoconstriction.

Sinus Tachycardia and Hypertension

I. Sinus tachycardia is herein defined as a heart rate above 160 bpm in the dog and 180 bpm in the cat.

    A. Hypertension is a mean blood pressure above 120 mm Hg or a systolic blood pressure above 160 mm Hg.

II. Sinus tachycardia is usually a sign of an underlying disease process that may need attention.

    A. Excessive sinus tachycardia (low 200s) may be associated with inadequate diastolic ventricular filling, resulting in insufficient cardiac output.

    B. Excessive hypertension may be associated with the following:

1. Increased workload (afterload) of the heart—arrhythmias and heart failure
2. Increased capillary hydrostatic pressure—cerebral and pulmonary edema
3. Retinal detachment

III. Causes of sinus tachycardia and hypertension
   A. Anesthesia level too light
   B. Sympathetic response to surgical stimulation
   C. An underlying complication such as hypoxia, hypercapnia, or hyperthermia
   D. Hypervolemia
   E. Certain drugs (sympathomimetics) and anesthetics (ketamine)
      1. Xylazine causes hypertension and bradycardia.
   F. Preexisting diseases—pheochromocytoma, hyperthyroidism, CNS ischemia, hypoxia, or elevated intracranial pressure.
      1. Patients with patent ductus arteriosus may be hypervolemic and may develop hypertension when the shunt is surgically occluded.
   G. Hypertension occasionally occurs 1–2 hours following the application of an appendage tourniquet.

IV. Treatment of sinus tachycardia or hypertension
   A. Specific treatment should be directed toward the underlying cause.
      1. It is unwise to attempt to override the hypertension with excessive anesthetic dosages.
   B. Vasodilator therapy may be necessary to obtain rapid control of blood pressure until the underlying disease process can be diagnosed and effectively treated.
      1. Nitroprusside and hydralazine can be used for this purpose.
      2. Calcium channel blockers and angiotensin-converting enzyme inhibitors have also been used.
   C. Furosemide

Peripheral Vasoconstriction

I. The signs of peripheral vasoconstriction are pale color, prolonged capillary refill time, cold extremities, anuria, and absence of bleeding at the operative site.
II. The importance of vasoconstriction is that it may be associated with inadequate blood flow to the peripheral tissues.
III. Vasoconstriction may be a compensatory response to hypovolemia.
   A. It may also be caused by surgical stimulation in the lightly anesthetized patient, hypothermia, alpha-receptor agonist therapy, the excitement stage of recovery, or postoperative pain.
IV. Treatment should be directed to the underlying disease process.

Premature Ventricular Contractions (PVCs)

I. Premature ventricular contractions in an animal with no previous heart problems signify the presence of an underlying complication that may lead to more serious arrhythmias or even to cardiac arrest if unchecked.

II. Causes of premature ventricular contractions
    A. Endogenous catecholamine release during light levels of anesthesia or during any stress such as hypoxemia, hypercapnia, or hypotension
        1. Exogenous catecholamine therapy
        2. Some anesthetics lower the threshold to catecholamine-induced arrhythmias (halothane, xylazine).
    B. Endogenous or exogenous toxemias such as the following:
        1. Severe acidosis or alkalosis
        2. Hypokalemia (potentiated by alkalosis, glucose, or insulin therapy)
        3. Hypercalcemia (potentiated by acidosis)
        4. Hypoxia or hypotension
        5. Visceral organ failure
        6. Severe hypothermia (<26°C; 79°F)
        7. Digitalis toxicity (potentiated by hypokalemia and hypercalcemia)
        8. Some anesthetics (thiopental)
    C. Direct endocardial stimulation (by long jugular catheters, endocarditis), myocardial stimulation (myocarditis), or epicardial stimulation (surgical manipulation of the heart)
        1. Myocardial stress resulting from excessive preload (high end-diastolic filling volume caused by fluid overload or congestive heart failure) or afterload (high diastolic arterial blood pressure caused by peripheral vasoconstriction)
III. Treatment of PVCs
    A. Treat anesthetic-induced abnormalities first.
        1. Eliminate obvious causes.
        2. Evaluate the level of anesthesia and make appropriate adjustments to the vaporizer setting.
        3. Maximize the inspired oxygen concentration.
        4. Provide ventilatory support.
        5. Check the anesthetic machine and ventilator to rule out machine-related causes of hypoxemia or hypercapnia.
        6. Begin rapid fluid administration.
        7. Discontinue administration of agents that may cause arrhythmias or lower the threshold to them.
    B. Specific antiarrhythmic therapy should be considered in the following situations:
        1. The PVC rate exceeds 180–200 per minute.
          a. When the rate of a paroxysmal rhythm would exceed 180–200 per minute if it were to continue for an entire minute;
        2. PVC frequency is increasing.
        3. The ectopic beat overrides the T wave of the preceding beat.
        4. The rhythm causes detectable cardiovascular deterioration.
    C. Specific antiarrhythmic therapy
        1. Lidocaine (1–5 mg/kg IV)
        2. Procainamide (1–5 mg/kg IV)
        3. Propranolol (0.05–0.3 mg/kg IV)

Central Venous Pressure (CVP)

I. Central venous pressure (CVP) is the luminal blood pressure of the intrathoracic vena cava.

A. It is regulated by central venous blood volume (venous return), venous tone, and cardiac output.

B. CVP is an estimate of the relationship between the blood volume and the blood volume capacity.

1. It should be measured when it is necessary to administer large volumes of fluids rapidly (as in cases of septic shock) and it is difficult to define an end point for the fluid administration by the physical signs alone.

2. When the CVP has been raised to a high-normal range by fluid therapy, it is generally assumed that therapy has been adequate to establish a reasonable preload.

C. CVP is also a measure of the relative ability of the heart to pump the quantity of fluids being returned to it.

1. It should be measured in animals when a component of heart failure is suspected.

D. If the preload is high and the forward-flow parameters such as cardiac output, pulse quality, arterial blood pressure, and tissue perfusion are unacceptable, it is assumed that the heart is failing to pump the available venous return.

1. Once organic causes such as pericardial tamponade or aortic stenosis are ruled out, systolic failure is expected and sympathomimetics are indicated.

II. CVP is a pressure measurement, not a flow or a volume measurement.

A. It is only indirectly influenced by flow (venous return) in that higher flows are often associated with higher pressures.

1. Venoconstriction can increase venous pressure while decreasing venous flow.

B. CVP is also only an indirect measure of volume.

1. Although higher pressures are associated with higher volumes, CVP may be high and end-diastolic ventricular volume (preload) low in conditions associated with decreased ventricular compliance (hypertrophic cardiomyopathy, fibrosis, pericardial tamponade) or tricuspid stenosis.

III. Catheters should be positioned via the jugular vein into the anterior vena cava.

A. Peripheral venous pressure is variably higher than CVP and does not reliably reflect CVP.

B. Contact with the endocardium of the right atrium or the right ventricle should be avoided, as such contact may stimulate ectopic pacemaker activity.

IV. Verification of a well-placed, unobstructed catheter can be ascertained by observing small fluctuations in the fluid meniscus within the manometer synchronous with the heartbeat and larger excursions synchronous with ventilation.

A. Very large fluctuations synchronous with each heartbeat may indicate that the end of the catheter is positioned within the right ventricle.

B. If the fluid meniscus in the column manometer falls very slowly and if there are no fluctuations in the meniscus, the tip of the catheter may be partially occluded and the measurement may be erroneously high.

C. CVP measurements should be made between ventilatory excursions as changes in pleural pressure affect the luminal pressure within the anterior vena cava.

V. The normal CVP in small animals is 0–10 cm H_2O. It may be 0 cm H_2O in an animal that is otherwise normal and may be 5 cm H_2O in an animal in hypovolemic shock, depending on other cardiovascular changes.

  A. High CVP measurements may be due to hypervolemia, poor cardiac output, or venoconstriction.

  B. Low CVP measurements may be due to hypovolemia, high cardiac output, or vasodilation.

Arterial Blood Pressure

I. Arterial blood pressure is the luminal pressure of the blood in a large artery.

  A. Arterial blood pressure is the product of cardiac output, vascular capacity, and blood volume.

  B. Digital palpation of the quality of the pulse amplitude in a peripheral artery reflects stroke volume and may not correlate at all to the arterial blood pressure.

   1. The weak, thready pulse that occurs with hypovolemia is due to a small stroke volume.

   2. Such patients may actually be normotensive, depending on other cardiovascular changes.

II. Arterial blood pressure is important for cerebral and coronary perfusion.

  A. Adequate cerebral and coronary perfusion is considered to require a mean systemic blood pressure of at least 50–60 mm Hg (assuming normal intracranial pressure).

  B. Arterial blood pressure is not, however, the only determinant of central organ perfusion.

   1. Organ perfusion pressure is determined by the difference between arterial blood pressure and intra-organ pressure (or post-organ venous pressure, whichever is greater).

    a. As an example, cerebral perfusion pressure is determined as mean arterial blood pressure minus intracranial pressure (which is normally about 10–15 mm Hg).

    b. In states of increased intracranial pressure, arterial blood pressure will have to increase proportionately in order to maintain adequate cerebral perfusion pressure.

  C. Arterial blood pressure is also not the main determinant of peripheral (visceral) organ perfusion; precapillary arteriolar vasomotor tone is.

  D. Arterial blood pressure is also not a measure of cardiac output, although it is influenced by it.

III. Arterial blood pressure can be measured indirectly or directly.

  A. Indirect sphygmomanometry involves the application of an occlusion cuff over an artery in a cylindrical appendage.

   1. The occlusion cuff should be placed snugly around the leg.

    a. If it is applied too tightly, the pressure measurements will be erroneously low.

    b. If it is applied too loosely, the pressure measurements will be erroneously high.

2. Inflation of the cuff applies pressure to the underlying tissues and will totally occlude blood flow when the pressure exceeds the systolic blood pressure.
    a. As the cuff pressure is gradually decreased, blood will begin to flow intermittently when the cuff pressure falls below the luminal systolic pressure.
3. The appearance of needle oscillations on the manometer during cuff deflation corresponds approximately to systolic blood pressure.
4. Digital palpation of a pulse distal to the cuff corresponds approximately to systolic blood pressure.
5. Doppler blood flow instrumentation involves the application of a small piezoelectric crystal over the artery.
    a. Energy is transmitted into the underlying tissue.
    b. The energy frequency reflected from moving tissues is shifted slightly from that which was transmitted, and this frequency difference is converted electronically to an audible signal.
    c. The first sounds heard as the cuff is slowly deflated correspond approximately to systolic blood pressure.
    d. At a lower cuff pressure there may occur a second sound associated with each pulse wave.
        (1) This second sound is that of a second forward flow associated with the dicrotic notch of the pulse pressure waveform.
        (2) It may approximate diastolic blood pressure.
6. Oscillometric technology involves simply the placement of a cuff around an appendage.
    a. The instrument automatically inflates and deflates the cuff.
        (1) Changes in intracuff pressure associated with each pulse wave are measured or computed.
        (2) Heart rate and systolic, diastolic, and mean blood pressure are displayed.
    b. This technology is very sensitive to motion artifact.
7. All external techniques are least accurate when vessels are small, when the blood pressure is low, and when vessels are constricted.

B. Direct measurements of arterial blood pressure are more accurate and continuous than indirect methods, but they require the introduction of a catheter into an artery by percutaneous or cutdown procedure.
1. The dorsal metatarsal artery is most commonly used for percutaneous catheterization.
    a. The backup artery is the femoral for percutaneous or cutdown introduction.
2. Once placed, the catheter must be flushed with heparinized saline at frequent intervals (hourly) or even continuously.
    a. Never allow blood to flow into the catheter as it will clot.
3. The catheter is then attached to the measuring device.
    a. A long fluid administration set can be suspended from the ceiling and operated like a CVP measuring device.
    b. The measuring device can also be an aneroid manometer attached to the arterial catheter via several lengths of extension tubing, with an inline three-way stopcock.
    c. The arterial catheter can be attached to a commercial transducer and recording system.

IV. Normal arterial blood pressures

	mm Hg
Systolic	100–160
Diastolic	60–100
Mean	80–120

A. Systolic pressures below 80 and mean pressures below 60 are assumed to result in inadequate cerebral and coronary perfusion and thus warrant therapy.

B. The zero level of the transducer must be set at heart level.

  1. The zero should be checked periodically.

C. The accuracy of the transducer or manometer could be checked against a mercury column if there is any question about it.

Hypotension

I. Hypotension may be due to hypovolemia, reduced cardiac output, or peripheral vasodilation.

A. Hypovolemia is the most common cause of hypotension.

  1. Extracellular fluid deficits may result from inadequate intake, diarrhea, vomiting, diuresis, or third-space fluid accumulations.

    a. Sometimes these fluid deficits are not readily apparent on the preanesthetic physical exam and are unmasked by induction of general anesthesia.

      (1) A preinduction loading dose of fluids may be indicated if there is a history of fluid losses even when there is no physical evidence of dehydration.

  2. Vascular volume deficiencies may, in addition, be due to whole blood or plasma losses or to hypoproteinemia.

  3. Bolus fluid therapy with crystalloids, colloids, or blood products should be administered.

B. Decreased cardiac output may be due to intrinsic or extrinsic myocardial failure, valvular disease, tamponade, or severe bradycardia, tachycardia, or arrhythmias.

  1. Decreased venous return may be caused by hypovolemia, surgical packing and obstruction of vena cava, positive pressure ventilation, gastric torsion, or pericardial tamponade.

C. Peripheral vasodilation may be caused by sepsis or drugs (acepromazine, bolus doses of most anesthetics, epidural or subarachnoid deposition of local anesthetics, specific vasodilators), or it may be a preterminal event of any disease process.

  1. Hypoxia, hypercapnia, hyperthermia, surface rewarming of hypothermic patients, and sepsis may also cause peripheral vasodilation.

  2. Fluid therapy to refill the expanded vascular volume is the primary focus of therapy.

  3. Alpha-receptor agonists may be indicated initially to pharmacologically support blood pressure and to provide time for blood volume restitution.

II. When hypotension occurs during general anesthesia, the first treatment should always be to decrease the quantity of anesthetic administered until the patient is anesthetized just enough to allow completion of the surgical procedure.

   A. It may be necessary to change to anesthetic agents that have less inherent cardiovascular depressant properties.

   B. A bolus volume of an isotonic replacement solution should be administered if the hypotension is deemed not to be due to heart failure.

      1. The volume to administer is determined by the magnitude of the hypotension (10–100 ml/kg in the dog and 5–60 ml/kg in the cat).

      2. Patients with normal hearts, lungs, and brains tolerate large fluid loads well.

         a. Patients with heart failure, pulmonary edema, or cerebral edema may be very sensitive to fluid loading.

      3. Colloids and red cells may need to be administered to maintain colloid oncotic pressure and hemoglobin concentrations.

   C. Sympathomimetics may be indicated if fluid therapy alone does not restore acceptable blood pressure and tissue perfusion.

      1. Agents that cause minimal peripheral vasoconstriction should be used.

         a. Dopamine is a good drug for improving arterial blood pressure.

            (1) Dosages of 1–3 μg/kg per minute increase renal blood flow (dopaminergic receptors) and may be useful in the treatment of acute renal failure.

            (2) Dosages of 3–7 μg/kg per minute increase heart rate, cardiac output, and arterial blood pressure (beta receptors).

            (3) Dosages in excess of 8 μg/kg per minute may be associated with excessive tachycardia and vasoconstriction (alpha receptors).

         b. Dobutamine is a good drug for improving myocardial contractility and peripheral blood flow.

            (1) Dosages of 5–15 μg/kg per minute are generally associated with minimal increases in arterial blood pressure but good enhancement of blood flow.

         c. Ephedrine is an indirect sympathomimetic that is less potent than either dopamine or dobutamine.

            (1) It is less likely to cause harm but also less likely to generate the desired effects.

            (2) The dosage is 0.1–0.5 mg/kg per dose (intravenously or intramuscularly).

Hypothermia

I. Hypothermia during general anesthesia is the almost inevitable consequence of the following:

   A. Decreased heat production resulting from anesthetic-induced decreases in basal metabolic rate and muscular activity

   B. Increased heat loss resulting from application and evaporation of antiseptic solutions, exposure to cold table surfaces, and exposure via open body cavities.

II. The main problem with hypothermia is the nonrecognition of it.

   A. The continued administration of normothermic quantities of anesthetics to hypothermic patients will result in an anesthetic overdose.

III. Consequences of hypothermia
  A. At 36°C (96°F) and above there is no effect except for postanesthetic shivering (which increases oxygen consumption and decreases ventilatory capacity).
  B. At 32–34°C (90–94°F) anesthetic requirements are reduced because of the hypometabolic effects of the hypothermia.
    1. Recovery may be prolonged, and thermoregulation may be impaired (artificial rewarming may be necessary).
  C. At 28–30°C (82–86°F) little or no anesthetic is required for the maintenance of anesthesia.
    1. Recovery will be prolonged.
    2. Patients must be artificially rewarmed.
    3. Metabolic acidosis resulting from inadequate tissue perfusion will occur upon rewarming.
  D. At 25–26°C (77–79°F) the following changes will occur:
    1. Cold-induced electrocardiographic changes
      a. Prolonged PR interval and widened QRS complexes
      b. Increased automaticity of heart
      c. Bradycardia in excess of the hypometabolism results in insufficient tissue perfusion.
    2. Microcirculatory sludging caused by excessive blood viscosity may occur.
  E. At 22°C (72°F) and below, the following changes will occur:
    1. Spontaneous ventilation ceases.
    2. Ventricular fibrillation occurs.
    3. Coagulation disorders occur.
IV. Prevention of hypothermia
  A. Prevention of heat loss
    1. Minimize the duration of the antiseptic preparation of the surgical site.
    2. Protect the animal from its cool environment with blankets or towels.
    3. Minimize the duration of the surgical procedure.
  B. Active warming of the animal or its immediate environment
    1. Circulating warm-water blankets
    2. Forced hot-air warming blankets
    3. Electric heating pads
      a. Electric heating pads are *dangerous*! They can easily overheat the body-surface contact area, causing burns and extensive skin sloughs.
      b. Either do not allow the pad to contact the patient, or insulate the pad with towels or newspapers and measure the temperature between the patient's skin and the blanket to make sure it is less than 42°C (108°F).
    4. Hot-water bottles may be placed around the patient and under the drapes.
      a. Hot-water bottles are *dangerous*! They can easily cause burns and extensive skin sloughs.
      b. Do not allow the bottle to contact the patient, or insulate the bottle with towels or newspapers and make sure that the water temperature is less than 42°C (108°F).
      c. The bottles should be changed when their measured temperature is

below core temperature, because at that point they will begin to reabsorb heat from the patient.

5. Infrared heat lamps may be used during or after the operative period.
   a. The optimum distance between the lamp and the patient is about 75 cm.
   b. Drying of the tissues at the operative site must be prevented.
   c. Radiant-heat infant warmers are also available commercially.
6. Open body cavities may be flushed with warm sterile saline (<42°C).
   a. Intravenous fluids may be warmed.
      (1) This will help prevent further hypothermia.
      (2) These fluids cannot, however, be administered in sufficient quantity to effectively increase core temperature.

Hyperthermia

I. Causes of hyperthermia
   A. Increased heat production resulting from increased metabolic rate secondary to increased muscular activity and light levels of anesthesia
   B. Decreased heat loss in large or obese patients, insulation by surgical draping, and breathing a fully humidified gas
   C. Malignant hyperthermia syndrome (MHS), a rapidly progressive hyperthermia often associated with the administration of halothane or succinylcholine (in people and swine, this disorder is related to a genetic functional defect within the sarcoplasmic reticulum)
      1. Muscular rigidity may or may not occur depending on cytoplasmic calcium concentrations.
II. The harmful effects of hyperthermia are primarily related to high metabolic activity and cellular oxygen consumption.
   A. When the body temperature rises above about 41°C (106°F), the hyperthermia-increased metabolic activity cycle becomes self-perpetuating.
   B. When oxygen utilization exceeds the oxygen supply, hypoxic cellular damage occurs.
   C. All body tissues are affected by the hypoxia, but the organs most likely to manifest insufficiencies are the brain, kidneys, liver, and blood (disseminated intravascular coagulation and hemolysis).
III. Treatment of hyperthermia
   A. General support
      1. Hyperthermic patients should breath an enriched oxygen mixture.
      2. Rapid administration of isotonic crystalloid fluids helps to restore an effective circulating blood volume and cool the patient.
      3. Corticosteroid and sodium bicarbonate therapy should be considered if the hyperthermia is severe or prolonged.
      4. Brain, liver, kidney, gastrointestinal, and endocrine function should be monitored by appropriate clinical and laboratory tests for several days following severe hyperthermic episodes.
   B. Active cooling techniques
      1. Evaporative heat loss can be enhanced by soaking the skin with water or alcohol.
      2. Conductive heat loss can be enhanced by immersing the patient in a cold-water (or ice-water) bath.

3. Infusion of cold fluids intravascularly or into an open body cavity may also be used, as well as ice-water enemas or gastric lavage.

4. Surface cooling techniques may have a substantial peripheral effect before much core cooling is measured by rectal thermometry.

    a. The core temperature will continue to decrease after the surface cooling technique is terminated as the core and peripheral temperatures equilibrate (afterdrop).

    b. Since the extent of the afterdrop is unpredictable, aggressive cooling techniques such as ice-water baths should cease as soon as the core temperature decreases to about 40°C (104°F).

    c. Additional cooling can be applied if necessary after the core and peripheral temperatures have equilibrated.

C. Antipyretics (aspirin, aminopyrine, dipyrone, phenylbutazone) may directly lower hypothalamic thermostatic settings or inhibit the release of pyrogens and thereby lower body temperature.

1. Dipyrone has caused excessive hypothermia in a few patients.

D. If malignant hyperthermia is suspected, the anesthetic agent should be terminated, the operative technique should be terminated, and aggressive attempts to lower the body temperature should be made.

1. Dantrolene may reduce mortality rate.

Anesthetic Emergencies and Complications

Cynthia M. Trim

COMPLICATIONS OCCURRING DURING INDUCTION OF ANESTHESIA

Anaphylactic, Anaphylactoid, and Allergic Reactions

I. Definition: *anaphylaxis* is circulatory failure resulting from an allergic reaction 1 minute to 1 hour after exposure. Anaphylactoid reactions (e.g., to contrast agents) do not involve the immune system but produce similar effects.

II. Clinical signs
   A. Cardiac arrest
   B. Muscle rigidity or flaccidity
   C. Hypotension
   D. Tachycardia
   E. Dysrhythmias
   F. Cyanosis
   G. Labored breathing
   H. Bronchospasm
   I. Laryngeal edema
   J. Urticarial rash (small localized areas of piloerection or large edematous plaques), hyperemia of the skin, thickening of lips, eyelids, and skinfolds
   K. Vomiting or retching
   L. Defecation

III. Causes
   A. Anesthetic drugs: atropine, morphine, meperidine, barbiturates, Cremophor EL (stabilizing agent for steroid anesthetics), tubocurarine, gallamine, procaine hydrochloride
   B. Antibiotics: penicillin, cephalosporins
   C. Dextran, blood or plasma transfusion
   D. Radiographic contrast media injected intravenously or intra-arterially

IV. Differential diagnosis
   A. Anaphylaxis or anaphylactoid reaction: history of recent drug administration, elimination of other possible causes
   B. Anesthetic overdose: occurs more frequently than anaphylaxis. Rapid intravenous injection of some drugs (e.g., morphine, meperidine) will cause circulatory collapse owing to direct effect on the cardiovascular system.
   C. Vagal reflex: traction or pressure on the eyeball, traction on ovaries
   D. Asthmatic or reflex bronchospasm
   E. Pneumothorax

V. Treatment
   A. Cardiopulmonary resuscitation should be instituted if the heart has arrested.

B. Epinephrine can be given intravenously if hypotension is severe and the patient is not breathing inhalation anesthetic agents.

C. Supply 100% oxygen. Intubate trachea. Institute controlled ventilation if breathing is inadequate. If patient is not yet anesthetized, it must be continuously monitored for signs of progressive airway obstruction

D. Antihistamine can be given: diphenhydramine (Benadryl) 2.2 mg/kg intravenously.

E. Treat hypotension by rapid intravenous infusion of lactated Ringer's solution or saline. Support mean arterial pressure by infusion of dopamine 7 μg/kg per minute or dobutamine 5 μg/kg per minute. Measure packed cell volume and plasma protein concentration frequently, and maintain normal values. Hemoconcentration despite infusion of a large volume of electrolyte solution is an indication for administration of colloid solution or plasma.

F. Administer aminophylline 6–10 mg/kg intravenously if bronchospasm is present. Methylprednisolone sodium succinate or dexamethasone can be used for long-term effects.

G. Continue to monitor following resuscitation for evidence of prolonged clotting time and disseminated intravascular coagulation; treat appropriately.

H. Administer antibiotic therapy if blood in feces or vomitus indicates mucosal damage.
  See Table 8–1 for a description of the drugs often used in emergencies.

Cyanosis

I. Causes
  A. Cardiac arrest
    1. Anesthetic overdose
  B. Apnea
    1. Thiopental or propofol
    2. Laryngospasm or airway obstruction
  C. Hypotension
    1. Thiopental or propofol
    2. Cardiac disease
  D. Pulmonary pathology
    1. Ruptured diaphragm
    2. Pulmonary edema
II. Treatment
  A. Administer oxygen via endotracheal tube. Artificially ventilate patient if it is apneic.
  B. Start cardiac massage if peripheral pulse is absent. Wait for anesthetic drug to redistribute if peripheral pulse is relatively strong. Do not administer further anesthetic agent until mucous membranes are pink.
  C. Treat hypotension.
III. Prevention
  A. Administer anesthetic agents for induction in increments.
  B. Administer propofol more slowly than thiopental, over 1–2 minutes.
  C. Consider supplying oxygen by face mask ("preoxygenation") immediately before and during induction of anesthesia with propofol.

Table 8–1. Pharmacology of Emergency Drugs

Drug	Indication	Dosage
Acetylcholine chloride and potassium citrate or potassium chloride	Chemical defibrillation; acetylcholine is a powder that must be dissolved before use	Ach 6 mg/kg and KCl 1 mg/kg IV; or Ach 3 mg/kg and KCl 0.5 mg/kg IC with aortic cross-clamping
Aminophylline	Pulmonary edema, bronchoconstriction	6–10 mg/kg IV
Atropine	Bradycardia, atrioventricular heart block, cardiac arrest	0.02 mg/kg IV; repeat in 5 min if necessary; 0.5 ml/10 kg (0.5 mg/ml)
Deferoxamine (Desferal)	Minimize reperfusion injury	30 mg/kg IM
Dobutamine (Dobutrex)	Hypotension, cardiac failure	2–5 µg/kg/min IV; 50 mg in 500 ml 0.9% saline (100 µg/ml)
Dopamine	Hypotension, oliguria	2–7 µg/kg/min IV
	Cardiac arrest, atrioventricular heart block	5–10 µg/kg/min IV; 50 mg in 500 ml 0.9% saline (100 µg/ml)
Doxapram (Dopram)	Respiratory depression, xylazine antagonist	1 mg/kg IV (inhalation anesthesia); 1–5 mg/kg IV (barbiturate anesthesia)
Epinephrine	Cardiac arrest, anaphylaxis	0.01–.02 mg/kg [dilute to 1:10,000 (0.1 mg/ml), 1 ml/10 kg] IV, intratracheally; if unsuccessful in 2 minutes, repeat with 0.05–0.1 mg/kg (undiluted, 1 mg/ml, 0.5–1.0 ml/10 kg) IV
Furosemide (Lasix)	Pulmonary edema, oliguria	2.2 mg/kg IV
Glycopyrrolate (Robinul)	Bradycardia	0.005 mg/kg IV; repeat in 2–5 min if necessary
Hypertonic (7.5%) saline	Hypotension associated with hemorrhage or sepsis	4 ml/kg IV over 10 minutes
Lidocaine	Premature ventricular contractions, ventricular tachycardia	1–2 mg/kg IV, 0.5–1.0 ml 2%/10 kg; 0.25–0.5 ml 4%/10 kg
Naloxone	Opioid antagonist	0.01–.02 mg/kg IV, IM
Propranolol	Ventricular tachycardia in cats	1 ml of 1 mg/ml and 3 ml saline; 0.2 ml bolus IV to effect
Sodium bicarbonate	Metabolic acidosis, prolonged hypertension	1.0–1.5 mEq/kg IV; may repeat after 10 minutes

D. Also consider such preoxygenation for patients with cardiac or pulmonary disease.

Inability to Intubate the Trachea

I. Causes

   A. Failure of anesthetist

      1. Inadequate positioning of patient

      2. Inadequate light to view the laryngeal entrance

      3. Inadequate anesthesia to provide muscle relaxation

   B. Abnormality in patient

      1. Laryngospasm

      2. Limited excursion of jaws

      3. Oral or pharyngeal tumors, retropharyngeal abscess, tissues distorted owing to changes following surgery

      4. English bulldogs: This breed has a small-diameter trachea in relation to its body weight, and some individuals have an anatomic distortion at

the laryngeal-tracheal junction. The anatomic abnormality requires that a smaller-diameter endotracheal tube than usual be passed. Occasionally only a 5–6 mm (internal diameter) tube can be inserted into an adult bulldog. A tube of this size increases resistance to airflow, so ventilation should be controlled throughout anesthesia to prevent hypoventilation.

  5. Narrowed tracheal lumen (partial obstruction of lumen or collapse from external pressure)

II. Treatment

  A. Ensure that patient's head and neck are extended so that the longitudinal axes of the oropharynx and the trachea are in a straight line.
  B. Provide adequate lighting.
  C. Administer anesthetic drug to produce relaxation of the jaws and abolish the swallowing reflex.
  D. Remove laryngospasm by topical application of lidocaine (without epinephrine) 1–2 mg/kg.
  E. A difficult intubation should be anticipated before induction of anesthesia.
    1. A mechanism for exerting tension or retraction on the jaws should be devised when jaw movements are restricted. This mechanism should be used carefully when fractures are present.
    2. Radiography before anesthesia may be helpful to determine the degree of airway obstruction present in patients with an oropharyngeal mass.
    3. Assistance may be needed in retracting tumors.
    4. Stiffening the endotracheal tube by inserting a metal stilette into it or using a fiberoptic endoscope and an endotracheal tube containing a metal spiral may facilitate tracheal intubation.
    5. Care should be taken not to rupture tissues or cause bleeding.
    6. Equipment to perform a tracheotomy should be present (see section on airway obstruction).

Perivascular Injection

I. Clinical signs
  A. Tissue swelling beneath the skin is observed.
  B. Patient shows signs of pain associated with injection. Note that intravenous injection of diazepam, ketamine, or etomidate may evoke this patient response.
  C. Less sedative or anesthetic effect than expected occurs from the dose administered

II. Treatment
  A. Thiopental: infiltrate tissues with lidocaine (without epinephrine) up to 2 mg/kg and saline. Use hot pack frequently.
  B. Ketamine: no treatment is needed.
  C. Sodium bicarbonate or 20–50% dextrose: infiltrate tissues with saline until tissues are moderately distended. Use hot pack frequently.

Vomiting or Regurgitation

I. General considerations
  A. *Vomiting* is the active process of moving gastric contents into the pharynx, whereas *regurgitation* is passive movement of gastric material into the

esophagus or pharynx. Regurgitation of gastric fluid into the pharynx occurs sometimes in dogs undergoing gastrointestinal surgery or upper abdominal surgery.

B. Reflux of gastric fluid into the esophagus occurs in some anesthetized dogs and cats but will not be observed by the anesthetist.

C. Stricture formation at the cardia, developing several weeks after anesthesia, has been attributed to esophagitis from gastric reflux.

II. Causes

A. Elevated intragastric pressure
   1. Recent feeding
   2. Delayed emptying: anxiety, cesarean section, trauma, intestinal obstruction
   3. Increased intra-abdominal pressure: pregnancy, gastrointestinal distention, surgical exploration of abdomen, tight abdominal bandage
   4. Muscle contractions after succinylcholine administration

B. Fluid sequestered in esophagus: megaesophagus, ruptured diaphragm

C. Relaxation of lower esophageal sphincter: atropine, xylazine, propofol, thiopental. Greater relaxation occurs during induction with propofol than with thiopental. Greatest relaxation occurs at induction of anesthesia and at the end of anesthesia.

D. Stimulation of vomiting reflex: morphine, apomorphine, oxymorphone, xylazine

III. Prevention

A. Withhold feed 12 hours before anesthesia and more than 12 hours for English bulldogs and for animals fed dry food.

B. Withhold water 2 hours before anesthesia.

C. Premedication with atropine or glycopyrrolate reduces gastrointestinal motility and the incidence of vomiting, especially during recovery from anesthesia. Premedication with atropine or glycopyrrolate decreases lower esophageal sphincter pressure and may predispose the patient to gastric reflux.

D. Premedication with a phenothiazine tranquilizer (acepromazine) may decrease the incidence of vomiting but not of regurgitation

E. Special considerations are necessary for the patient with a high probability of vomiting.
   1. Premedication with glycopyrrolate (at least 1 hour before induction of anesthesia) should be considered to reduce the acidity of gastric fluid.
   2. Some patients may benefit from pretreatment with cimetidine (Tagamet) 10 mg/kg orally, intravenously, or intramuscularly, which decreases gastric acid secretion. Biotransformation of some drugs (lidocaine, diazepam, morphine) is impaired by concurrent administration of cimetidine.
   3. Opioids increase gastroesophageal sphincter pressure and decrease peristalsis. Premedication with one of these drugs (except morphine or oxymorphone, which may cause vomiting) may decrease the incidence of vomiting and regurgitation. Of the opioids commonly used, butorphanol or buprenorphine are less likely to induce vomiting.
   4. Anesthesia should be induced with the patient in a sternal, head-up position, the trachea intubated with an endotracheal tube, and the cuff inflated before the patient is allowed to assume lateral recumbency.
   5. Cricoid pressure may be effective in interrupting regurgitation. Before and during induction of anesthesia, an assistant should apply thumb

pressure on the left side of the patient's neck over the cricoid cartilage, thus collapsing the esophagus between thumb and larynx.

IV. Treatment

    A. Vomition or regurgitation during induction of anesthesia

        1. Lower the patient's head below the level of its body to encourage food and fluid to drain from the mouth.

        2. Clean pharynx with a gauze square folded and held in forceps. When the pharynx is observed to be clean, insert an endotracheal tube.

        3. If pulmonary aspiration has occurred, the following procedures should be used:

            a. Attempt to aspirate material from trachea by suction. To avoid creating hypoxia, use a catheter less than half the diameter of the trachea, and apply suction for no more than 5 seconds at a time. Bronchoscopy may be used to remove large particulate matter. Bronchial lavage should not be done.

            b. Administer oxygen.

            c. Postpone surgery if possible, and allow the patient to recover from anesthesia. It has been demonstrated in dogs that endotracheal intubation and halothane anesthesia suppress the clearance mechanisms of the lung for several hours. Recovery from aspiration of gastric fluid is jeopardized if surgery immediately continues.

            d. Bronchospasm should be treated with intravenous aminophylline.

            e. Administer systemic antibiotics.

            f. Corticosteroid treatment is controversial.

            g. Maintain intravascular fluid volume by intravenous infusion of electrolyte fluids.

    B. Regurgitation during anesthesia and surgery

        1. Consider passing a stomach tube to drain fluid from stomach.

        2. At the end of anesthesia, wipe fluid from pharynx and around epiglottis.

        3. At the end of anesthesia, suction nasal passages.

        4. Do not extubate until swallowing reflex has completely returned. Extubate with the patient's head lowered.

CENTRAL NERVOUS SYSTEM COMPLICATIONS DURING ANESTHESIA

Anesthetic Overdose

I. General considerations

    A. Anesthetic drug administration that has resulted in deep anesthesia, without cardiac arrest, is discussed here.

II. Clinical signs

    A. Fixed, dilated pupils

    B. Profound respiratory depression or respiratory arrest

    C. Signs not specific to anesthetic overdose: palpebral and pedal reflexes absent, hypotension, prolonged capillary refill time

III. Causes

    A. Absolute drug overdose

        1. Miscalculation of dosage, inaccurate estimation of patient's body weight,

incorrect evaluation of depth of anesthesia, failure to monitor depth of anesthesia frequently

2. Vaporizer malfunction, overfilling or jostling of anesthesia machine resulting in spillage of liquid anesthetic into the oxygen line

B. Relative drug overdose

1. Patient has a reduced requirement for anesthetic drugs because of old age, advanced pregnancy, hypothyroidism, hypoadrenocorticism, disease-induced central nervous system (CNS) depression, or individual variation.

2. Patient has reduced volume for redistribution of anesthetic drug because of hypovolemia, obesity, or hypercalcemia.

3. Activity of drug is increased above normal by altered ionization or protein binding; activity of barbiturates is increased by acidosis or hypoproteinemia.

IV. Treatment

A. Barbiturate, propofol, or ketamine overdose

1. Intubate trachea and institute controlled ventilation with 100% oxygen.

2. If circulatory depression is severe, infuse dopamine or dobutamine (see section on hypotension for details).

3. If circulatory depression is life-threatening, and an opioid was given for premedication, inject naloxone intravenously. If xylazine or medetomidine was given for premedication, inject yohimbine (Yobine) or atipamezole (Antesedan), respectively.

4. Expand plasma volume by infusing balanced electrolyte solution (lactated Ringer's solution) 10–20 ml/kg over 10 minutes. Dextrose-containing fluids should not be used because they may increase the action of barbiturate.

5. Xylazine and barbiturates can be antagonized by doxapram (Dopram). Inject doxapram, 1–5 mg/kg intravenously. Doxapram causes release of norepinephrine and may result in tachycardia and dysrhythmias. Consequently, the dosage should not exceed 1 mg/kg when an inhalation agent has been administered.

6. Infusion of sodium bicarbonate, 1 mEq/kg intravenously will alter blood pH and ionization of barbiturate and decrease its activity.

7. Maintain body temperature to maintain metabolic rate. Turn animal hourly to minimize hypostatic congestion. Apply eye ointment to prevent corneal drying.

B. Halothane, isoflurane, or sevoflurane overdose

1. Turn vaporizer to zero, discontinue nitrous oxide administration, and empty rebreathing bag and refill it with oxygen. Although most of the inhalation anesthetic is eliminated via the lungs, simply discontinuing anesthetic administration may not prevent progression to respiratory and cardiac arrest.

2. Institute controlled ventilation; deep anesthesia results in decreased ventilation, and elimination of anesthetic gas will be slow.

3. If depth of anesthesia is life-threatening and an opioid has been used, its effects should be reversed by injection of naloxone, 0.02 mg/kg intravenously.

4. Empty rebreathing bag of a circle circuit and refill it with oxygen every few minutes until depth of anesthesia has lightened.

5. Support cardiovascular function.

INADEQUATE DEPTH OF ANESTHESIA

I. General considerations
  A. Investigations of anesthetized humans indicate that hearing is the first sense to return as the depth of anesthesia lightens. A person may be aware of surroundings but may or may not feel the pain of surgery. Conversely, reflex movement can also occur during anesthesia when the depth of anesthesia is adequate. These findings in humans may be relevant for animals as well.

II. Clinical signs
  A. Movement of limbs, chewing on the endotracheal tube, and shivering.
  B. Pupillary dilation
  C. Tachycardia
  D. Hypertension
  E. Increased respiratory rate, and panting
  F. Breath-holding
  G. Vocalization
  H. Salivation: awareness during neuromuscular blockade

III. Causes
  A. Insufficient drug administration
    1. Equipment failure: separation of inner tube of Bain circuit, endotracheal tube cuff deflated, or tube disconnected
    2. Anesthetist-originated: perivascular injection, endotracheal tube in esophagus or in one bronchus, vaporizer empty or setting too low
    3. Low inspired anesthetic concentration: a large dog and a low oxygen flow results in a rebreathing-bag anesthetic concentration that is 20–50% lower than the vaporizer setting.
  B. Impaired drug uptake
    1. Poor absorption following an intramuscular injection: part of dose deposited in fascia
    2. Hypoventilation: limits uptake of an inhalation anesthetic
  C. Incomplete transfer from one anesthetic drug to another: a return to consciousness from redistribution of thiopental or propofol before sufficient uptake of inhalation anesthetic has occurred
  D. Waning effect of premedicant drugs: oxymorphone or butorphanol may have to be "topped up" during surgery
  E. Acute change in anesthetic requirement: at the start of surgery, an abrupt increase in the intensity of surgical stimulus

IV. Differential diagnosis
  A. Inadequate depth of anesthesia
    1. Observe patient for signs of a light plane of anesthesia. These signs are, except in ketamine anesthesia, a strong palpebral reflex with the eyeball centrally located in the orbit, pupillary dilation, increased heart rate, and usually, but not always, a strong arterial pulse. Respiratory rate may increase. Signs of returning consciousness during ketamine anesthesia include increased muscle movement, particularly of the facial muscles, and spontaneous swallowing.
  B. Deep anesthesia
    1. May produce tachycardia, pupillary dilation, a centrally placed eyeball, labored breathing, and opening of the jaws on inspiration. Deep anes-

thesia is differentiated by the absence of a palpebral reflex and limb movement and, usually, by the presence of hypotension.

C. Hypercarbia or hypoxemia

1. May produce cardiovascular stimulation with tachycardia and increased blood pressure

D. Movement initiated by the surgeon

1. Total body movement in response to traction on the abdominal wall or on a limb.

2. Muscle contraction when a nerve is severed

E. Hyperthermia

1. Characterized by panting and confirmed by high rectal or oral temperature

V. Treatment

A. Barbiturate, propofol, or ketamine anesthesia

1. Check placement of intravenous catheter.

2. Inject more drug.

3. Inject butorphanol 0.05–0.1 mg/kg or oxymorphone 0.025–0.05 mg/kg intravenously if appropriate for the patient.

4. Add inhalation anesthesia.

B. Inhalation anesthesia

1. Check placement and connections of endotracheal tube and circuit hoses.

2. Check vaporizer fluid level.

3. If movement corresponded to an increase in surgical stimulus, increase vaporizer setting.

4. Assess rate and, particularly, depth of breathing. Institute controlled ventilation if hypoventilation is moderate to severe.

5. In some surgical procedures, a dog may continue to respond despite a high vaporizer setting (2% halothane or 3% isoflurane). An alternative to increasing the vaporizer setting is to inject a small dose of opioid intravenously, for example, oxymorphone (Numorphan) 0.02–0.05 mg/kg

RESPIRATORY EMERGENCIES AND COMPLICATIONS

Airway Obstruction

I. General considerations

A. Airway obstruction can occur both at the beginning of and during anesthesia. Patients most likely to develop obstruction (brachycephalic breeds and animals with pharyngeal, tracheal, or cervical tumors) should have been identified before induction of anesthesia. Special preparations or techniques for these patients include (1) preoxygenation; (2) assembling a selection of tube sizes with a stilette and laryngoscope; (3) inserting a tracheostomy tube using local analgesia or assembling the equipment for performing a tracheostomy in case the need should arise; and (4) performing orotracheal intubation in the partially conscious patient using neuroleptanalgesia. All personnel working with anesthetized animals should regularly practice intubation of normal dogs and cats so that failure to intubate in an emergency will not occur because of inexperience.

II. Clinical signs

  A. Paradoxic breathing: during inspiration the thoracic wall is sucked inward, whereas the abdominal wall expands

  B. During inspiration the mouth opens, the lower jaw is pulled in, and the neck is flexed.

  C. In the absence of an endotracheal tube, inspiratory "crowing noise" (stridor) indicates partial laryngeal obstruction.

  D. Prolonged inspiratory time

  E. Exaggerated lift to chest wall

  F. Bronchial stridor or wheezing.

  G. Cyanosis (may not be present if patient has been breathing oxygen)

  H. Hypotension

III. Causes

  A. Obstruction in traumatized patients: swelling of tongue and pharyngeal tissues, accumulated blood and saliva, tracheal compression from cervical swelling (bite wound), ruptured trachea

  B. Abnormalities of the head and neck: limited movement of temporomandibular joints, occlusion of laryngeal opening by soft-palate and pharyngeal tissue in brachycephalic breeds, laryngeal paralysis, laryngospasm (often occurs in cats; may be triggered by saliva), ventricular sac eversion (bulldogs), soft-palate entrapment of epiglottis (beagles), pharyngeal or tracheal tumors, tracheal collapse

  C. Aspiration of solid object: gauze packing, blood clot, loose tooth, food material

  D. Complications with the endotracheal tube: tube in the esophagus or one bronchus, kinked tube, cuff overinflated with constricting lumen of tube, bevel of tube against wall of trachea, lumen obstructed by a mucus plug or dried K-Y lubricant (especially in cats and small dogs)

  E. Problems with the anesthesia machine: rebreathing bag empty so that the patient has no air to breathe; pop-off valve on circle closed, resulting in high circuit pressure and expiratory obstruction, hose(s) of anesthesia circuit kinked

  F. Bronchial obstruction: bronchospasm (aspiration, allergic reaction)

IV. Differential diagnosis

  A. Anesthetic overdose: evaluate signs for depth of anesthesia, breathing usually irregular, breathing by diaphragmatic effort only.

  B. Localized airway obstruction: failure of airflow with inspiratory stridor indicates obstruction is at the level of the vocal cords and above; with inspiratory and expiratory stridor it indicates obstruction is lower in respiratory tract.

  C. Generalized airway obstruction: bronchospasm, indicated by wheezing sounds heard on auscultation of the lungs, may be associated with aspiration of gastric reflux or signs of allergic reaction.

V. Treatment

  A. Airway obstruction anticipated from history and physical examination:

    1. Preparation for tracheostomy (see section IV) should be made when there is a high probability that orotracheal intubation cannot be accomplished.

    2. The anesthetist should be prepared with a laryngoscope—or a good light source and a tongue depressor—and a selection of small-diameter endotracheal tubes.

3. The patient should be kept quiet before induction of anesthesia because the increase in intrathoracic negative pressure generated during forced breathing from excitement may cause airway obstruction.

4. Preanesthetic sedation may precipitate complete obstruction; therefore, the patient should be under continuous observation after any drug has been injected.

5. Give the patient oxygen to breathe by mask for several minutes before induction of anesthesia and during intravenous induction to increase the arterial oxygen concentration (preoxygenation). This will delay the onset of hypoxemia during a difficult intubation.

6. Transtracheal ventilation may be used in patients with partial upper airway obstruction.

7. If a smaller than normal tube is inserted, controlled ventilation should be used to offset the increased resistance to spontaneous breathing.

8. The patient should be evaluated at the end of anesthesia, before extubation, for the potential ability to breathe adequately after extubation.

B. Unexpected airway obstruction

1. The head and neck should be extended, the mouth opened widely, and the tongue pulled rostrally. The trachea should be intubated if the obstruction persists.

2. Partial laryngospasm should be treated by topical application of lidocaine 2 mg/kg and oxygen by face mask. The trachea should be intubated if laryngospasm is complete.

3. The endotracheal tube and anesthesia hoses should be checked for kinks, and the rebreathing bag should be checked to see that it is not overdistended.

4. Deflate the endotracheal tube cuff, and reposition the tube.

5. A small-diameter endotracheal tube may become plugged with mucus; extubation may be necessary for diagnosis.

6. A bitten off piece of endotracheal tube that has been aspirated can sometimes be grasped with forceps. Alternatively, it may be retrieved by inserting a smaller endotracheal tube inside the broken piece, inflating the cuff, and slowly withdrawing the tube. The dog or cat will have to be reanesthetized for this procedure. Endoscopy may be necessary.

7. Other objects, such as gauze or a tooth, may be grasped by forceps, facilitated by an endoscope if available. Suction may be used to remove large blood clots.

8. A tracheostomy may be necessary to improve access to the foreign body if an endoscope is unavailable or to relieve the obstruction temporarily.

9. Treat bronchospasm (see section so named).

VI. Tracheostomy

A. An emergency tracheostomy should be a rare occurrence. Usually airway obstruction is anticipated, and the tracheostomy is performed aseptically under local or general anesthesia. One technique for tracheostomy is illustrated in Figure 8–1.

B. The animal should be positioned on its back, with a sandbag or roll of towels placed under its neck and its forelimbs pulled caudally (Fig. 8–1 A). The skin should be incised midline over the first to the eighth tracheal rings and the trachea exposed by separation of the sternohyoid muscles. The trachea may be incised between the third and fourth or fourth and fifth tracheal rings (Fig. 8–1 B) to approximately 40% of the circumference. A suture placed around the distal tracheal ring, or on each of the

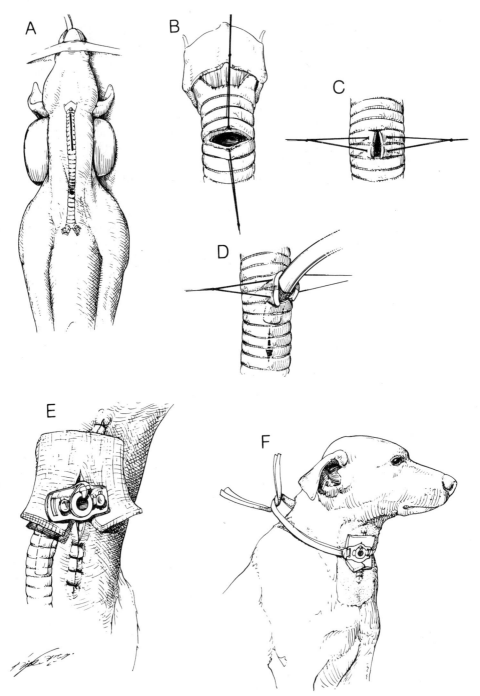

Figure 8–1. Tracheostomy: see text for description of technique. (From Aron DN, Crowe DT: Upper airway obstruction. Vet Clin North Am 15:891, 1985.)

proximal and distal rings, will be helpful in manipulating the trachea during insertion of the tracheostomy tube. Alternatively, two tracheal rings may be incised longitudinally. Short transverse incisions may be included at each end to form an "H" (Fig. 8–1 *C, D*). Stay sutures should be placed to prevent the tracheal cartilage from inverting when the tube is inserted.

C. The incision should remain open to avoid subcutaneous emphysema. If the incision is exceptionally long, a few sutures may be placed at either end (Fig. 8–1 E). Sterile gauze may be used to provide some protection for the wound.

D. The tracheostomy tube is usually secured by nonadhesive tapes tied around the neck (Fig. 8–1 F). Ideally, the tracheostomy tube should have a high-volume cuff that, when inflated, will distribute the pressure evenly and over a wider area of the tracheal mucosa than a low-volume cuff would, causing less damage. Postoperative nursing care will be easier if a tracheostomy tube with an inner cannula is used (Fig. 8–2). The diameter of the tube should be only slightly smaller than the size normally used for orotracheal intubation. The tube should be inserted gently and secured so that it cannot move. The external end of most tracheostomy tubes will connect directly to an anesthesia circuit. Care should be taken to prevent the weight of the breathing circuit from rotating the tracheostomy tube, which will abrade the tracheal mucosa.

Apnea

I. General considerations
   A. Breathing may cease (apnea) in an anesthetized animal from a number of causes. The duration of apnea may be transient (40 seconds) in response to traction on an ovary, or the apnea may be a sign of a serious complication.
II. Clinical signs
   A. No thoracic movement is visible.
   B. Cyanosis will not develop for several minutes if the animal has been

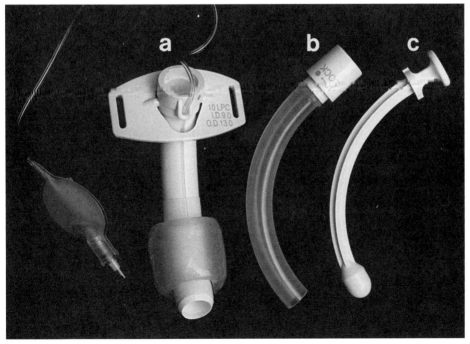

Figure 8–2. Tracheostomy tube (a) with an inner cannula (b). The inner cannula can be removed for cleaning without removing the tracheostomy tube from the trachea. A stilette (c) provides stiffness for initial placement of the tube.

breathing oxygen. The arterial carbon dioxide (CO_2) concentration begins to increase from the onset of apnea and may cause severe cardiovascular depression before hypoxemia develops.

III. Causes

A. Failure of oxygen delivery to brain may be due to cardiac arrest, hypotension (from anesthetic drugs or hemorrhage), or hypoxemia.

B. The major stimulus for breathing is CO_2. Anesthetic drugs depress the sensitivity of the brain respiratory centers to CO_2, so that CO_2 must accumulate in the blood to a higher concentration than normal (hypercarbia) before breathing is stimulated. Thus apnea may occur after induction of anesthesia with thiopental or propofol, and several minutes may elapse before sufficient CO_2 has accumulated for breathing to occur. Opioids severely change the threshold of the respiratory centers to CO_2 but, rather than apnea, opioids usually cause slow breathing or panting, which result in hypoventilation.

C. Lower than normal arterial P_{CO_2} (hypocarbia, hypocapnia) may result from insufficient CO_2 to stimulate breathing. This insufficiency of CO_2 may occur after a hyperventilatory response by the patient to a painful stimulus, after the patient has been "sighed," or at the termination of controlled ventilation.

D. Reflex suppression of respiration may be caused by traction on ovaries or tracheal mucosa stimulation.

E. Paralysis of muscles of respiration may be caused by neuromuscular blocking drugs (e.g., succinylcholine, pancuronium, atracurium, vecuronium).

F. Mechanical obstruction to breathing may result from continuous high pressure in the anesthesia circuit produced by a closed pop-off valve and resulting in maximal lung inflation.

IV. Diagnosis and treatment (see Fig. 8–3)

A. If respiratory failure was caused by hypoxemia, breathing may not resume immediately after the cause (airway obstruction, hypotension) has been corrected. Controlled ventilation with oxygen will be necessary for several minutes.

Bronchospasm

I. Clinical signs

A. Labored breathing

B. Wheezing

C. Cyanosis may or may not be present.

II. Causes

A. Hyperactivity of the airways may exist for several weeks after symptomatic recovery from an airway viral infection.

B. Reflex bronchospasm may be triggered by endotracheal intubation or large lung inflations in asthmatic patients.

C. Bronchospasm may be triggered by a variety of biochemical mediators, including histamine and arachidonic acid derivatives.

D. Aspiration of gastric contents may be causative.

E. Anaphylaxis may cause bronchospasm.

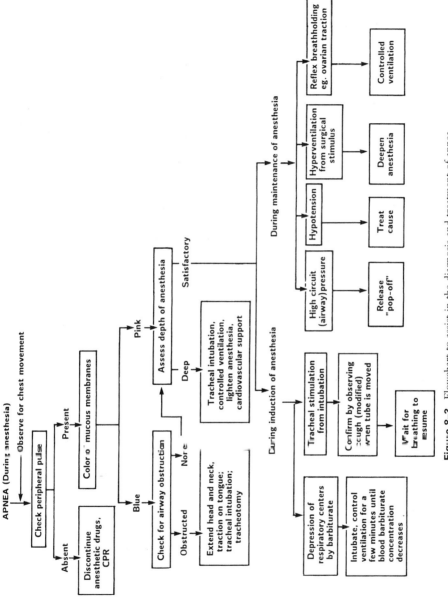

Figure 8–3. Flowchart to assist in the diagnosis and treatment of apnea.

161

III. Differential diagnosis
   A. Mechanical obstruction of the endotracheal tube: exaggerated chest movements without air flow
   B. Endobronchial intubation: chest excursion will be increased, but wheezing should be absent. Anesthesia may be inadequate despite a usually adequate vaporizer setting
   C. Pulmonary edema: fluid pulmonary sounds on auscultation
   D. Tension pneumothorax: chest movements will be exaggerated, lungs will not deflate, and high inspiratory pressure will be required to achieve positive pressure ventilation.

IV. Prophylaxis and treatment
   A. Anticholinergic drugs are effective in preventing and reversing allergic and reflex bronchospasm, although premedicant doses may not be sufficiently large. Atropine is also effective when administered into the trachea.
   B. Anesthetic drugs may influence the development of bronchospasm. The use of opioids is controversial, but it is unlikely that they produce bronchoconstriction. Thiopental leaves airway reflexes intact, allowing bronchoconstriction to occur. Ketamine would seem to be a better drug in a patient at risk, as it has prevented bronchoconstriction in experimental dogs with allergic asthma. Halothane and enflurane will reverse allergic bronchoconstriction in dogs, and isoflurane has been demonstrated to be almost as effective. Intravenous injection of lidocaine 2 mg/kg before tracheal intubation will prevent reflex bronchoconstriction in dogs.
   C. Increase inspired oxygen concentration to 100%.
   D. Bronchoconstriction during anesthesia can be treated with intravenous aminophylline 6 mg/kg injected slowly.
   E. Antihistamines are relatively ineffective in the treatment of allergic bronchospasm because histamine is not the only mediator involved. Antihistamines will not block reflex bronchoconstriction.
   F. Aspirated gastric contents should be removed by suction of the trachea and bronchi. Antibiotics should be administered parenterally. Anesthesia should be terminated as soon as possible.
   G. See discussion of treatment for anaphylaxis.

Hiccups

I. Clinical signs
   A. Jerky inspiration resembling hiccups in humans.
II. Treatment
   A. Squeeze reservoir bag on anesthesia machine, and hold lungs inflated for 5 seconds. This maneuver may have to be repeated several times. Allow arterial pressure to restabilize between inflations.

Hypoventilation

I. General considerations
   A. Hypoventilation occurs when alveolar ventilation decreases, resulting in an increase in arterial carbon dioxide tension (Pa_{CO_2}) above normal. Normal Pa_{CO_2} of conscious dogs has been reported as 34 ± 3 mm Hg and of cats as 34 ± 7 mm Hg.
   B. When the animal is breathing air, mild hypoventilation causes little change

in the oxygen saturation of hemoglobin, because of the shape of the oxyhemoglobin dissociation curve. Consequently, the mucous membranes may remain pink despite hypoventilation and an increase in Pa_{CO_2}. More severe hypoventilation will result in hypoxemia caused by alveolar collapse and, when the animal is breathing air, by the displacement of oxygen by carbon dioxide in the ventilated alveolae.

   C. Mild increases in Pa_{CO_2} directly activate the central nervous system (CNS) to increase cardiac output and heart rate. Catecholamines may be released and result in arrhythmias. Carbon dioxide has a direct effect of dilating peripheral arterioles and depressing myocardial contractility.

II. Clinical signs

   A. Decreased rate of breathing or rapid, shallow breathing may be observed.

   B. Bright-red mucous membranes from vasodilation may be observed when the Pa_{CO_2} is high.

   C. Cyanosis may or may not be present.

   D. A mild increase in heart rate and blood pressure occurs in most patients. Tachycardia and hypertension occasionally develop, and severe cardiovascular depression is produced in a few patients.

   E. Electrocardiographic (EKG) changes are an increase in size of the T wave or a change in polarity (Fig. 8–4).

   F. Premature ventricular depolarizations may occur.

III. Causes

   A. Anesthetic drugs

      1. Hypoventilation is common in dogs anesthetized with halothane or isoflurane after opioid premedication, and in cats anesthetized with halothane or isoflurane after ketamine.

   B. Neurologic disease

      1. Decreased neuromuscular function (myasthenia gravis, Guillain-Barré disease)

   C. Restricted air flow

      1. Partial airway obstruction (anatomic, pathologic, or produced by obstructed endotracheal tube or kinked anesthesia machine hoses)

   D. Movement of ribs restricted

      1. External pressure (surgeon leaning on thorax, instruments resting on a small animal)

      2. Fractured ribs

      3. Neuromuscular blocking drugs

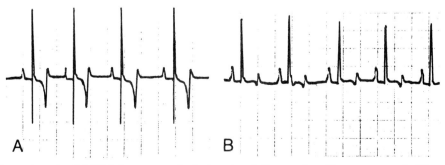

Figure 8–4. Lead II EKG from an anesthetized terrier. *A*, Dog was breathing spontaneously. Note the large inverted T wave. *B*, Recording 2 minutes after the start of artificial ventilation. The vaporizer setting was unchanged. Paper speed was 25 mm/second. (The trace was inked for clarity of reproduction.)

E. Diaphragm excursion limited
  1. Increased abdominal pressure (obesity, pregnancy, prone position, gastrointestinal distension, abdominal surgery, colonoscopy)
  2. Impaired function (ruptured diaphragm, neuromuscular blocking drugs)
F. Movement of lungs restricted
  1. Reduced intrathoracic space (pneumothorax, chylothorax, tumor, abdominal organs in thorax due to a ruptured diaphragm)
G. Lung disease
  1. Increased P_{CO_2} produced from ventilation-perfusion mismatch or shunt (pulmonary contusions, pulmonary edema, or anesthesia-induced lung collapse).
H. Anesthesia machine malfunction
  1. One-way valve on circle circuit is wet and therefore stuck in open position. Exhaled gas is no longer forced through the carbon dioxide absorber, and so the patient inhales carbon dioxide.
  2. Soda lime or Baralyme is exhausted and needs to be changed. Patient inhales carbon dioxide.

IV. Diagnosis
A. It may be suspected from the history or physical examination (neurologic disease, movement of ribs, diaphragm, or lungs restricted).
B. It may be suspected from the slow respiratory rate (fewer than 8 breaths per minute in a dog) or from rapid, shallow breathing.
C. Tidal volume can be measured by attaching a respirometer to the endotracheal tube or circle circuit.
D. Hypoventilation can be confirmed by Pa_{CO_2} of greater than 40 mm Hg in arterial blood (blood gas analysis).
E. Capnography measures CO_2 concentration in exhaled gas. Arterial P_{CO_2} is usually about 4 mm Hg higher than the concentration measured at the end of exhalation (end-tidal concentration). End-tidal CO_2 of 60 mm Hg indicates severe hypoventilation, and artificial ventilation should be started.

V. Treatment
A. Spontaneous ventilation can be allowed to continue if hypoventilation is mild and patient is young and healthy.
B. Lighten the level of anesthesia.
C. Institute controlled ventilation when breathing is moderately or severely depressed.
D. Institute controlled ventilation in geriatric and sick patients and in those with depressed cardiovascular function.

Hypoxemia

I. General considerations
A. Cyanosis has been defined as the presence of more than 5 g desaturated hemoglobin per 100 ml of blood. Cyanosis of mucous membranes may be difficult to determine when the patient has a low hemoglobin concentration, is covered with drapes, or is in poor lighting.
II. Definition
A. Arterial blood oxygen tension of less than 60 mm Hg and blood oxygen saturation of less than 90%
III. Clinical signs

To my wife Chris and our daughter Julie
Both have blessed my life every single day

NOTICE

Veterinary Medicine is an ever-changing field. Standard safety precautions must be followed, but as new research and clinical experience broaden our knowledge, changes in treatment and drug therapy become necessary or appropriate. Readers are advised to check the product information currently provided by the manufacturer of each drug to be administered to verify the recommended dose, the method and duration of administration, and the contraindications. It is the responsibility of the treating veterinarian, relying on experience and knowledge of the animal, to determine dosages and the best treatment for the animal. Neither the Publisher nor the editor assumes any responsibility for any injury and/or damage to animals or property.

THE PUBLISHER

THE NEW YORK PUBLIC LIBRARY   MM
MID-MANHATTAN LIBRARY   HIC
455 FIFTH AVENUE
NEW YORK, NEW YORK 10016

HIC REFERENCE

Contents

NO REFERENCE

Preanesthetic Physical Examination and Evaluation

Robert R. Paddleford

I. General considerations

Careful preanesthetic evaluation is essential for selection of drug regimen, monitoring requirements, and other supportive measures (e.g., fluid administration, ventilation).

A. Patient identification

1. Patient identification is extremely important. Measures such as neck banding with case number or the owner's and patient's names should be part of every patient's hospitalization.

2. Signalment

a. Species

Dogs and cats, which are the most common species in small animal practice, differ considerably in anatomy, physiology (e.g., normal arterial concentrations of carbon dioxide, nutritional requirements), pharmacologic responses, requirements for restraint techniques, and the types of diseases that commonly need surgery. *A cat is not a small dog.* Pets of other species (e.g., birds, snakes, turtles, rabbits, guinea pigs, hamsters, gerbils) also differ, one from another and from dogs and cats.

b. Breed

Several breed groups have anatomic or pharmacokinetic variations that markedly affect the choice of anesthetic regimens and surgical management.

(1) Brachycephalic breeds such as English bulldogs, Pugs, Pekingese, Boston terriers, French bulldogs, and Persians are extremely prone to airway obstruction. They generally require minimal premedication, rapid induction and intubation, oxygen administration, and rapid recovery from anesthesia.

(2) Two other breeds that have some of the characteristics of the brachycephalic breeds (long soft palates; redundant pharyngeal-laryngeal tissue; shortened muzzles) are the Chow Chow and the Chinese Shar pei. These two breeds may have upper airway obstruction problems.

(3) "Sight hounds" such as Greyhounds, Borzois, Afghans, Salukis, and Irish wolfhounds often exhibit prolonged recoveries following thiobarbiturate anesthesia because of their decreased body fat. Alternative induction techniques such as methohexital, propofol, or neuroleptanesthesia and inhalational maintenance should be considered.

(4) Chinese Shar peis, collies, German shepherds, Boxers, Golden

retrievers, Belgian breeds, Great Danes, Soft Coated Wheaten terriers, Neopolitan Mastiffs, black-and-tan dog breeds, and the Siamese, Himalayan, and Maine coon cats are all breeds that have been anecdotally associated with idiosyncratic reactions or increased sensitivity to central nervous system (CNS) depressants and general anesthetics.

  (i) No formal studies support these reports.

  (ii) Nevertheless, because of the anecdotal evidence, one should use caution when anesthetizing these breeds.

c. Age

  (1) Neonates are generally thought to metabolize and excrete drugs less efficiently than adults. It is suggested that premedication be minimal and that short-acting or antagonizable agents be used. Inhalational anesthetics are preferable to injectable anesthetics. Perioperative hypoglycemia should be prevented or rapidly detected and treated. Neonates are also very susceptible to hypothermia, and every effort should be made to prevent hypothermia. Neonates are also very susceptible to fluid imbalances.

  (2) Geriatric patients, like neonates, are thought to have a decreased anesthetic requirement and a decreased ability to metabolize and excrete injectable agents, especially longer-acting ones such as the phenothiazines. In general, such long-acting and nonantagonizable drugs should be avoided. Fluid therapy is very important in these patients because they may have subclinical renal impairment.

d. Sex

  The sex of the animal is usually significant only in pregnancy. Anesthesia should generally be avoided during pregnancy because of potential teratogenic or abortifacient effects. Anesthesia for cesarean section is discussed elsewhere.

e. Body weight

  An accurate body weight is important in determining drug doses (most drug dosages are given in mg/kg or mg/lb), fluid therapy, and anesthetic circuit selection.

  (1) Obese patients are usually given a reduced dose or one calculated on their ideal weight. Obese patients are much more likely to exhibit poor ventilation or hypoxemia during or following anesthesia than those of normal weight.

  (2) Cachetic patients may have impaired hepatic function and thus tolerate injectable agents poorly. Body positioning and padding are important to minimize hypothermia and to prevent pressure on nerves (such as the radial nerves).

f. Temperament

  (1) Every breed has its good-tempered and bad-tempered individuals.

  (2) Many individuals are well-mannered and easy to handle.

  (3) Some breeds (Chow Chows, Chinese Shar peis, German shepherds, and Rottweilers) are more likely to be aggressive or to be fear biters.

  (4) Aggressive, vicious, or unmanageable individuals may be impossible to evaluate prior to anesthesia. These animals are therefore at greater anesthetic risk because of the lack of evaluation and the stress of restraint.

B. Client complaint and history

1. The duration and nature of illness determine what procedures should be done and therefore the duration and type of anesthesia required. The duration and nature of illness also determine whether certain undesirable effects of the agents used might occur and what monitoring or supportive measures will be required.

2. Concurrent disease
   a. Diarrhea can produce dehydration and hypovolemia as well as loss of electrolytes.
   b. Acute vomiting can also result in dehydration and chloride loss, which may result in metabolic alkalosis. Chronic vomiting often produces metabolic acidosis.
   c. Any patient with a history or symptoms suspect of epilepsy should not be given agents that can lower the seizure threshold, such as the phenothiazines, methohexital, and enflurane. Virtually all anesthetic agents affect the electroencephalogram (EEG). Therefore, the agents used and the depth of anesthesia should be considered in EEG evaluation.
   d. Patients in heart failure are very poor anesthetic risks. Therapy with diuretics or inotropes should be instituted and the heart failure corrected before any elective procedures are done. Patients with a history of cardiac failure require close monitoring, anesthetic regimens that are minimally cardiac depressant, and careful fluid administration.
   e. Patients in renal failure are greater anesthetic risks because of uremic toxicity and fluid and electrolyte imbalance. Appropriate agent selection and monitoring are essential. Patients who have a history of renal failure or who are likely to go into renal failure will also require close monitoring to ensure that neither hypovolemia nor hypotension occurs in the perianesthetic period.

3. The level of activity should be determined. Very excitable or aggressive patients will usually benefit greatly from premedication, whereas depressed patients will need little if any. Any neurologic deficit should be noted so that its presence during recovery is not unwarrantably attributed to anesthetic management. The patient's exercise tolerance can help predict how cardiopulmonary depression from anesthesia will be tolerated.

4. Previous and current administration of drugs may affect the anesthesia regimen.
   a. Organophosphates have various characteristics that must be considered.
      (1) Organophosphate toxicity may be potentiated by phenothiazines because they compete for esterases.
      (2) Organophosphates are cholinesterase inhibitors, so the decrease in plasma cholinesterase activity will markedly prolong the action of succinylcholine.
      (3) Flea collars impregnated with dichlorvos were once thought to potentiate barbiturate anesthesia, but this connection has been disproved.
   b. Sulfonamides can prolong sleep time from pentobarbital in laboratory rodents, presumably by displacing protein-binding sites.
   c. Chloramphenicol is a hepatic microsomal enzyme inhibitor and can thus prolong barbiturate (thiobarbiturates and pentobarbital) anesthesia.
   d. Streptomycin, neomycin, and polymyxin B all have neuromuscular-

blocking properties that can potentiate muscle paralysis produced by agents such as pancuronium or atracurium. This blocking property can be especially important if the antibiotics are given in the recovery period, as they may interfere with antagonism of or decline in the relaxant's activity, causing paralysis to persist or recur.

e. Digitalis glycosides can cause many types of arrhythmias and may potentiate the dysrhythmic effects of agents such as xylazine, the thiobarbiturates, and halothane.

f. Beta-adrenergic blocking agents will markedly potentiate the cardiovascular depressant actions of general anesthetics. Thus, these agents can produce significant decreases in cardiac output.

g. Phenobarbital enhances hepatic microsomal enzyme activity. It may increase the clearance of some drugs.

h. H2 blockers such as cimetidine reduce hepatic microsomal enzyme activity. This action may slow the metabolism of some injectable anesthetics and thus prolong their effects.

i. Carbonic anhydrase inhibitors are used in some ophthalmology cases. They can produce metabolic acidosis and hence a more profound or an increased duration of effect from some injectable anesthetics.

j. Calcium channel blockers are highly protein bound. They can produce smooth-muscle dilation and neuromuscular blockade. They can potentiate the hypotension and bradycardia that sometimes occur with opioids, alpha-2 agonists, and inhalant anesthetics. They can also potentiate muscle relaxants.

5. Previous anesthetic reactions should be given serious consideration. Although they can frequently be explained (for example, prolonged recovery in a dog premedicated with acetylpromazine can be explained by the dog's age if the dog is very old), care should be taken to avoid the previous problem. It is extremely important in this regard to obtain "informed" consent from the owner.

6. Recent feeding will increase the risk of vomiting after induction of anesthesia and in the recovery period and thus increase the risk of tracheal aspiration. Fasting of most small animal patients for 8–12 hours is recommended. Diabetic and very young animals at risk for hypoglycemia should be monitored for vomiting or given parenteral dextrose to help prevent hypoglycemia.

II. Current physical examination

It is extremely important that a physical examination be performed before administering any premedication or anesthetic agent to the patient.

A. General body condition

1. Obesity is an increasingly common finding in pets and can increase anesthetic risk. It can also make venipuncture, catheter placement, and monitoring more difficult.

2. Cachexia is usually a sign of underlying disease. It may be associated with decreased glycogen reserves and thus increase the risk of unrecognized intraoperative hypoglycemia. It also makes assessment of hydration more difficult as patients with cachexia commonly have poor skin elasticity with "tenting."

3. Pregnancy affects many different organ systems and the patient's response to anesthetics. For example, minimal alveolar concentration (MAC) of inhalational agents is decreased during pregnancy, apparently well before term. Other changes in maternal physiology are discussed elsewhere in this text.

4. Dehydration can have many causes, but it always increases the risk of anesthesia as it may indicate current or impending hypovolemia. Every effort should be made to correct fluid deficits prior to anesthesia induction.

B. Cardiovascular status evaluation

1. Heart rate and rhythm vary among species.

   a. Dog: 70–180 beats/min. Rates are generally inversely related to size. Sinus arrhythmia is not considered pathologic in the dog.

   b. Cat: 145–200 beats/min.

2. Simultaneous assessment of heart and pulse rate and quality can reveal pulse deficits (such as from premature ventricular contractions). Poor pulse quality can result from hypovolemia, peripheral vasoconstriction, or other cardiovascular abnormalities.

3. Capillary refill time (CRT) is easily assessed in nonpigmented mucous membranes. Prolonged CRT usually indicates peripheral vasoconstriction or decreased tissue perfusion.

4. Auscultation for cardiac murmurs is important, although the presence of a murmur does not necessarily correlate with risk of anesthesia. Murmurs, if present, should be evaluated in conjunction with other cardiovascular findings.

C. Pulmonary testing

Pulmonary testing as is commonly done in human patients is difficult to do in animals because of their lack of cooperation. Nonetheless, it is extremely important to assess the patient's respiratory system.

1. Respiratory rate and depth should be noted. It is important to differentiate between tachypnea (panting) and dyspnea (difficult or labored breathing). Cats are primarily nasal breathers, so open-mouthed breathing in this species indicates dyspnea.

2. Mucous membrane color should be assessed in nonpigmented areas in the presence of adequate lighting.

   a. Pallor usually indicates anemia but can also be seen with vasoconstriction caused by pain or cold.

   b. Cyanosis indicates hypoxemia but can be detected only if there is more than 5 g/dl of unoxygenated hemoglobin. Severely anemic patients can therefore be hypoxemic but not cyanotic. The ability to detect cyanosis can vary greatly from one observer to the next.

3. Auscultation for breath sounds should be performed over the lung fields on both sides of the chest and is most readily done with a calm, cooperative patient.

4. Upper airway obstruction can result from stress or drug administration and can cause severe hypoxemia within 90 seconds in a patient who has been breathing room air. The brachycephalic breeds are most prone to upper airway obstruction, but it can occur in other breeds as a result of laryngeal or pharyngeal masses. The routine examination should include palpation of the trachea (which will help in selecting an appropriate size of endotracheal tube), observation of whether the animal can breathe comfortably with the mouth closed, and verification that the mouth can be opened easily for intubation.

5. Percussion of the chest can be useful in diagnosing pneumothorax, hydrothrax, pneumonia, and so forth.

D. Hepatic function

Hepatic function is important not only for anesthetic metabolism and excretion but because of its influence on other body systems. Any patient who appears jaundiced or whose blood fails to clot normally should be checked for hepatic disease.

E. Renal disease

Renal disease should be suspected in patients showing anuria, oliguria, or polyuria/polydipsia. Palpation of a kidney of abnormal size or shape should be followed by appropriate diagnostic tests. Preexisting renal disease can be exacerbated by anesthesia or surgical stress.

F. Gastrointestinal disease

Gastrointestinal disease is very common in small animals. Diarrhea and vomiting cause the fluid and electrolyte imbalances noted previously. Parasites can cause diarrhea, anemia, or obstructions. Abdominal distention is of concern because of its ability to impair ventilation and, if severe (as in gastric dilatation or volvulus), depress cardiac output.

G. Neurologic dysfunction

Patients presenting with the extremes of neurologic dysfunction have differing but equally important problems.

1. Seizures
   a. The need to avoid epileptogenic agents in patients with a history of seizures has been discussed.
   b. Drugs such as phenobarbital, which are used to treat seizure disorders, can activate hepatic enzymes. This reaction generally poses no problem in clinical practice, but it is thought to increase the metabolism of methoxyflurane into free fluoride ion, which is nephrotoxic in humans.
   c. Patients who are having seizures have an increased oxygen requirement yet have impaired ventilation. Therefore, hypoxemia is probable (if the patient is breathing room air). In addition, prolonged or very frequent seizures can produce hyperthermia.
   d. Drugs such as diazepam given parenterally to control seizures will potentiate the effects of anesthetic agents.

2. Coma
   a. Comatose patients do not need anesthesia but frequently require monitoring and cardiopulmonary support.
   b. Comatose patients are at risk for tracheal aspiration.

H. Metabolism
   1. Hyperthermia will increase the patient's oxygen requirement.
   2. Hypothermia will potentiate the effects of anesthesia.

I. Integument
   1. Elasticity of the skin is decreased in dehydrated patients.
   2. If the patient has cutaneous neoplasia, the possibility of pulmonary metastases should be considered.
   3. Subcutaneous emphysema usually indicates pneumomediastinum or pneumothorax and may accompany fractured ribs.
   4. Parasite (fleas, mites) infestation can cause anemia.
   5. Burns, especially if extensive, can cause severe fluid and electrolyte loss.
   6. Trauma can cause laceration or bruising of the skin.

J. Musculoskeletal system
   1. Weakness may be due to neurologic abnormalities, electrolyte imbalances, hypoglycemia, or poor cardiac output. If weakness is severe, the respiratory muscles may also be affected, causing hypoventilation.

    c. Ways to minimize exposure to waste anesthetic gases

       (1) Avoid mask and chamber inductions when possible. Work in a well-ventilated area and under a fume hood with these techniques when possible.

       (2) Use properly fitting masks when masking is required.

       (3) The vaporizer and N_2O should be turned off if the breathing system is not connected to the patient.

       (4) Endotracheal tubes should be used with the cuff inflated to prevent leakage during anesthesia.

       (5) The reservoir bag should be emptied into the scavenging system before the patient is disconnected from the breathing system.

       (6) Minimize spillage of liquid anesthetic by using appropriate spouts for filling vaporizers. Refill vaporizers at the end of the day when most personnel have gone. Fill vaporizers in a well-ventilated location.

       (7) Assure that scavenging systems are in proper working condition.

       (8) Routinely evaluate all anesthetic equipment (machines, breathing systems, and scavenging systems) to assure proper function and to detect and correct leaks (e.g., high-pressure leaks from N_2O cylinders). A regular log of equipment checkout and maintenance procedures is ideal.

       (9) Personnel at special risk (e.g., pregnant women) should seek the advice of their physician about exposure to waste anesthetic gases. They should consider wearing activated charcoal masks if they must work in close proximity to anesthesia machines. Remember, activated charcoal is not effective in scavenging N_2O.

    d. It is prudent to establish a consistent program for monitoring exposure to waste gases. Economical monitoring systems are available.

K. Evaluating an anesthesia machine: checkout recommendations

    1. Anesthesia machines should be evaluated before use each day and before use with each patient. Evaluations help to assure that the machine and breathing system will be safe for the patient and that no hazards exist for personnel working in the vicinity of the machine. The Food and Drug Administration has published *Anesthesia Apparatus Checkout Recommendations* suggesting that the following practices or their equivalents be followed.[12, 13] Guidelines for the checkout specifically of veterinary anesthesia machines have also been published.[11]

    2. Evaluation procedures may include the following:

      a. Central O_2 and N_2O supplies should be checked for quantity and pressure.

      b. All parts of the anesthesia machine should be visually inspected for defects or improper connections.

      c. The absorbent for CO_2 should be evaluated and changed if necessary.

      d. The scavenging system should be evaluated for proper connections, and charcoal canisters, if used, should be confirmed to be functional.

      e. The flow-control valves for the flowmeters should be "off."

      f. The vaporizer should be filled, sealed, and "off."

      g. Oxygen cylinders on the machine should be evaluated. With the central O_2 "off," the cylinder valve should be opened slowly to assure a minimum pressure of 500 psi. With the cylinder valve "on" and the flowmeter control "off," the cylinder should be checked for slow leaks (e.g., a drop in pressure over a period of 10 minutes).

   h. The N_2O cylinders should be checked the same way as the O_2 cylinders.

   i. Starting in the "off" position, flowmeter indicators should be checked for sticking or erratic movement through their full range.

   j. With the small cylinders on the machine "off," central supplies of O_2 and N_2O should be checked by adjusting flows to mid-range and assuring that the line pressure remains at 50 psi.

   k. With the vaporizer "off," no odor of anesthetic should be present when the O_2 flowmeter is turned "on."

   l. On a circle system, the function of the one-way valves should be checked. They should be properly assembled, with all parts in place. Wearing a surgical mask, the operator can exhale through the Y-piece to check the movement of the expiratory valve. With the pop-off valve "closed" and the Y-piece "open," compression of the reservoir bag should confirm the function of the inspiratory valve.

   m. The circle and the anesthesia machine should be tested for leaks.

     (1) With the pop-off valve closed and the Y-piece occluded, the system is filled with O_2, and the O_2 flow is set at 5 L/min. When the system pressure reaches 20 cm of H_2O, the O_2 flow is gradually decreased until the pressure no longer rises. Any leak should be negligible.

     (2) Squeeze the reservoir bag to produce a pressure of 40–50 cm of H_2O, and assure that the system is tight.

     (3) One recommendation is that at a pressure of 30 cm of H_2O in the circle system, the leak rate should be less than 250 ml/min and that the pressure should remain at 30 cm of H_2O for at least 10 seconds.[2]

     (4) When the pop-off valve is opened slowly, the pressure in the system should decline. With the Y-piece occluded and the pop-off valve open, only negligible positive or negative pressures should develop at O_2 flows of zero and 5 L/min.

     (5) The open pop-off valve should provide pressure relief when the flush valve is activated.

   n. Bain circuits and other pediatric noncircle (non-rebreathing) systems should be evaluated before use.

     (1) For the complete system evaluation of a Bain circuit, the patient port is occluded, the relief valve or port is closed, and the reservoir bag is distended. The bag should remain distended, and the pressure should not decrease.

     (2) In addition, the inner tube of the Bain coaxial system should be checked for leaks by briefly occluding the inner tube at the patient end of the system while the O_2 flow is set at 1–2 L/min. With an intact system, the O_2 flow indicator should fall in the flow tube.

     (3) The complete system check in item "(1)" is appropriate for other pediatric systems (e.g., Ayre's T-piece system).

3. Between patients anesthetized on the same day, abbreviated evaluations may suffice, but operators should assure maximum safety for each patient. Generally, the breathing system should be checked before each patient, and the vaporizer should be refilled and gas cylinders replaced if necessary.

4. Other checkout recommendations may be explained in the operations

Contributors

Sandee M. Hartsfield, DVM, MS

Professor and Associate Department Head, Department of Veterinary Small Animal Medicine, College of Veterinary Medicine; Chief of Veterinary Anesthesiology, Veterinary Teaching Hospital, Texas A&M University, College Station, Texas

Anesthetic Equipment

Steve C. Haskins, DVM, MS

Professor, Department of Surgery and Radiological Sciences; Director, Small Animal Intensive Care Unit, Veterinary Medical Teaching Hospital, University of California, Davis, School of Veterinary Medicine, Davis, California

Controlled Ventilation and Mechanical Ventilators; Perioperative Monitoring; Fluid, Electrolyte, and Acid-Base Balance: Maintenance in the Perioperative Period

Charles J. Sedgwick, DVM, DACLAM, DACZM

Director of Animal Health Services, Los Angeles Zoo, Los Angeles, California

Anesthesia for Small to Medium Sized Exotic Mammals, Birds, and Reptiles

Cynthia M. Trim, BVSc, MRCVS, DACVA, DECVA

Professor in Anesthesiology, College of Veterinary Medicine, University of Georgia, Athens, Georgia

Anesthetic Emergencies and Complications; Postanesthetic Care and Complications

Preface

Since the first edition was published a decade ago, knowledge of the anesthetic process has expanded at an unprecedented rate, and the information available to veterinarians has also expanded. New drugs, equipment, and techniques have become available, and the busy small animal practitioner, on the one hand, has been overwhelmed with a new body of anesthesia information and, on the other, has been expected to have readily available the knowledge and expertise of that expanded armamentarium. To keep abreast of all the anesthesia research and clinical literature, however, has become a luxury for most small animal veterinarians.

To meet this need, we have developed a manual in a concise outline format that allows us to offer information in the most easily retrievable form. The contributors have provided the most pertinent information from their own clinical experience and have given the reader a synthesis of the current literature and clinical research. This is not an all-encompassing textbook, but rather a practical clinical guide of small animal anesthetic principles and techniques.

I am grateful to the contributors, all recognized authorities in veterinary anesthesia, for their excellent chapters. Without their efforts, *Manual of Small Animal Anesthesia* would not have been possible.

The staff at the W.B. Saunders Company deserves special thanks for their efforts in the production of this book. The desire for a high quality, professional product of benefit to the veterinary profession is representative of the high standards at the W.B. Saunders Company. They have always been a leader in books for the veterinary profession.

I would like to extend special thanks to Ray Kersey for his excellent help and assistance in the preparation of this book. Without Ray's guidance and suggestions, this book would not have been possible. Additionally, I would like to thank the editorial and production staff of the W.B. Saunders Company for their excellent assistance, guidance, and professionalism.

Finally, I would like to thank Dr. Charles E. Short, my teacher, my colleague, and most importantly, my friend, whose training, advice, and encouragement allowed me to undertake this volume.

ROBERT R. PADDLEFORD, D.V.M.

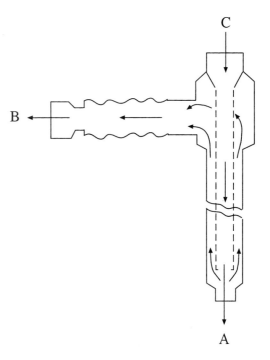

Figure 5–3. Diagram of Universal F System (an alternative to the traditional inspiratory and expiratory breathing tubes of a circle system). Arrows show the direction of gas flow—from C to A on inspiration and from A to B on exhalation.
A = endotracheal tube connector (15 mm i.d.)
B = connector (22 mm i.d.) to the expiratory one-way valve of the circle system
C = connector (22 mm i.d.) to the inspiratory one-way valve of the circle system

circle system. The patient must inspire through the vaporizer; it must be of a low-resistance type.

b. Only fresh gas flow rate determines whether a circle system is classified as closed, low-flow, or semiclosed. A common mistake is to base this classification on the patency of the pop-off valve, but the pop-off valve (a safety feature) should be open in all circles except during artificial ventilation.

(1) The consumption of O_2 in an anesthetized patient is variable, depending on such factors as the patient's body weight and surface area and the anesthetic itself. Reported values for O_2 consumption in anesthetized dogs range from 3 ml/kg to 11 ml/kg pcr minute.[1]

(2) In a closed circle, the fresh gas flow matches the patient's metabolic consumption of O_2 and anesthetic. As O_2 consumption is variable, common practice is to use a fresh gas inflow that keeps the reservoir bag approximately three fourths full. N_2O should not be used in closed circle systems.

(3) A low-flow circle uses a fresh gas inflow that is greater than the patient's metabolic O_2 consumption, but less than traditional higher flows (<22 ml/kg per minute) for semiclosed circle systems.[9] Generally, N_2O is not recommended for use in low-flow circle systems without continuous monitoring of inspired and expired gases (O_2).

(4) Traditional semiclosed circles use fresh gas flow rates (22–44 ml/kg per minute) that significantly exceed the patient's metabolic O_2 consumption.[9] Commonly, three times the patient's O_2 consumption has been recommended.[5] N_2O oxide can be used safely in semiclosed circle systems; N_2O flow is added to the calculated O_2 flow to achieve the desired concentration of N_2O.

(5) Many of the recommendations about closed and low-flow circles are primarily for maintenance of anesthesia. Often, semiclosed

circle flow rates are suggested for induction, for the first 10 minutes after induction, and for crises (e.g., the depth of anesthesia becomes too light during maintenance) when VOC vaporizers are in use.

(6) The minimum fresh gas flow to a circle system may be limited by the minimum flow required by the vaporizer. Most VOC vaporizers are linear in output above carrier gas flows of 300–500 ml/min. In addition, flowmeters for O_2 and N_2O may not be accurate at very low flows.

(7) Guidelines for low-flow and closed-circle systems with VOC and VIC vaporizers have been published.[9]

4. Pediatric, noncircle breathing systems include those systems commonly called "non-rebreathing systems," and they have been classified as Mapleson systems.[5] True non-rebreathing systems were designed with valves to route exhaled gases to the atmosphere (e.g., the Stephens-Slater valve). Other pediatric systems, used with very high fresh gas flows, essentially produce non-rebreathing because of the rapid washout of CO_2; these systems do not use soda lime for absorption of CO_2. Because pediatric systems may be operated with moderate flow rates, some rebreathing may occur. Modifications of the Ayre's T-piece system and Bain circuits seem to be most prevalent.

   a. Application, advantages, and disadvantages of noncircle pediatric systems:

   (1) These systems are usually used for patients weighing less than 7 kg; however, some veterinary anesthesiologists use them only for patients weighing less than 3 kg.

   (2) They induce less resistance to breathing and contain slightly less mechanical dead space than circle systems. Less inspiratory effort is required than with circle systems.

   (3) The concentration of inhalant anesthetic in the system can be changed rapidly, making alteration of the depth of anesthesia easy.

   (4) Compared with circle systems, noncircle systems are relatively inexpensive to purchase and maintain, but they are expensive to use because of the higher fresh gas flows. Higher flow rates mandate the use of an efficient scavenging system.

   (5) The higher flows with these systems, as compared against circle systems, cause greater loss of heat and humidity through the patient's respiratory system.

   (6) They are lightweight systems (e.g., Bain circuits are mostly plastic) that are less cumbersome for small patients.

   b. A Bain valveless, coaxial system (Fig. 5–4) is a modified Mapleson D system.

   (1) The smaller internal tube delivers fresh gases to a point near the endotracheal tube connector, which minimizes mechanical dead space by rapidly washing out CO_2, between exhalation and the next inspiration.

   (2) The external corrugated tube transports exhaled gases and excess fresh gases from the patient end of the Bain system to the reservoir (bag).

   (3) The overflow port may be built into the reservoir bag, or the Bain's corrugated outer tube may attach to a metal block with a

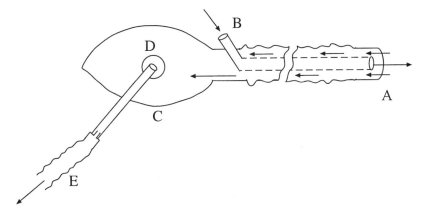

Figure 5–4. Diagram of Bain circuit. Arrows indicate the flow of gases during the period between exhalation and inhalation.
A = connector (15 mm i.d.) to the endotracheal tube connector (15 mm o.d.)
B = fresh gas inlet into the Bain circuit (continuous high flow to assure washout of CO_2)
C = reservoir bag
D = overflow outlet
E = corrugated tubing to the scavenging system

pop-off valve, a reservoir bag, and a manometer. In either case, the overflow port is connected to a scavenging system.

(4) Recommended total fresh gas flow rates (O_2 flow, or O_2 flow plus N_2O flow if N_2O is used) into a Bain circuit are quite variable.

   (i) To assure no rebreathing of CO_2 in essentially all patients, a total flow rate of two to three times the minute volume is required, but other guidelines are often used. These guidelines have been reviewed.[5]

   (ii) During spontaneous ventilation, a total flow of 100–130 ml/ kg per minute has been recommended.[10] Total flow rates of 440–660 ml/kg per minute will assure that there is essentially no rebreathing of carbon dioxide. Other researchers have recommended flow rates that are between these values.[5]

   (iii) With controlled ventilation, a total fresh gas flow of 100 ml/ kg per minute may be adequate.[10]

   (iv) Generally, the total flow rate for a Bain circuit is above 500 ml/min, even with very small patients.

c. Ayre's T-piece, Norman Elbow, Jackson-Rees, and similar Mapleson systems are common and have been described.[1, 2, 4, 5] These systems are used like Bain systems, but total fresh gas flow rates of two to three times the patient's minute volume are recommended to prevent rebreathing of CO_2.

5. Scavenging systems are used to eliminate excess anesthetic gases from the environment of the operating room and thus minimize the exposure of personnel to waste anesthetic gases. Because potential health hazards have been associated (though with little proof of a cause-and-effect relationship) with exposure to the inhalant anesthetics, scavenging should be employed whenever inhalant anesthetics are used.[11]

a. Potential health hazards associated with exposure to inhalants

   (1) Short-term—headaches, fatigue, lethargy, depression, pruritis, and decreased performance and mental acuity

   (2) Long-term—spontaneous abortions (known effect of exposure to

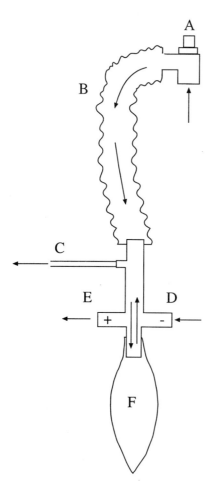

Figure 5–5. Diagram of a simple scavenging system for use with a high-pressure vacuum system. A similar setup can be used effectively with low-pressure vacuum systems or passive scavenging systems.
A = pop-off (APL) valve from a circle breathing system
B = corrugated tubing from the pop-off valve to the interface of the scavenging system
C = hose to a high-pressure vacuum system (often a flow-control valve is present on this line)
D = negative pressure-relief valve (allows entrainment of room air if needed)
E = positive pressure-relief valve (allows escape of gases if the scavenging system should overfill)
F = reservoir bag of the scavenging system (functions as a storage area for excess gases that are entering the scavenging system faster than they can be removed by the vacuum system)

N_2O), congenital abnormalities, neoplasia, hepatic disease, and renal disease

b. Components of a scavenging system (Fig. 5–5)
   (1) Gas-capturing assembly (scavenging pop-off valve) and transfer tubing
   (2) Interface system and transfer tubing
       (i) Positive and negative pressure-relief valves
       (ii) Reservoir bag
       (iii) Vacuum regulator
   (3) Gas-disposal system
       (i) Active system
           • High-pressure dedicated vacuum system
           • Low-pressure dedicated vacuum system
           • Non-recirculating air-conditioning system (effective with 12–15 air changes per hour)
       (ii) Passive system
           • Passively venting gases to the floor is not effective.
           • Conduit through an outside wall is effective.
           • Activated charcoal canister is effective. It should be changed every 8 hours. It is ineffective with N_2O.

manuals for specific anesthesia machines, and other tests should be used when mechanical ventilators are to be used.[1, 2, 5]

III. Supplemental equipment

   A. Induction chambers or closed containers are useful for oxygenation and inhalant inductions in small patients. The main benefit is that induction can be completed without much physical restraint. Cats, small laboratory animals, and some small exotic and wild species accept induction in closed containers.

      Induction chambers should be essentially airtight except for the inlet for O_2 and anesthetic and the outlet for scavenging of excess gases. Complete control of waste gases would require concurrent use of a fume hood. The chamber should be clear for observation of the patient during induction; most are constructed of glass or Plexiglas. The primary concern is the patient's airway during the short period of struggling that may accompany the excitatory phase of induction. A 5-minute period of oxygenation before introducing the inhalant anesthetic is ideal.

      For most small animals, the fresh gas flow rate should be 2–5 L/min in a chamber that is relatively close to the size of the patient. Faster fresh gas flows are associated with more rapid inductions. Increasing the inhalant concentration at 0.5% increments about every 10 seconds until 4–4.5% isoflurane is being delivered seems to be accepted very well. Once the animal is induced to light anesthesia, the induction should be completed with a face mask. Unless there are specific medical contraindications to its use, N_2O can be delivered with both chamber and mask inductions, generally in concentrations of 50–60%.

   B. Face masks are used to preoxygenate animals prior to induction and to facilitate inhalant inductions in sedated, depressed, or very tractable animals. The flow rates and concentrations discussed for chambers are appropriate for mask inductions; higher flows promote the establishment of effective anesthetic concentrations, shorten induction, and dilute exhaled CO_2 under the mask. The mask should fit snugly over the nose and mouth to prevent leakage, entrainment of room air, and prolonged induction.

      Masks should be attached to a breathing system to provide the reservoir of gases needed to (1) meet tidal volume and minute volume demands and (2) provide a scavenging system for excess gases. Although many types of masks are functional, clear plastic masks with rubber diaphragms offer the advantages of a tight fit with minimal leakage and an unimpaired view of breathing during the induction process. Like the chamber, masking is associated with some leakage of anesthetic gases and so is best utilized under a fume hood.

   C. Endotracheal tubes should be used in essentially all patients that are to be maintained with inhalant anesthetics. Not only does an endotracheal tube offer the obvious advantages of providing a patent airway and a means for controlling ventilation, but a properly sized tube with a correctly inflated cuff is necessary to prevent contamination of the workplace with inhalant anesthetic.

      1. For small animal use, two basic styles of tubes are available. A Murphy-style tube (Fig. 5–6) has the same lumen size from the proximal to the distal end (patient end or beveled end). It has a side hole (Murphy eye) located opposite the bevel near the distal end of the tube to provide patency should the end hole become occluded. Most Murphy-style tubes are fitted with built-in cuffs, pilot lines, pilot balloons, and self-sealing valves for inflation and deflation of the cuffs. Uncuffed tubes are still marketed, though, and may be advantageous for very small patients.

        A Cole tube has two lumen sizes with the proximal end being larger

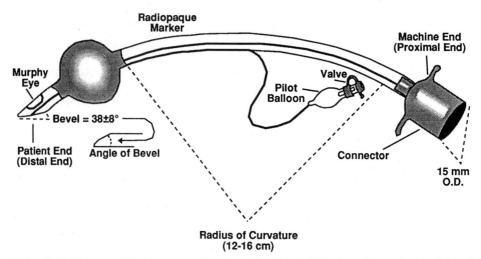

Figure 5-6. Diagram of Murphy-type endotracheal tube. The dark line from the proximal to the distal end of the endotracheal tube is the radiopaque marker. (From Hartsfield SM: Airway management and ventilation. In Thurmon JC, Tranquilli WJ, Benson GJ, eds. Lumb and Jones' Veterinary Anesthesia, 3rd ed. Baltimore: Williams & Wilkins, 1996, p. 517.)

than the distal end, creating a "shoulder" at the junction. The distal end fits into the larynx and trachea. This laryngotracheal part of the tube must be the correct size for the patient to protect the airway from foreign material and to create a seal to allow artificial ventilation. The proximal end of either style of endotracheal tube is fitted with an adapter/connector. The connector (15 mm o.d.) portion accepts the patient end of a breathing system (e.g., the Y-piece of a circle system).

2. Cuffed tubes are safest if the cuffs are of the "high-volume, low-pressure" design, allowing the cuff to be filled with enough air to seal the airway without creating a high pressure that might impair circulation to the tracheal mucosa. Generally, a cuff is inflated with enough volume to prevent leakage of gases around the cuff when a pressure of 20–25 cm of H_2O is applied to the respiratory system.

3. Most contemporary, high-quality endotracheal tubes are made from polyvinyl chloride or silicone rubber. Because of the propensity to cracking, difficulty with cleaning and sterilization, and opacity, red rubber tubes are no longer recommended. Clear endotracheal tubes allow easy inspection for patency so that, for example, accumulation of respiratory secretions can be seen. Silicone tubes are relatively soft, and they appear to traumatize tissues minimally. Endotracheal tubes for special purposes are available. For example, armored tubes with helical wire or plastic implanted within the wall facilitate procedures requiring extreme flexion of the head and neck.

4. In general, a variety of sizes of endotracheal tubes should be available—from 2.5 mm i.d. to 14 mm i.d.—in a mixed small animal practice. Cole tubes are advantageous for very small patients and some exotic species, and sizes from 5-French to 20-French can prove useful. French units on endotracheal tubes refer to outside diameter. An endotracheal tube should be of a length that allows the adapter/connector to be at the level of the patient's incisors and the cuff to be near the thoracic inlet. Very long tubes should be shortened (at the proximal end) to prevent intubation of one bronchus or creation of unnecessary mechanical dead space.

5. The markings or labels on endotracheal tubes follow:

    a. Manufacturer's name

    b. Internal diameter (i.d. in mm) (oral size)

    c. Outside diameter (o.d. in mm or in French units) (nasal size)

    d. Length markers from the distal end (cm)

    e. I.T., Z79, or F29 (indicating that the material has been implantation tested)

6. Endotracheal tubes should be clean, dry, and preferably sterile before use. Tubes should be inspected for patency, the adapter should be firmly seated into the proximal end of the tube, and the cuff system should be tested. A small amount of sterile, water-soluble lubricant placed on the distal end of the tube just before use is beneficial.

7. Once the endotracheal tube is in place, it should be secured to the patient to prevent movement of the tube or inadvertent extubation; movement of the tube within the trachea may irritate the mucosa.

D. Stylets are intended for stiffening endotracheal tubes to allow easier intubation. Commercially available stylets are malleable but rigid. They are usually made of wire coated with a plastic material. Such stylets are less likely to damage endotracheal tubes or tissues than stylets made from coat hangers or other wire. A stylet is not a guide tube; that is, a stylet should be placed entirely within the lumen of the endotracheal tube to provide rigidity and should not extend past the patient end of the endotracheal tube.

E. A guide tube facilitates passage of an endotracheal tube through the glottis and larynx and into the trachea. A guide tube can be placed through the lumen of the endotracheal tube so that a few centimeters of the guide tube extend beyond the patient-end of the endotracheal tube. The small diameter of the guide tube facilitates its introduction into the airway; then the guide tube directs the passage of the endotracheal tube into the larynx and trachea.

    For small animals, polyethylene urinary catheters, with the blunted end passing into the respiratory system, make excellent guide tubes. For medium to large dogs, 8-French to 10-French catheters work well as guide tubes. Smaller catheters should be chosen for animals requiring smaller endotracheal tubes. The guide tube should not occlude the lumen of the endotracheal tube. Guide tubes are especially useful in patients with oropharyngeal or laryngeal pathology. Often a guide tube can be passed under direct vision using a laryngoscope, whereas an endotracheal tube being passed alone would obstruct the view of the glottis.

F. Fiberoptic endoscopes or bronchoscopes can be used to expedite endotracheal intubation. An endoscope facilitates viewing of the larynx while passing either an endotracheal tube or a guide tube. Such ancillary equipment may be most useful in animals that are unable to open their mouths and in animals with laryngeal or tracheal lesions that could be adversely affected by blind passage of a guide tube or endotracheal tube.

G. Mouth specula can be used to facilitate endotracheal intubation, especially when the operator is working alone. Spring-type specula are quite useful. When specula are used, they should not be left in place with the patient's mouth opened widely for long periods. If specula are needed throughout anesthesia, they should be positioned so that the patient's mouth is not opened maximally.

H. Laryngoscopes are valuable for examination of the larynx, pharynx, and oral cavity. Although they are not essential for endotracheal intubation in most cases, laryngoscopes can be life-saving. Veterinarians should use laryngoscopes in enough normal patients to be proficient with them in life-threatening situations.

1. The parts of a typical laryngoscope include a handle (with batteries), a

blade, and a light source near the end of the blade. In a laryngoscope with a snap-on blade, the light comes on when the blade is extended to an angle of 90° to the handle. Before induction of anesthesia, the function of the laryngoscope should be assured (i.e., batteries and bulb should be checked).

2. Many styles of laryngoscope blades are available, including the Miller, the MacIntosh, and the Bizarri-Guiffrida. Sizes vary, and it is appropriate to have small, medium, and long blades (typically 205 mm for large dogs) for patients of various sizes. Blades of sizes 0 (very small), 2, and 4 provide a good variety to meet the needs of small animals.

3. Laryngoscopes facilitate intubation when they are used correctly, but they can be a hindrance when used improperly. Laryngoscopes work best when an assistant holds the patient's maxilla and tongue. The operator should place the distal tip of the blade at the base of the epiglottis to tip the epiglottis rostral and expose the glottis. The blade should be positioned flat on the tongue; a common mistake is to allow the handle and blade to rise away from the tongue, impairing the operator's field of view.

IV. Determining the cost of inhalation anesthesia
  A. Calculate the cost of O_2 and, if used, N_2O:
    1. Cost/Cylinder ÷ Liters/Cylinder = Cost/Liter
    2. Liters/Minute × 60 Minutes/Hour = Liters/Hour
    3. Cost/Liter × Liters/Hour = Cost/Hour
  B. Calculate the cost of the primary inhalant anesthetic:
    1. Cost/Bottle ÷ Milliliters/Bottle = Cost/Milliliters of Liquid
    2. Percent Concentration × Fresh Gas Flow in Liters/Hour = Liters of Vapor/Hour
    3. Liters/Hour × 1000 Milliliters/Liter = Milliliters of Vapor/Hour
    4. Milliliters of Vapor/Hour ÷ Milliliters of Vapor/Milliliters of Liquid = Milliliters of Liquid/Hour
    5. Cost/Milliliters of Liquid × Milliliters of Liquid/Hour = Cost/Hour
  C. At 20°C:[3]
    1. Desflurane: 1 ml of liquid = 207 ml of vapor
    2. Enflurane: 1 ml of liquid = 196 ml of vapor
    3. Halothane: 1 ml of liquid = 226 ml of vapor
    4. Isoflurane: 1 ml of liquid = 195 ml of vapor
    5. Methoxyflurane: 1 ml of liquid = 204 ml of vapor
    6. Sevoflurane: 1 ml of liquid = 182 ml of vapor

V. Sources of anesthetic equipment
  A. Anesco
    PO Box 492
    115 Etter Lane
    Georgetown, KY 40324
    502-867-0784
    800-416-9018

  B. Anesthesia Equipment Service and Supply
    1941 East 129th Street
    Thornton, CO 80241-1907
    800-809-8499

  C. Bivona Inc.
    5700 West 23rd Ave.
    Gary, IN 46406
    219-989-9150

D. Critical Care Products
   507 Garden Oaks Blvd.
   Houston, TX 77018
   800-392-6749

E. DRE, Inc.
   106 Watterson Trail
   Louisville, KY 40243
   800-477-2006

F. Matrx Medical, Inc.
   145 Mid County Drive
   Orchard Park, NY 14127
   716-662-6650

G. Summit Hill Laboratories
   Navesink, NJ 07752
   201-291-3600

References

1. Dorsch JA, Dorsch SE: Understanding Anesthesia Equipment, 2nd ed. Baltimore: Williams & Wilkins, 1984.
2. Dorsch JA, Dorsch SC: Understanding Anesthesia Equipment, 3rd ed. Baltimore: Williams & Wilkins, 1994.
3. Ehrenwerth J, Eisenkraft JB: Anesthesia Equipment: Principles and Application. St. Louis: CV Mosby, 1993.
4. Hartsfield SM: Machines and breathing systems for administration of inhalation anesthetics. In Short CE (ed): Principles and Practice of Veterinary Anesthesia. Baltimore: Williams & Wilkins, 1987, p. 395.
5. Hartsfield SM: Anesthetic machines and breathing systems. In Thurmon JC, Tranquilli WJ, Benson GJ (eds): Lumb and Jones' Veterinary Anesthesia, 3rd ed. Baltimore: Williams & Wilkins, 1996, p. 366.
6. Soma LR: Systems and techniques for inhalation anesthesia. In Soma LR (ed): Textbook of Veterinary Anesthesiology. Baltimore: Williams & Wilkins, 1971, p. 201.
7. Ludders JW: Vaporizers used in veterinary anesthesia. Semin Vet Med Surg (Small Anim) 8:72, 1993.
8. Bednarski RM, Gaynor JS, Muir WW III: Vaporizer in circle for delivery of isoflurane to dogs. J Am Vet Med Assoc 202:943, 1993.
9. Wagner AE, Bednarski RM: Use of low-flow and closed-system anesthesia. J Am Vet Med Assoc 200:1005, 1992.
10. Manley SV, McDonell WN: Clinical evaluation of the Bain breathing circuit in small animal anesthesia. J Am Anim Hosp Assoc 15:67, 1979.
11. Hartsfield SM, Cornick-Seahorn J, Cuvelliez S, Gaynor J, McGrath C: Commentary and recommendations on control of waste anesthetic gases in the workplace. J Am Vet Med Assoc 209:75, 1996.
12. Anesthesia apparatus checkout recommendations; availability. Washington, DC: Fed Reg 52:5583, 1987.
13. March MG, Growley JJ: An evaluation of anesthesiologists' present checkout methods and the validity of the FDA checklist. Anesthesiology 75:724, 1991.
14. Mason DE: Anesthesia machine checkout and troubleshooting. Semin Vet Med Surg (Small Anim) 8:104, 1993.

Controlled Ventilation and Mechanical Ventilators

6

Steve C. Haskins

GENERAL COMMENTS ABOUT VENTILATORS

I. An automatic ventilator is analogous to a mechanical hand squeezing the rebreathing bag.

II. Should I buy an automatic ventilator?

    A. Yes! (and then you should use it!) An automatic ventilator will do the following:

        1. Allow you to ventilate a patient without tying up expensive personnel.

        2. Provide proper and adequate ventilatory support to patients that might be marginal "pulmonary performers" (automatic ventilators take some of the worry out of using general anesthesia in critical patients).

        3. Smooth out anesthetic experiences in which the anesthetic depth is variable because the uptake of inhalational anesthetic is variable owing to the animal's variable alveolar minute ventilation.

    B. Personnel working around a ventilator should understand well its operations and idiosyncracies.

        1. Learn how to operate it using a rebreathing bag as an artificial lung.

        2. Monitor its function and the appropriateness of its settings for each patient.

    C. Ventilator sources

        1. New ventilators

            a. Bear Medical Systems, 2085 Rustin Ave., Riverside, CA 92507; 800-331-Bear

            b. Bird Corporation, Palm Springs, CA 92263; 714-327-1571

            c. Bourns, 9335 Douglas Dr., Riverside, CA 92503; 714-781-5060

            d. Engler Engineering Corp, 1099 East 47th St., Hialeah, FL 33013; 800-445-8581

            e. Hallowell Corp, 74 North St., Ste 214, Pittsfield, MA 01201-5116; 413-445-4263

            f. Puritan-Bennet (Nelcor), 1639 Eleventh St., Santa Monica, CA 90406

            g. Seimens-Elma, 2360 North Palmer Dr., Schaumburg, IL 60173-3887

        2. Previously owned ventilators (and equipment of all kinds)

            a. Universal Hospital Services, 4220 West Old Shakopee Rd., Bloomington, MN 55437; 612-721-3374

            b. Hospal Medical Corp, 4100 East Dry Creek Rd., Littleton, CO 80122; 202-770-2700

    c. A bank of large ("G" or "H") compressed-gas cylinders attached to a manifold provides a reasonably economical and convenient way of supplying medical gases. A system of variable diameters and thread types allows large cylinder valve bodies to accept only specific connectors from the manifold and regulator, preventing the inadvertent interchange of medical gases.

  4. Portable sources of medical gases

    a. Small cylinders ("E") of O_2 and N_2O attach to hanger yokes on anesthesia machines. Hanger yokes are pin-coded (pin-indexed safety system) to prevent inadvertent interchange of gases. The pin spacing differs for each gas. Two pins and a nipple on the hanger yoke correspond to two holes and the valve port on the valve body.

    b. Small cylinders on the anesthesia machine supply gases primarily for transport and emergencies (e.g., failure of the central supply). Veterinary machines may use small cylinders as the only gas source, requiring a ready supply for replacement of "E" cylinders when the pressure decreases (usually <500 psi).

D. A pressure gauge is needed for each gas supplied to a machine. The gauge indicates the cylinder pressure when the valve is open. Gauges are color-coded and labeled with the symbol of the gas. Generally, pressure gauges indicate the pressure on the cylinder side of the regulator. Pressure gauges may be present at other locations to indicate pipeline pressure (typically, 50 psi).

E. Regulators for compressed-gas cylinders

  1. Pressures in gas cylinders are high (cylinder to regulator equals a high-pressure system) and must be reduced and regulated to provide safe, efficient supplies of gases to the flowmeters. A regulator facilitates a constant pressure and flow to the flowmeter despite the continual drop in pressure as the gas in the cylinder is depleted. A lower, constant pressure downstream from the regulator decreases the sensitivity of the flowmeter control knob to manual adjustments.

  2. Typically, regulators on veterinary anesthesia machines have been set at about 50 psi (regulator to flowmeter and flush valve equals an intermediate-pressure system). Newer machines may utilize lower pressures (i.e., 37–45 psi) to assure preferential delivery of gases from the hospital's pipeline system (commonly set at 50 psi). Contemporary anesthesia machines for human use may be regulated to an even lower pressure.

F. The O_2 flush valve (Fig. 5–1) activates O_2 flow from the intermediate-pressure area ($\approx$50 psi) to the common gas outlet, bypassing the flowmeter and any vaporizer located outside the breathing system (VOC) in contemporary machines. The flush valve delivers a high, unmetered flow (35–75 L/min) of O_2 for refilling the circle system quickly in emergencies. In older veterinary machines, the flow through the flush valve may not bypass VOC vaporizers, which may deliver high anesthetic concentrations to the patient. The flush valve should not be activated with small-volume, pediatric breathing systems (e.g., Bain circuit); there is danger of over-pressurization and barotrauma. A flush valve should be recessed or protected to prevent inadvertent activation.

G. Flowmeters for medical gases

  1. Flowmeters for each medical gas measure and indicate the rate of flow to the common gas outlet. Flowmeters precisely control O_2 and N_2O flow rates. They assure that the appropriate amount of O_2 (total O_2 in ml/min) is delivered to meet the patient's metabolic demands and that

the delivered concentration (F_IO_2) will be sufficient for proper saturation of hemoglobin.

2. Gas enters a flowmeter through a needle valve and passes through a tapered tube, exiting at the top. An indicator rises in the tube as flow increases. Indicators are read at the top, except for ball-shaped indicators, which are read in the center. It is important to read the indicator correctly; a misreading can cause a difference of more than 0.5 L/min in some cases. The control knobs for flowmeters should be adjusted carefully and should not be tightened excessively. The lowest mark on the flowmeter's scale is the minimum accurate flow; lower flows should not be extrapolated.

3. Standard guidelines to help prevent adjustment of the wrong flowmeter:
   a. The control knob for O_2 should be as large or larger than the other flowmeter control knobs.
   b. The O_2 control knob should be fluted to differentiate it from other knobs in a cluster of control knobs.
   c. The O_2 flowmeter control knob should be to the right of other flowmeters in a cluster; O_2 is delivered downstream from other gases.

4. The controls for flowmeters should be "off" when the flowmeters are not in use. Pressure (turning "on" the cylinder valve) should not be applied to an open flowmeter.

H. Vaporizers
  1. Vaporizers are designed to change a liquid anesthetic into its vapor and to add a controlled amount of vapor to the flow of gases to the patient.[2] Relative accuracy is implied. Accuracy is important because vapor pressures of the inhalant anesthetics are high. Without controlled delivery, many times the minimum alveolar concentration (MAC) of the inhalant could be delivered, potentially with lethal consequences.
  2. Vaporizers have been classified using many schemes, and no single method is fully descriptive. The following classifications[2] (which are listed with an example vaporizer for each class) may be used:
     a. Method of output regulation
        (1) Variable-bypass or concentration-calibrated—Tec 3
        (2) Measured-flow—Vernitrol
     b. Method of vaporization
        (1) Flowover—Tec 3
        (2) Bubble-through—Copper Kettle
        (3) Injection—Tec 6
     c. Location of the vaporizer in relation to the breathing system
        (1) VOC = vaporizer out-of-the-circle (Fig. 5–1)—Tec 3
        (2) VIC = vaporizer in-the-circle (Fig. 5–2)—Ohio #8
     d. Method of temperature compensation
        (1) Thermocompensation
           (i) Bimetallic strip valve—Tec 3
           (ii) Silicone cone—Vapor 19.1
        (2) Supplied heat—Tec 6
     e. Specificity
        (1) Agent-specific—Tec 3
        (2) Multipurpose—Vernitrol
     f. Resistance

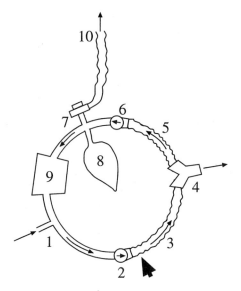

Figure 5–2. Diagram of the basic parts of a traditional circle breathing system. Small arrows show the direction of gas flow. If an anesthesia machine is equipped with a VIC vaporizer, it will be located at the large arrow between 2 and 3.
1 = fresh gas inlet (usually connected to the common gas outlet [Fig. 5–1] by rubber tubing)
2 = inspiratory one-way valve
3 = inspiratory breathing tube
4 = Y-piece
5 = expiratory breathing tube
6 = expiratory one-way valve
7 = pop-off (APL) valve
8 = reservoir bag
9 = absorbent canister
10 = corrugated tubing to the scavenging system
(see Fig. 5–5)

    (1) High-resistance or plenum—Tec 3
    (2) Low-resistance—Ohio #8
3. Most modern vaporizers are positioned outside the breathing circuit (VOC). Indeed, only VOC vaporizers are presently manufactured for use in human anesthesia. VOC vaporizers are considered to be precision vaporizers; they are flow-, temperature-, and back-pressure-compensated and are intended for use with a single anesthetic agent.
  a. VOC vaporizers have outputs that approximate the setting on the control dial. Therefore, the operator can make adjustments on the basis of MAC values as well as the clinical depth of anesthesia. Compared to VIC vaporizers, output from VOC vaporizers is less affected by changes in ventilation and flow.[6]
    (1) Changes in ventilation do not affect vaporizer output.
    (2) Higher fresh gas flows produce a faster achievement of the selected vaporizer concentration in the breathing system.
    (3) Artificial ventilation can be used safely (with no effect on the output of the vaporizer).
    (4) Because vaporizer output is relatively constant, increased ventilation will reduce the inspired concentration in a circle system as patient uptake of anesthetic increases.
    (5) Lower fresh gas flows can be used to improve economy.
    (6) Lower fresh gas flows are not associated with potentially unsafe increases in inspired anesthetic concentration.
  b. Tec-type vaporizers (Fluotec, Isotec, Pentec, Sevotec) are very common in veterinary anesthesia. Tec 3 vaporizers are available but are no longer being manufactured. Yet Tec 3 vaporizers consistently perform better than earlier models. Tec 2 vaporizers are unreliable at lower flow rates and are not recommended. Tec 3 vaporizers are described as concentration-calibrated, flowover with a wick, VOC, temperature-compensated (by a bimetallic strip valve), agent-specific, back-pressure-compensated (small vaporization chamber), and high-resistance.
  c. Newer Tec vaporizers (Tec 4, Tec 5, and Tec 6) are concentration-

calibrated vaporizers that are common in human anesthesia and are now being sold with veterinary anesthesia machines. Their construction and functional characteristics have been described.[2, 3]

(1) Tec 4 vaporizers are described as concentration-calibrated, flow-over with a wick, VOC, automatically thermocompensated, agent-specific, back-pressure-compensated, and high-resistance. The Tec 4 was designed to prevent the operation of more than one Tec 4 vaporizer at a time when multiple vaporizers are mounted on the same anesthesia machine.[2] The manufacturer recommends yearly service.

(2) Tec 5 vaporizers are described as concentration-calibrated, flow-over with a wick, VOC, automatically thermocompensated, agent-specific, back-pressure-compensated, and high-resistance. Compared to Tec 4 vaporizers, Tec 5 vaporizers have a larger capacity for liquid anesthetic. Output is more linear over a wider range of flows, and some functional characteristics of the control dial are better.[3] The manufacturer recommends service every three years.

(3) Tec 6 vaporizers were designed specifically for desflurane. They are classified as concentration-calibrated, injection, VOC, thermo-compensated (by supplied heat), agent-specific, unaffected by back pressure, and high-resistance. Tec 6 vaporizers are very expensive. They should be serviced annually at an authorized service center.[2]

d. Ohio concentration-calibrated vaporizers are common in veterinary anesthesia. They are described as concentration-calibrated, flowover with a wick, VOC, temperature-compensated (by a change in flow regulated by a temperature-sensitive bellows), agent-specific, back-pressure-compensated, and high-resistance.

e. Drager vaporizers (Vapor 19.1) have been common in veterinary anesthesia but are no longer being manufactured. They are described as concentration-calibrated, flowover with a wick, VOC, temperature-compensated (by an expandable silicone cone regulating flow through the vaporization chamber), agent-specific, back-pressure-compensated (by a long spiral inlet), and high-resistance.

f. Measured flow vaporizers (Copper Kettle and Vernitrol) are no longer manufactured but are available on reconditioned anesthesia machines. Output regulation is by calculation. Two flowmeters are used. One is for the flow of carrier gas through the vaporization chamber, where it becomes fully saturated with anesthetic. The other supplies gases to dilute the anesthetic to the desired concentration.

Calculators similar to slide rules are supplied to facilitate determination of flows. Gases exiting the vaporization chamber are fully saturated with anesthetic because the carrier gas (O_2) is bubbled through the liquid anesthetic after being dispersed through a diffuser. Measured-flow vaporizers are thermostable by virtue of their construction materials (silicon-bronze or copper); if necessary, flows are changed manually to maintain a constant output in response to a thermometer in the vaporizer. These vaporizers can be used to deliver any of the volatile liquid inhalant anesthetics if they are properly maintained. Back-pressure compensation is by means of a check valve. Measured-flow vaporizers are high-resistance, VOC vaporizers.

(1) Calculations of flow settings for measured-flow vaporizers follow:

(i) Lethal concentrations of inhalant anesthetic can be delivered from measured-flow vaporizers. Both the flow to the vaporization chamber and the diluent flow must be set correctly.

   (ii) The fastest and perhaps most reliable way to calculate the flows necessary for delivery of an accurate concentration of an inhalant anesthetic is to use a slide rule–like calculator. The flow of carrier gas to the vaporizer can be determined accurately with the calculator and the following information:

    • Identity of the anesthetic agent

    • Temperature of the liquid anesthetic

    • Total gas flow requirement for the patient

    • Desired delivered concentration

  (2) Estimates of the flow requirements for measured-flow vaporizers can be made. As an example, the following would allow approximation of the flow needs if isoflurane (at a vapor pressure of 240 mm of Hg at sea level and a vaporizer temperature of 70–75°F) is used with a total fresh gas flow of 3 L/min to produce a concentration of 2% isoflurane:

   (i) A flow of 60 ml/min of isoflurane gas is required (3000 ml/min $\times$ 0.02 = 60 ml/min).

   (ii) The vapor pressure (VP) of isoflurane is 240 mm of Hg, and barometric pressure is 760 mm of Hg (240 $\div$ 760 mm of Hg = 0.32). Therefore, the flow entering the vaporizer must be 120 ml/min for 60 ml/min of isoflurane to exit the vaporizer (60 ml/min $\approx$ 0.32 $\times$ 180 ml/min). Thus, the total flow exiting the vaporizer is 180 ml/min.

   (iii) The total flow of 3 L/min is provided as follows: 180 ml/min from the vaporizer and 2820 ml/min from the primary oxygen flowmeter.

  (3) Specific formulas for calculation of flow rates and outputs for measured-flow vaporizers are available.[7]

 g. Variable-bypass, concentration-calibrated vaporizers should be serviced and recalibrated periodically by a qualified vaporizer technician. Manufacturers and anesthesia equipment service companies recommend specific intervals (often every 6 months or every year) for replacement of worn parts and recalibration. The recalibration should be complete, including assurance of temperature compensation. Vaporizers for halothane and methoxyflurane (with nonvolatile preservatives, thymol and butylated hydroxytoluene, respectively) may need more frequent service than vaporizers for anesthetics without preservatives.

4. Vaporizers positioned within the breathing circuit (VIC) were very common when methoxyflurane was the prevalent inhalant anesthetic in veterinary medicine. Because methoxyflurane has a very low VP, it is perhaps the safest of the inhalants for VIC vaporizers. VIC vaporizers are nonprecision and low-efficiency units; they are not temperature-, flow-, or back-pressure-compensated. VIC vaporizers are considered to be multipurpose (suitable for various anesthetics), but special precautions are needed with highly volatile, very potent anesthetics (e.g., removal of the wick from the vaporization chamber).[8]

 a. In contrast to VOC vaporizers, the output from VIC vaporizers and the concentration of anesthetic in the circle system are affected significantly by ventilation, fresh gas flows, and other factors.[6]

  (1) Increased spontaneous ventilation increases vaporizer output.

  (2) Sudden increases in ventilation can produce dangerous increases in vaporizer output.

(3) Artificial ventilation at any vaporizer setting will increase vaporizer output.

(4) Higher fresh gas flows are associated with lower inspired anesthetic concentrations; fresh gases (O_2) dilute the gases returning to the vaporizer.

(5) Lower fresh gas flows are associated with increased economy.

(6) Potentially, low fresh gas flows may be associated with very high inspired anesthetic concentrations.

b. An Ohio vaporizer is called a drawover vaporizer.[6] The patient pulls gas through the vaporizer on inspiration. The setting of the control lever ("off" and "full," with numbered gradations between) indicates the percentage (0–100%) of gas entering the vaporizer that is being diverted through the vaporization chamber to become partially or fully saturated with anesthetic vapor. As the output of the vaporizer is unknown, the operator adjusts the control lever in response to changes in the patient's anesthetic depth. This vaporizer is no longer being manufactured and is considered obsolete in human anesthesia. An Ohio vaporizer is described as variable-bypass (not concentration-calibrated), flowover with a removable wick, VIC, not temperature-compensated, multipurpose (methoxyflurane is delivered with the wick in place, although the use of this vaporizer for the delivery of isoflurane to small animals has been described with the wick removed),[8] not back-pressure-compensated, and low-resistance.

c. Another VIC vaporizer, the Stephens Universal Vaporizer, can be purchased on new veterinary anesthesia machines. The settings on the control dial indicate the fraction (in increments of one eighth) of gas entering the vaporization chamber to be partially or fully saturated with anesthetic. The vaporizer is described as variable-bypass (not concentration-calibrated), flowover with a removal wick, VIC, not temperature-compensated, multipurpose (the manufacturer recommends that the wick be used for methoxyflurane but not for halothane or isoflurane), not back-pressure-compensated (the vaporizer has a relatively small vaporization chamber, which may be advantageous), and low resistance. The manufacturer provides relatively detailed directions for use of the vaporizer.

d. VIC vaporizers may retain nonvolatile preservatives from methoxyflurane or halothane. The preservatives create a yellowish color in the liquid and can collect on the wick, which may interfere with vaporization. The wicks can be cleaned with alcohol or ether and allowed to dry in a well-ventilated area.

I. Common gas outlet

1. The common gas outlet (Fig. 5–1) is where the mixture of anesthetic gas(es) and O_2 exits the anesthesia machine and enters a conduit (usually rubber tubing) to the fresh gas inlet of the breathing system.

2. The common gas outlet is the location for attachment of the pediatric breathing systems that are often used in lieu of adult or standard small animal circle systems for small patients.

3. Simple veterinary anesthesia machines utilize rubber tubing to connect the outlet of the VOC vaporizer to the fresh gas inlet of the breathing system. Essentially, the outlet of the vaporizer becomes the common gas outlet.

4. The common gas outlet or the outlet from the vaporizer is a site for disconnections and should be examined during preanesthetic evaluation

of the machine. Contemporary guidelines for human anesthesia machines require a secure attachment at the common gas outlet.

J. Breathing systems

1. Breathing systems deliver inhalant anesthetic(s), supply O_2, remove CO_2, and provide a mechanism for assisted or controlled ventilation.[4, 5]

2. The classification of breathing systems has been "a favorite pastime of anesthesiologists." Nevertheless, naming the system (e.g., circle), describing the patient (e.g., according to body weight or metabolic rate), and stating the fresh gas flow (O_2 and N_2O flow rates) provide an excellent description of the use of a breathing system in a particular patient. Other classifications are cumbersome and easily misunderstood. As an exception, the terms "semiclosed" and "closed" for circle systems will be retained because of their prevalence in the scientific literature.

3. Circle systems are called "rebreathing systems" because all or part of the expired gases (after the chemical removal of CO_2) is recirculated to the patient. Yet, it is possible for most of the exhaled gases to be eliminated from the circle if very high fresh gas flow rates are used, making "rebreathing system" an inexact term. For many small animals, circle systems with dimensions intended for human adults work well. Some pediatric circle systems (with smaller dimensions and volumes) are available for the smallest veterinary patients.

    a. Components of circle systems and their arrangement may vary depending on the manufacturer; the basic parts follow (Fig. 5–2):

        (1) The fresh gas inlet accepts gases from the common gas outlet of the machine. The fresh gas inlet is usually located on the inspiratory side of the circle, between the CO_2-absorbent canister and the inspiratory one-way valve.

        (2) The inspiratory one-way valve, in concert with the expiratory one-way valve, promotes the flow of gases in a single direction around the circle. The inspiratory one-way valve opens during inspiration and closes during expiration. Properly functioning valves are essential; incompetent valves may increase dead space, cause rebreathing of CO_2, or increase resistance to ventilation.

        (3) The inspiratory breathing tube conducts gases from the inspiratory one-way valve to the Y-piece. The internal diameter (i.d.) of a breathing tube is either 22 mm (human adult) or 15 mm (pediatric).

        (4) The Y-piece connects the inspiratory and expiratory breathing tubes and attaches to the endotracheal tube connector. The outside diameter (o.d.) of the Y-piece is either 22 mm (human adult) or slightly greater than 15 mm (pediatric). The i.d. of the Y-piece is 15 mm to fit the endotracheal tube connector. The Y-piece contains the only mechanical dead space in a properly functioning circle system.

        (5) The expiratory breathing tube conducts gases from the Y-piece to the expiratory one-way valve. It has the same dimensions as the inspiratory breathing tube.

        (6) The expiratory one-way valve closes during inspiration and opens during expiration to promote the flow of gases in only one direction around the circle.

        (7) The pop-off, or adjustable pressure-limiting (APL), valve is an essential safety feature of a circle system. It vents excess gas (inflow greater than the patient's O_2 consumption) and prevents the devel-

opment of excessive pressure. Pop-off valves should remain open, except during purposeful application of positive pressure to the respiratory system. Modern pop-off valves have an exit portal (19 mm o.d.) that fits standard scavenging tubing.

(8) The reservoir bag provides for the patient's tidal volume and minute volume during ventilation. A guideline for the minimum size of a reservoir bag is six times the patient's tidal volume (V_T is approximately 11 ml/kg, or 5 ml/lb). A larger bag can be selected if it facilitates manual ventilation, but a larger bag adds volume and slows the equilibration of anesthetic concentration after changes in settings on the vaporizer.

(9) The canister for CO_2 absorbent (e.g., soda lime) should have a volume of approximately twice the patient's tidal volume, because the gas space around the granules of absorbent is about half the volume of the canister. Unfortunately, canister size on most veterinary machines cannot be changed from patient to patient.

    (i) CO_2 absorbents (soda lime, barium hydroxide lime) chemically remove CO_2 from expired gases. The absorbent must be fresh and functional to prevent rebreathing of CO_2.

    (ii) The simplified equation for CO_2 absorption by soda lime is as follows:

$$2\ NaOH + 2\ H_2CO_3 + Ca(OH)_2 \rightarrow CaCO_3 + Na_2CO_3 + 4\ H_2O + Heat$$

    (iii) Color indicators (e.g., white to blue or purple) show when the absorbent has been exhausted. The color change may regress when the system is not in use. Absorbents are soft and will crumble in the functional state but become hard when they are exhausted. Heat production occurs during active absorption of CO_2, and a heat line is detectable on the canister.

    (iv) Absorbents should be changed regularly, usually when about one half to two thirds of the absorbent in the canister has been consumed.

(10) A scavenging system should be attached to a circle system to eliminate waste gases from the operating room environment. The scavenging system (to be discussed shortly) attaches to the exit portal of the pop-off valve through corrugated tubing (19 mm i.d.).

(11) Other components of circle systems

    (i) The Universal-F rebreathing circuit (Fig. 5–3) is a tube-within-a-tube apparatus that replaces the traditional Y-piece and breathing tubes. It has an inner inspiratory tube of 15 mm and an outer expiratory tube of 25 mm. The manufacturer recommends the circuit for patients weighing up to 136 kg (300 lb).

    (ii) A manometer is a pressure gauge, usually attached to the absorber and calibrated in centimeters of H_2O to measure the amount of pressure in the circle system. It is particularly useful during manual ventilation and "sighing" to evaluate the pressure being applied to the respiratory system.

    (iii) An air-intake (negative pressure-relief) valve is present on some circles. It allows inspiration of room air if the fresh gas supply to the circle fails.

    (iv) When present, a VIC vaporizer is an integral part of the

2. Electrolyte imbalances, especially hypokalemia, will affect cardiac as well as skeletal muscle.

3. Whether the patient is ambulatory or not is important. Nonambulatory patients may have lung congestion if they are allowed to lie on one side for prolonged periods of time. They may develop decubitus ulcers, which can be difficult to heal and can have serious sequelae.

4. Fractures may cause significant hemorrhage at the fracture site. Compound fractures increase the risk of infection. Cranial fractures can cause CNS depression. Spinal fracture cases should be handled very carefully, and patients with cervical fractures should be intubated with as little movement of the neck as possible.

III. Presurgical laboratory workup

A. Controversy exists over what, if any, laboratory testing is required for all patients. Determination of packed cell volume (PCV) and plasma protein (PP) concentration is relatively quick, simple, and inexpensive. These two tests can provide significant information both pre- and intraoperatively.

1. PP concentration is a useful indicator of the state of hemoconcentration and is considered to be a more sensitive index than PCV.

a. Hyperproteinemia can indicate hemoconcentration and dehydration.

b. Hypoproteinemia may result from disease states but can also be caused by iatrogenic hemodilution with large amounts of crystalloid infusions.

c. The albumin fraction of the proteins accounts for approximately 80% of the effective oncotic pressure of plasma. Since edema can occur when the albumin drops below 1.0 g/100 ml, it is recommended that the total plasma proteins be maintained above 3.5 g/100 ml.

d. Drug responses can be affected by hypoproteinemia, because a great many drugs (e.g., barbiturates, benzodiazepine tranquilizers) are reversibly bound to albumin, and only the unbound fraction is pharmacologically active. Thus, induction of anesthesia with barbiturates in a hypoproteinemic patient should be done very cautiously.

2. The PCV provides an index of the body's oxygen-carrying capacity.

a. It has been recommended that preoperative PCV be 27–30% and intraoperative and postoperative PCV be kept above 20%.

b. As blood viscosity is doubled and cardiac output is halved when the PCV is 60%, it is suggested that the hematocrit be kept below this level.

3. The hemoglobin level is important because it affects oxygen-carrying capacity. Such capacity will influence the choice of inspired oxygen concentration and method of ventilation (i.e., spontaneous versus assisted or controlled).

B. Additional tests may be indicated depending on the patient's age and disease (Table 1–1).

1. A complete blood count provides additional information.

a. The red blood cell count gives additional information on oxygen-carrying capacity.

b. The white blood cell count and differential can give indications of stress or infection. With infection, pyrexia may develop, which will increase both the oxygen and anesthetic requirements of the patient. Inapparent clinical infections may be exacerbated following the stress of anesthesia and surgery, according to some evidence suggesting that general anesthesia may be immunosuppressive. The extent of anesthetic-induced immunosuppression is not currently known, but

Table 1–1. Suggested Diagnostic Screening Tests Based on Physical Status and Age

	Age		
Physical Status	***Less Than 4 Months****	***Range of 4 Months to 5 Years****	***More Than 5 Years****
I, II	PCV, TP, glucose	PCV, TP, BUN	PCV, TP, BUN, creatinine, UA, EKG
III	CBC, UA, glucose, BUN, creatinine	CBC, UA, surgery profile,† EKG	CBC, UA, complete profile,‡ EKG
IV, V	CBC, UA, complete profile‡	CBC, UA, complete profile,‡ EKG	CBC, UA, complete profile,‡ EKG

PCV = packed cell volume
TP = total protein
BUN = blood urea nitrogen
EKG = electrocardiogram
CBC = complete blood cell count: white blood cell count and differential, red blood cell count and indices, platelet count, hematocrit, hemoglobin, plasma protein
UA = urinalysis: color, transparency, specific gravity, protein, glucose, ketones, bilirubin, occult blood, urobilinogen, pH, nitrate, sediment

*Additional tests may be indicated based on the specific circumstances of each patient.
†Glucose, BUN, creatinine, ALT, total CO_2, sodium, potassium, and chloride. Different laboratories may include different tests in their chemistry profiles.
‡Surgery profile, plus total protein, albumin, AST, ALP, calcium, phosphorus, anion gap, and T. bilirubin. Different laboratories may include different tests in their chemistry profiles.

Note: Trauma patients (especially those hit by cars) should have an EKG done to help determine the presence of myocardial contusions. Thoracic radiographs should also be done to determine any chest trauma.

patients with potential infections or metastatic conditions should be anesthetized with caution.

c. Eosinophilia may indicate a heartworm infection, and the patient should be specifically tested for this disease. Heartworm-infected dogs have an abnormal cardiopulmonary system and occasionally will show arrhythmias. The presence of arrhythmias will influence the choice of anesthetic regimen.

2. Monitoring of arterial blood gases provides immeasurably useful information to the anesthesiologist.
   a. The Pa_{CO_2} is used to determine the adequacy of ventilation, which can be extremely difficult to assess visually. Many of the other tests of respiratory function used in human medicine are not feasible in the veterinary patient, so blood gas determinations become even more important. It is necessary to determine the patient's respiratory function level preoperatively, because virtually all anesthetics depress respiration.
   b. The Pa_{O_2} is used to assess the adequacy of oxygenation. When all other organ systems are normal, the brain will tolerate a Pa_{O_2} as low as 36 mmHg. In the majority of clinical patients, however, hypoxemia (Pa_{O_2} <60 mm Hg) will cause damage. "Shunting," or an increased A–aDO_2, increases under anesthesia. Shunting may also be affected by the patient's positioning and by manipulations during surgery. The adequacy of oxygenation will influence the decision on whether to assist or control ventilation and on what the desired inspired oxygen concentration should be.
   c. Arterial pH is a very important factor. It affects the oxyhemoglobin dissociation curve. Acidosis decreases protein binding and thus reduces the dosage of barbiturates required for a given level of anesthesia.

Acidosis also depresses the myocardium. Acidosis may result from the patient's disease, from administration of certain drugs, or from inadequate tissue oxygenation. The base excess is merely a figure calculated to describe the metabolic component of the acid-base state of the patient.

3. Tests of clotting function

   Anesthesiologists are concerned primarily with acute bleeding disorders that occur intraoperatively.

   a. Coagulation deficiencies may occasionally be the result of dilution of the patient's clotting factors following massive transfusion or fluid administration.

   b. The syndrome of disseminated intravascular coagulopathy will usually result in multiple factor abnormalities and prolonged partial thromboplastin time (PTT) and prothrombin times. Alterations in the fibrinogen level may also help establish the diagnosis. More sophisticated tests, such as measurement of fibrin degradation product levels or the thromboelastogram, can lead to an accurate diagnosis, but these tests are not readily available in most veterinary facilities. In an acute situation, monitoring the platelet count and the activated clotting time (ACT) may be more practical. In theory at least, the ACT of whole blood should reveal severe deficiencies of any procoagulant other than factor VII. This test is especially useful when a reliable coagulation laboratory is not available. The normal ACT is 60–90 seconds. ACTs greater than 120 seconds are considered prolonged.

C. Blood chemistries can help in the assessment of various organ functions or diseases.

   1. A normal electrolyte balance is necessary for optimal physiologic function.

      a. Sodium, which is the major cation in the extracellular fluid compartment, is very important in determining the osmolality of the patient. Hyponatremia may prolong the patient's recovery from anesthesia. It is recommended that the serum sodium concentration be greater than 130 mEq/L.

      b. Chloride ion affects how sodium is reabsorbed by the renal tubule; hypochloremia can cause hypokalemia and alkalosis.

      c. Potassium levels are extremely important for the anesthesiologist to know because the intracellular versus extracellular levels of potassium figure in the maintenance of a proper transmembrane electronegativity.

         (1) Hyperkalemia can lead to bradycardia and arrest, whereas hypokalemia can lead to an irritable myocardium and ventricular ectopic beats. Hyperkalemia levels of 5.5–6.0 mEq/L can be increased by anesthetic techniques to the point of cardiac standstill or fibrillation—for example, by the use of succinylcholine, which results in potassium release.

         (2) Hypokalemia potentiates and prolongs the effects of competitive-muscle relaxants.

   2. The blood urea nitrogen (BUN) measurement provides a crude index of glomerular filtration rate.

   3. The creatinine measurement may be more reliable prognostically, as it is not affected by dietary protein, protein catabolism, age, or sex, and levels are elevated only when renal function is impaired.

   4. Alanine aminotransferase levels can indicate recent hepatic cell destruc-

tion. Other commonly used tests of hepatic function are alkaline phosphatase levels (in dogs), serum bilirubin (total and indirect), and Bromsulphalein excretion (BSP). Abnormal levels of albumin and globulin can also indicate hepatic disease. All of the tests have limitations, however, in view of the fact that experimentally as much as 85% of the liver can be removed before any abnormality shows up on laboratory tests. Nonetheless, it is important to be aware of any evidence of impaired hepatic function, because the liver plays a highly significant role in drug metabolism. Although some authorities believe that liver disease must be very severe before biotransformation of anesthetic drugs is influenced, it is well to remember that the great majority of these agents are detoxified by the liver.

  D. Urinalysis can also provide useful information.
    1. Specific gravity can reflect the patient's hydration and the ability of the kidneys to concentrate the urine if necessary.
    2. The pH should be determined and the urine tested for protein, acetone, bilirubin, and blood.
    3. Microscopic evaluation of urine sediment will help determine whether renal disease is present.

IV. Diagnostic tests
Additional and extremely useful diagnostic tests are electrocardiography and radiography.
  A. Electrocardiography
    1. Recently traumatized patients should be checked for related myocarditis, as this condition can be exacerbated by many anesthetic agents (xylazine, thiobarbiturates, halothane).
    2. Patients with suspected or known heart disease should have an electrocardiographic evaluation.
    3. Electrolyte abnormalities may be revealed on an electrocardiogram.
  B. Radiography
    1. Thoracic radiographs are used to detect and evaluate congenital and acquired cardiopulmonary diseases. They will show abnormalities in approximately one third of dogs traumatized by automobiles. Such abnormalities (e.g., pneumothorax, diaphragmatic hernia, pulmonary contusions) can increase the risk of anesthetic morbidity and mortality.
    2. Abdominal films can aid in the diagnosis and assessment of various hepatic, gastrointestinal, and urinary diseases, which in turn can markedly affect the outcome from anesthesia.

V. ASA physical status
  A. The classification system used by the American Society of Anesthesiologists (ASA) can be used with small animal patients.
  B. The ASA classification for small animals is based primarily on the presence and severity of systemic disease.
    1. ASA I (excellent anesthetic risk): normal, healthy patients with no organic disease. Patients undergoing elective procedures such as ovariohysterectomies, castrations, or declawings would be classified ASA I.
    2. ASA II (good anesthetic risk): neonatal or geriatric patients or patients with mild systemic disease, mild to moderate obesity, simple fractures, compensated cardiac disease, or conditions requiring uncomplicated ocular surgery.
    3. ASA III (fair anesthetic risk): patients with moderate systemic disease, low to moderate fever, moderate dehydration and hypovolemia, anorexia,

cachexia, anemia, chronic heart disease, chronic renal disease, complicated fractures, or mild to moderate chest trauma.

4. ASA IV (poor anesthetic risk): patients with severe systemic disease that is a constant threat to life. Patients with shock, high fever, uremia, toxemia, severe dehydration and hypovolemia, morbid obesity, severe anemia, emaciation, diabetes, gastric dilatation-volvulus, decompensated cardiac/renal/hepatic disease, severe pulmonary disease, severe chest trauma, or diaphragmatic hernia would be classified ASA IV.

5. ASA V (guarded anesthetic risk): moribund patients not expected to survive 24 hours. Patients with advanced multiorgan system failure, severe shock, major trauma, or DIC would be classified ASA V.

6. Emergency operations are designated by an "E" after the numeric classification.

Suggested Readings

Blue JT, Short CE: Preanesthetic evaluation and clinical pathology. In Short CE (ed): Principles and Practice of Veterinary Anesthesia. Baltimore: Williams & Wilkins, 1987, pp. 3–7.

Collins VJ: Preanesthetic evaluation and preparation. In Principles of Anesthesiology, 2nd ed. Philadelphia: Lea & Febiger, 1976.

Heavner JE: Drug interactions. In Thurmon JC, Tranquilli WJ, Benson GJ (eds): Lumb and Jones' Veterinary Anesthesia. Baltimore: Williams & Wilkins, 1996, pp. 34–39.

Roizen MF: Routine perioperative evaluation. In Miller RD (ed): Anesthesia, 2nd ed. New York: Churchill Livingstone, 1986, pp. 225–254.

Thurmon JC, Tranquilli WJ, Benson GJ: Considerations for general anesthesia. In Lumb and Jones' Veterinary Anesthesia. Baltimore: Williams & Wilkins, 1996, pp. 5–34.

Chapter 2 | Preanesthetic Agents

Robert R. Paddleford

I. Preanesthetic agents are drugs given to a patient prior to administration of an anesthetic for one or more of the following reasons:
   A. To sedate and calm a patient and thus prevent struggling from fear during anesthetic induction
   B. To relieve pain preoperatively
   C. To be used as adjuncts to local or regional anesthesia to prevent movement of the patient
   D. To reduce the amount of general anesthetic needed
   E. To decrease salivary secretions, decrease gastric and intestinal motility, and prevent bradycardia
   F. To provide for a smooth recovery from anesthesia
II. Classifications of preanesthetic agents
   A. Anticholinergics
      1. Atropine sulfate
      2. Glycopyrrolate (Robinul-V)
   B. Tranquilizers/sedatives/hypnotics
      1. Phenothiazine derivatives
      2. Butyrophenone derivatives
      3. Benzodiazepine derivatives
      4. Alpha-2 agonists
      5. Pentobarbital
   C. Narcotic analgesics
   D. Neuroleptanalgesics
III. Anticholinergics
   A. Anticholinergics are used for the following reasons:
      1. To reduce secretions of the salivary glands and mucous glands of the respiratory tract
      2. To reduce gastric and intestinal motility
      3. To block the vagal nerves and thus help prevent or counteract sinus bradycardia
   B. Atropine sulfate
      1. Mechanism of action
         a. Atropine is a belladonna alkaloid.
         b. Atropine blocks acetylcholine at the postganglionic terminations of cholinergic fibers in the autonomic nervous system.
         c. Atropine does not inhibit acetylcholine release.
      2. Dose and route of administration
         a. Refer to Table 2–1.
         b. Atropine may be given subcutaneously, intramuscularly, or intravenously.

Table 2–1. Suggested Dosages for Preanesthetic Medications
in the Dog and Cat

Drug	Dose Dog	Cat	Duration of Action
Anticholinergics			
Atropine	0.02 mg/lb SC, IM 0.01 mg/lb IV	Same	1–1½ hours
Glycopyrrolate (Robinul-V)	0.005 mg/lb SC, IM, IV	Same	2–3 hours
Tranquilizers/Sedatives/Hypnotics			
Acetylpromazine or acepromazine	0.05–0.1 mg/lb SC, IM, IV, to a maximum total dose of 3 mg	Same	3–6 hours
Chlorpromazine (Thorazine)	0.1–0.2 mg/lb SC, IM, IV	Same	4–6 hours
Promazine (Sparine)	0.25–0.5 mg/lb SC, IM, IV	Same	4–6 hours
Droperidol (Inapsine)	1 mg/lb IM 0.25–0.5 mg/lb IV	Same	Up to 12 hours
Lenperone (Elanone-V)	0.1–0.4 mg/lb IV 0.2–0.8 mg/lb IM	Same	2–4 hours
Diazepam (Valium)	0.2 mg/lb IM, IV to a total dose of 10 mg	0.2 mg/lb IM, IV	1–3 hours
Midazolam (Versed)	0.05–0.1 mg/lb IM, IV	Same	1–2 hours
Xylazine (Rompun)	0.1–0.5 mg/lb IM, IV	0.1–0.5 mg/lb IM, IV	1–2 hours
Medetomidine (Domitor)	0.005–0.02 mg/lb IM, IV	Approved for dogs only	1–2 hours
Narcotic Analgesics			
Morphine	0.05–3 mg/lb SC/IM	0.05 mg/lb SC	3–6 hours
Meperidine	0.5–3 mg/lb IM, IV	0.5–3 mg/lb IM, IV	2–4 hours
Oxymorphone	0.1 mg/lb IM, IV to a maximum total dose of 3 mg	0.1 mg/lb IM, IV	2–4 hours
Fentanyl (Sublimaze)	0.001–0.003 mg/lb IV 0.003–0.01 mg/lb IM	Not recommended	30–45 minutes
Pentazocine (Talwin)	0.5–1.5 mg/lb IM, IV	Same	1–2 hours
Butorphanol (Torbugesic)	0.05–0.2 mg/lb IM, IV	Same	Up to 4 hours
Buprenorphine (Buprenex)	0.003–0.005 mg/lb IM, IV	Same	6–8 hours

    c. With extremely low doses of atropine, less than 0.003 mg/lb, central vagal stimulation may occur.

    d. Atropine's duration of action is 1–1.5 hours.

    e. Atropine may initially increase vagal tone both centrally and peripherally when given intravenously.

3. Cardiovascular effects

    a. Atropine may increase heart rate.

    b. Cardiac output may increase if the heart rate increases.

    c. Atropine has minimal effects on systolic or diastolic blood pressure at therapeutic doses.

       d. It may lower the ventricular fibrillation threshold.

       e. It helps prevent the vasovagal response.

    4. Respiratory effects

       a. Atropine decreases salivary and airway secretions.

       b. It increases the viscosity of the secretions.

       c. It decreases airway resistance and increases anatomic dead space resulting from dilation of the bronchi.

       d. It helps prevent bronchospasm.

    5. Other physiologic effects

       a. Atropine decreases gastric and intestinal motility.

       b. It reduces tear formation.

       c. It crosses the blood-brain barrier.

       d. It can prolong thiobarbiturate anesthesia.

    6. Metabolism and elimination

       a. The dog excretes part of the atropine intact via the kidneys; the remainder undergoes hepatic metabolism.

       b. The cat metabolizes the majority of the atropine in the liver via atropine esterase.

    7. Uses and contraindications

       a. The routine use of atropine as a preanesthetic agent has decreased in recent years.

       b. It is indicated for decreasing salivary and respiratory secretions and to counteract sinus bradycardia.

       c. Its selective use is still recommended when potent vagotonic preanesthetic and anesthetic drugs are used.

       d. It is contraindicated for patients with preexisting tachycardia.

    8. Atropine overdose is characterized by one more of the following:

       a. Dry mucous membranes

       b. Thirst

       c. Dilation of the pupils

       d. Tachycardia

       e. Vomiting

       f. Seizures

C. Glycopyrrolate (Robinul-V)

    1. Mechanism of action

       a. Glycopyrrolate is a synthetic quaternary ammonium anticholinergic drug.

       b. Its mechanism of action is similar to that of atropine, but its effect lasts longer.

    2. Dose and route of administration

       a. Refer to Table 2–1.

       b. Glycopyrrolate can be given subcutaneously, intramuscularly, or intravenously.

       c. Its effect peaks at 30–45 minutes after subcutaneous or intramuscular injection and lasts for 2–3 hours. Its antisialagogue effect may persist for 6–8 hours.

    3. Cardiovascular effects

       a. At recommended doses, glycopyrrolate has minimal effects on blood pressure or heart rate.

      b. It seems less likely than atropine to produce sinus tachycardia.
  4. Respiratory effects
      a. Glycopyrrolate decreases salivary and respiratory secretions.
      b. It produces some dilation of the bronchi.
  5. Other physiologic effects
      a. Glycopyrrolate decreases the volume and acidity of gastric secretions.
      b. It decreases intestinal tone and contraction.
      c. It does not cross the blood-brain barrier.
  6. Uses and contraindications
      a. Uses and contraindications for glycopyrrolate are the same as for atropine.
      b. Glycopyrrolate seems less likely than atropine to produce tachycardias.
      c. Its effects last longer than those of atropine.

IV. Phenothiazine tranquilizers

  A. The phenothiazine tranquilizers include, among others, acetylpromazine, promazine, chlorpromazine, propiopromazine, and triflupromazine.
  B. Acetylpromazine is probably the most common phenothiazine tranquilizer used in small animal practice.
  C. Dose and route of administration
    1. Refer to Table 2–1.
    2. The phenothiazine tranquilizers may be given orally, subcutaneously, intramuscularly, or intravenously.
    3. Their duration of action is 3–6 hours, but it may be much longer in patients with hepatic dysfunction.
  D. All the phenothiazine tranquilizers have the same physiologic effects on a patient, varying only in potency and duration of action.
  E. CNS effects
    1. Phenothiazine derivatives cause CNS depression by affecting the basal ganglia, hypothalamus, limbic system, brain stem, and reticular activating system.
    2. They lack any generalized hypnotic effect, and they do not produce analgesia.
    3. They block dopamine receptors and the action of 5-hydroxytryptamine.
    4. Most phenothiazine derivatives are potent antiemetics. They act centrally on the chemoreceptor zone as well as on the vomition center in the medulla.
    5. They depress the thermoregulation center.
    6. They produce peripheral anticholinergic, antiadrenergic, and antiganglionic activities.
    7. The phenothiazine derivatives lower the threshold to seizures.
  F. Cardiovascular effects
    1. The phenothiazine derivatives have the ability to produce hypotension.
    2. The hypotension produced is somewhat dose-independent and is due to alpha-1-adrenergic blockade, peripheral antiadrenergic activity, and direct vasodilatory action.

3. Hypotension may cause a reflex sinus tachycardia in patients receiving a phenothiazine derivative.

4. Phenothiazine derivatives have a antidysrhythmic effect resulting from either a quinidine-like effect or a local anesthetic effect on the myocardium.

5. They inhibit myocardial sensitization to catecholamines.

6. They produce a negative inotropic effect.

7. In patients with elevated catecholamine levels, they may cause a significant fall in blood pressure because of alpha-1-adrenergic blockade in the presence of beta-2 receptor stimulation.

G. Respiratory effects

1. At therapeutic doses, the phenothiazine derivatives produce negligible respiratory effects.

2. They may cause a decrease in respiratory rate, but this is usually compensated for by an increase in tidal volume, resulting in a normal minute ventilation.

3. The phenothiazine derivatives do not delay respiratory center response (threshold) to increases in Pa_{CO_2}, although the maximum ventilatory response (sensitivity) may be decreased.

4. Large doses can depress respiration.

5. Respiratory depression may also occur when phenothiazine derivatives are used in combination with hypnotics or narcotics. This respiratory depression is due to an additive effect.

H. Other physiologic effects

1. The phenothiazine derivatives produce some skeletal-muscle relaxant activity.

2. They cause delayed gastric emptying and prolonged intestinal transit times.

3. Decreases in packed cell volume and total plasma proteins, and increases in plasma volume, have been reported to occur as a result of hypotension and subsequent shifts of extravascular water into the vascular space.

4. Phenothiazine derivatives can cause a fall in body temperature resulting from peripheral vasodilation, a reduction in skeletal-muscle activity, and depression of the thermoregulation center.

I. Metabolism and excretion

1. The liver is the major site of detoxification.

2. The metabolic pathway varies with the particular phenothiazine derivative.

3. Metabolites are identifiable in the urine for several days after a single dose.

J. Advantages

1. They decrease the amount of general anesthetic needed.

2. They sedate and calm the patient prior to anesthesia.

3. They have minimal respiratory depressant effects.

4. They may help prevent cardiac dysrhythmias.

K. Disadvantages

1. The effects of phenothiazine tranquilizers are irreversible. No specific antagonist is available to counteract their effects.

2. They can cause hypotension.

3. They can produce hypothermia.

4. They are nonanalgesic.

5. They can potentiate seizures.

V. Butyrophenone derivatives

   A. The three butyrophenone derivatives used in veterinary anesthesia are droperidol (Inapsine), azaperone (Stresnil), and lenperone HCl (Elanone-V).

   B. Droperidol (Inapsine)

      1. Droperidol's main use is in combination with the narcotic fentanyl citrate to form Innovar-Vet.

      2. It has little or no effect on cardiac output, but it decreases arterial blood pressure, total peripheral resistance, and heart rate.

      3. It can depress respiration.

      4. It appears to produce antishock and adrenolytic activity.

      5. Its duration of action is approximately 2 hours.

      6. It is detoxified in the liver.

   C. Azaperone (Stresnil)

      1. Azaperone's physiologic effects are similar to those of droperidol.

      2. Its primary use has been in swine.

   D. Lenperone HCl (Elanone-V)

      1. Lenperone is approved for use in both dogs and cats.

      2. Its physiologic effects are similar to those of droperidol.

VI. Benzodiazepine tranquilizers

   A. The primary benzodiazepine derivatives used in small animal anesthesia are diazepam (Valium) and midazolam (Versed).

   B. Benzodiazepine-derivative tranquilizers are considered minor tranquilizers.

   C. Diazepam (Valium)

      1. Dose and route of administration

         a. Refer to Table 2–1.

         b. Diazepam may be administered orally, intramuscularly, or intravenously.

         c. Intravenous diazepam should be injected slowly to prevent venous thrombus.

         d. Diazepam is not water-soluble and is dissolved in propylene glycol; thus its absorption from intramuscular injection sites may be unpredictable and erratic.

         e. Propylene glycol is a cardiopulmonary depressant. Rapid intravenous administration may cause hypotension, bradycardia, and apnea.

         f. Considerable variation exists in individual responses to the sedative effects of diazepam.

      2. CNS effects

         a. Diazepam acts primarily on parts of the limbic system, the thalamus, and the hypothalamus.

         b. It produces a calming, or taming, effect in animals. In humans it also produces amnesia.

         c. Fear and anxiety are reduced without marked sedation.

         d. High-affinity benzodiazepine receptors exist in the CNS.

e. Benzodiazepine receptors appear to have widespread distribution in the brain; however, these receptors appear to be lacking in the white matter.

f. Diazepam has broad-spectrum anticonvulsant activity.

g. It has been proposed that a number of neurotransmitter systems may be involved in the CNS effects produced by the benzodiazepines. These include acetylcholine, catecholamines, serotonin, glycine, and gamma-aminobutyric acid (GABA).

h. The muscle-relaxant properties of diazepam occur at the spinal cord level and at the reticular formation of the brain stem.

3. Cardiopulmonary effects

a. Diazepam has minimal cardiopulmonary depressant effects at clinically used doses.

b. High intravenous doses can cause a decrease in respiration and blood pressure.

4. Other physiologic effects

a. Diazepam is an anticonvulsant.

b. It produces skeletal-muscle relaxation.

c. After diazepam administration, paradoxic excitement and aggression have both been reported in the dog and the cat. The addition of other CNS depressants, i.e., opioids, will help attenuate this effect.

5. Metabolism and excretion

a. Up to 96% of diazepam is protein bound.

b. Diazepam is metabolized in the liver to N-desmethyldiazepam, 3-hydroxydiazepam, and oxazepam. These metabolites are pharmacologically active.

c. The majority of the metabolites are excreted in the urine.

6. Advantages

a. Diazepam has minimal cardiopulmonary depressant effects.

b. It may be especially useful in patients with CNS dysfunction—especially epileptics.

c. It may be useful as a preanesthetic in old or debilitated patients.

d. Its effects can be antagonized by flumazenil (Romazicon).

7. Disadvantages

a. Diazepam may cause paradoxic excitement and aggression, especially when given intravenously in the absence of other CNS depressants.

b. Intravenous diazepam must be given slowly to prevent venous thrombosis and cardiopulmonary depression caused by the propylene glycol.

c. In healthy patients it may not produce significant CNS depression or tranquilization.

d. It produces variable responses among individuals.

D. Midazolam (Versed)

1. Dose and route of administration

a. Refer to Table 2–1.

b. Midazolam may be administered intramuscularly or intravenously.

c. It is water-soluble and has a more predictable effect than diazepam when given intramuscularly.

2. CNS effects

   a. CNS effects of midazolam are similar to those of diazepam.

   b. Midazolam can produce behavioral changes in the dog and cat just as diazepam can. Cats and dogs may become restless, pace, vocalize, and become difficult to handle following midazolam administration.

   c. The behavioral changes can be attenuated if other CNS depressants, i.e., opioids, are used in combination with midazolam.

3. Cardiopulmonary effects

   a. Cardiopulmonary effects of midazolam are similar to those of diazepam.

   b. Midazolam may cause more respiratory depression than diazepam.

4. Metabolism and excretion

   a. Metabolism and excretion of midazolam are similar to that of diazepam.

   b. Complete recovery period for midazolam is no shorter than for diazepam; however, midazolam's duration of action is shorter, with a rapid elimination half-life and total body clearance.

5. Advantages

   a. Advantages of midazolam are similar to those of diazepam.

   b. Its effects are more predictable than those of diazepam when given intramuscularly.

6. Disadvantages

   a. Midazolam may produce undesirable behavioral changes, especially when given intravenously in the absence of other CNS depressants.

   b. It may produce more respiratory depression than diazepam.

E. Flumazenil (Romazicon)

1. Flumazenil is a specific antagonist for the benzodiazepine tranquilizers.

2. It has a very high affinity for benzodiazepine receptors and will reverse all the CNS effects of diazepam and midazolam.

3. See Table 2–2 for dose and route of administration.

4. It will antagonize the effects of the benzodiazepines within 2–4 minutes following intravenous administration.

   a. Reversal is not accompanied by tachycardia, hypertension, agitation, or anxiety.

   b. Its antagonistic dose lasts only about 60 minutes.

   c. It may require redosing to antagonize large doses of benzodiazepine tranquilizers.

VII. Alpha-2 agonists

A. The alpha-2 adrenoceptor is a distinct subclassification of alpha-adrenergic receptors. Alpha-2 receptors can produce analgesic, sedative, anticonvulsant, and calming effects.

B. The alpha-2 adrenoceptor is further divided into subtypes of alpha-2A, alpha-2B, alpha-2C, and alpha-2D.

C. Clonidine is the prototype compound of the alpha-2 agonists.

1. Xylazine (Rompun), medetomidine (Domitor), and detomidine (Dormosedan) are currently being used in veterinary anesthesia.

2. Other alpha-2 agonists currently under investigation for use in hu-

Table 2–2. Various Antagonists: Their Dosages and Duration of Action

Antagonist	Dose	Antagonizes the Effects of	Duration of Action
Levallorphan (Lorfan)	0.01 to 0.1 mg/lb IV	Narcotic agonist-antagonist	1.5–3 hours
Nalorphine (Nalline)	0.5 mg/lb IV, IM, SC	Narcotic agonist-antagonist	1.5–3 hours
Naloxone (Narcan)	0.01 to 0.05 mg/lb IV, IM, SC	Pure narcotic antagonist	15–45 minutes
4-Aminopyridine	0.15 mg/lb IV	Partial antagonist for alpha-2 agonists	
Flumazenil (Romazicon)	0.01 to 0.05 mg/lb IV	Benzodiazepine derivatives	1 hour
Yohimbine (Yobine)	0.05 to 0.1 mg/lb IV	Alpha-2 agonist	
Atipamezole (Antisedan)	0.1 to 0.2 mg/lb IV (cat) 0.08 to 0.12 mg/lb IV (dog)	Alpha-2 agonist	
Tolazoline (Priscoline)	0.1 mg/lb IV (cat) 0.25 to 0.5 mg/lb IV (dog)	Alpha-2 agonist	

mans and animals include dexmedetomidine, romifidine, azepexole, milvazerol and oxymetazoline.

   D. Alpha-2 receptors are found in the CNS, gastrointestinal tract, uterus, kidney, and platelets.

      1. Prejunctional inhibitory receptors exist within the sympathetic nervous system.

      2. Alpha-2 receptors produce smooth-muscle mediated vasoconstriction and endothelial-dependent mediated vasodilation.

      3. Alpha-2 receptors produce analgesia and sedation effects similar to those of opioid receptor stimulation in the CNS.

         a. Alpha-2 and opioid receptors are found in similar regions of the brain and on some of the same neurons.

         b. Mu-opioid receptors and alpha-2 receptors produce similar effects when activated.

         c. When mu-opioid agonists or alpha-2 agonists bind to their specific receptors, the membrane-associated G proteins are activated, causing the same chain of events to occur.

         d. When membrane-associated G proteins are activated, they open potassium channels in the neuronal membrane, causing the cell to lose potassium. The cell becomes hyperpolarized (more negatively charged), making it unresponsive to excitatory input; thus, the transmission pathway is blocked.

         e. Alpha-2 agonists and mu-opioid agonists produce the same pharmacologic effects for the following reasons:

           (i) Even though the receptors are different, they are found in the same areas of the brain and on the same neurons.

           (ii) Both types of receptors are connected to the same signal transducer.

           (iii) The same effector mechanism is used by both types of agonists.

   E. Xylazine (Rompun)

      1. Xylazine is a thiazine derivative that has sedative, analgesic, and muscle-relaxant properties.

2. Dose and route of administration
   a. See Table 2–1 for dose.
   b. Xylazine may be administered intramuscularly or intravenously.
   c. Effects are seen in 3–5 minutes following intravenous administration and in 10–15 minutes following intramuscular administration.
3. CNS effects
   a. The sedative and analgesic effects of xylazine are due to alpha-2 adrenergic stimulation in the brain and xylazine's ability to block the release of norepinephrine.
   b. Its muscle-relaxation effect is produced by inhibition of interneural transmission at the spinal cord.
   c. It produces selective activation and inhibition of the parasympathetic and sympathetic systems.
   d. It produces depression of the vasomotor centers in the brain stem and increases central vagal and baroreceptor activity.
   e. Its analgesic effects may be relatively short-lived (15–30 minutes). Its sedative effects last 1–2 hours.
   f. Sedation lasting as long as 6–10 hours has been reported in the dog and cat.
   g. Transitory personality changes have been reported in the dog and cat following its use.
4. Cardiovascular effects
   a. Xylazine has a variable effect on the cardiovascular system.
   b. Initially there may be an increase in arterial blood pressure that may be followed by hypotension.
   c. Xylazine appears to sensitize the myocardium to catecholamines, thus making dysrhythmias more likely.
   d. Bradycardia, sinoatrial block, first and second atrioventricular block, atrioventricular dissociation, and pronounced sinus arrhythmia can be produced by xylazine. These conditions are most likely caused by increased vagal activity and can be counteracted with atropine.
   e. Xylazine can cause marked vasoconstriction.
5. Respiratory effects
   a. Xylazine has a variable effect on the respiratory system.
   b. In some animals little or no respiratory depression occurs, whereas in other animals marked decreases in respiratory rate and depth occur.
   c. Respiratory rates usually decrease with clinically used doses of xylazine, although arterial pH, Pa_{O_2}, and Pa_{CO_2} often remain virtually unchanged.
   d. When large doses of xylazine are used or when additional CNS depressants (tranquilizers, opioids, injectable general anesthetics, inhalant anesthetics) are used with xylazine, *significant* respiratory depression may occur.
   e. Xylazine causes relaxation of the larynx and suppresses the cough reflex.
6. Other physiologic effects
   a. Xylazine occasionally causes emesis in dogs and frequently causes emesis in cats as a result of activation of central alpha-2 receptors.
   b. Acute abdominal distension has occurred in large dogs following

xylazine administration. The bloat is apparently due to aerophagia or parasympatholytic activity and may occur several hours after the xylazine has been administered.

   c. Xylazine decreases gastroesophageal sphincter pressure and may increase gastric reflux.

   d. It depresses the thermoregulation center of the brain and can cause hypothermia.

   e. Hyperglycemia and hypoinsulinemia can be caused by stimulation of the alpha-2-adrenergic receptors in pancreatic beta cells that inhibit insulin release.

   f. Administration of xylazine to very excited or unmanageable animals has resulted in a paradoxic increase in excitement.

7. Metabolism, elimination, and antagonism

   a. Xylazine undergoes extensive biodegradation in the liver.

   b. Metabolites are excreted in the urine.

   c. The effects of xylazine can be antagonized by using specific alpha-2 antagonists, namely, yohimbine, atipamezole, tolazoline, and idazoxan (see Table 2–2).

8. Uses

   a. Xylazine is used as a preanesthetic sedative prior to local, regional, or epidural anesthesia. It has also been used prior to injectable or inhalant general anesthesia.

   b. It has been used as the sole agent for minor diagnostic procedures or manipulative procedures.

   c. It has been combined with opioids to produce profound sedation and analgesia.

9. Precautions and contraindications

   a. Xylazine should not be used in combination with tranquilizers.

   b. The marked additive depressant effects of xylazine and general anesthetics and other CNS depressants cannot be overemphasized. When other CNS depressants and general anesthetics are used in combination with xylazine, their doses can be greatly reduced. Barbiturate doses may be reduced by as much as 80–90% and inhalant anesthetic concentrations as much as 40–50%.

   c. Xylazine should be used with caution in breeds of dogs susceptible to bloat, e.g., Irish Setters, Great Danes, Basset Hounds, Saint Bernards.

   d. It should be used with extreme caution in debilitated animals with dysfunction of the cardiovascular, respiratory, hepatic, or renal systems.

   e. It has caused early parturition and abortion in cattle and therefore may be contraindicated in the pregnant small animal.

   f. The administration of an anticholinergic prior to administering xylazine should be considered because of xylazine's marked vagotonic effect.

   g. Care should be exercised by persons administering xylazine as it can be absorbed through breaks in the skin or mucous membranes.

F. Medetomidine (Domitor)

1. Medetomidine is one of the newest alpha-2 agonists approved for veterinary use.

2. It is more potent than other alpha-2 agonists for the following reasons:

   a. It is lipophilic and is rapidly eliminated.

   b. Medetomidine's alpha-2 to alpha-1 receptor selectivity binding ratio is 1620 compared against 260 for detomidine and 160 for xylazine. This means it is approximately 10 times more potent than xylazine.

  3. See Table 2–1 for dose and route of administration.

  4. Physiologic effects

   a. The cardiopulmonary effects of medetomidine are similar to those of xylazine, although they may be more pronounced.

   b. *Significant* bradycardia or vagal-induced dysrhythmias may be produced by medetomidine.

   c. The administration of an anticholinergic agent *prior* to the administration of medetomidine may be more effective in preventing bradycardia than an attempt to reverse it after it occurs.

   d. Atropine may be more effective than glycopyrrolate in preventing medetomidine-induced bradycardia.

   e. Significant respiratory depression may occur in some patients following medetomidine administration. This respiratory depression is especially likely if higher doses of medetomidine are used or if medetomidine is used in combination with other CNS depressants.

   f. Medetomidine seems to produce less variation than xylazine in potency and efficiency among patients.

  5. Metabolism, elimination, and antagonism

   a. Metabolism, elimination, and antagonism of medetomidine are similar to those of xylazine.

   b. The effects of medetomidine can be antagonized by yohimbine, tolazoline, or atipamezole. Atipamezole may be the most effective of the three because of its high alpha-2 to alpha-1 selectivity ratio.

  6. Medetomidine is approved for use only in the dog.

   a. It is recommended for use in only young, healthy, exercise-tolerant dogs.

   b. It is recommended for use as a sole agent, not in combination with other CNS depressants.

   c. It should not be used in patients with cardiopulmonary problems or in debilitated patients.

  7. The precautions and contraindications for medetomidine are the same as for xylazine.

 G. Alpha-2 antagonists

  1. Specific alpha-2 antagonists have been developed that will reverse the physiologic effects of alpha-2 agonists.

  2. Alpha-2 antagonists include yohimbine, tolazoline, idazoxan, and atipamezole.

  3. Tolazoline has the least specificity for alpha-2 receptors of all the alpha-2 antagonists.

   a. It is a potent H2 receptor agonist and has been associated with gastrointestinal bleeding in human patients.

   b. It has also been implicated in the production of abdominal pain, nausea, and diarrhea.

  4. Yohimbine has been shown to be an effective alpha-2 antagonist, although it has less specificity than atipamezole. Yohimbine also affects dopaminergic, serotonergic, and GABAergic receptors.

5. Atipamezole is the most selective of the alpha-2 antagonists.
   a. Its alpha-2 to alpha-1 selectivity ratio is 200 to 300 times higher than the ratio of idazoxan or yohimbine.
   b. Atipamezole has no activity at beta, histaminergic, serotonergic, dopaminergic, GABAergic, opioid, or benzodiazepine receptor sites.
   c. Atipamezole's half-life is nearly twice that of medetomidine.
6. Hypotension and tachycardia have occurred following the rapid intravenous administration of alpha-2 antagonists. On rare occasions, patients have died following the rapid intravenous administration of yohimbine and tolazoline.
   a. Therefore, intravenous alpha-2 antagonists should be administered slowly to get the desired antagonistic effect, or the alpha-2 antagonists should be given intramuscularly.
   b. The use of more specific alpha-2 antagonists, such as atipamezole, also helps to decrease undesirable reactions.

VIII. Pentobarbital
   A. Pentobarbital can be used as a sedative.
   B. The usual dose is 1–2 mg/lb intramuscularly.
   C. Pentobarbital is discussed under injectable general anesthetics.

IX. Narcotic analgesics
   A. Several narcotic analgesics have been utilized in the small animal patient, including morphine, meperidine, oxymorphone, fentanyl, pentazocine, butorphanol, and buprenorphine.
   B. Specific opiate receptors have been identified in the brain, spinal cord, myenteric plexus of the gastrointestinal tract, heart, kidney, adrenal glands, and joint capsules.
   C. CNS effects
      1. Narcotic analgesics produce their CNS effects by occupying stereospecific opioid receptors in the brain and spinal cord. The opioids have three sites of action in the CNS:
         a. Inhibition of pain transmission in the dorsal horn
         b. Inhibition of somatosensory afferents at supraspinal levels
         c. Activation of descending inhibitory pathways
      2. Several distinct opioid receptors with differing physiologic actions appear to exist.
         a. Mu receptor—responsible for supraspinal analgesia, respiratory depression, euphoria, and physical dependence.
         b. Kappa receptor—responsible for spinal analgesia, miosis, sedation, and dysphoria.
         c. Sigma receptor—once thought to be responsible for dysphoria, hallucinations, and respiratory and vasomotor stimulation. Evidence now suggests these may not be opioid receptors and should be classified instead as nonopioid or phencyclidine receptors.
         d. Delta receptor—modifies mu-receptor activity. Mu and delta receptors form a molecular complex and interact.
      3. Depending on the drug used, the dose administered, and the species of animal receiving the drug, narcotic analgesics may produce CNS depression or excitement.
      4. Species that show CNS depression from narcotic analgesics have at

least two times more opioid receptors in the amygdala and frontal cortex than species that show CNS excitement when given opiates.

5. CNS excitation caused by some narcotic analgesics may also be caused in part from alteration in the functioning of brain dopaminergic or noradrenergic systems resulting in increased CNS dopamine levels. Therefore, dopaminergic and noradrenergic blocking agents, such as phenothiazine tranquilizers and droperidol, may prevent opioid excitation.

6. The analgesic effects of the narcotics involve three mechanisms:
   a. Inhibition of pain transmission in the dorsal horn
   b. Inhibition of somatosensory afferents at supraspinal levels
   c. Activation of descending inhibitory pathways

7. Narcotic analgesics depress the respiratory, cough, and vasomotor centers in the medulla.

8. Depending on the species and the specific narcotic analgesic, the vomition center is usually stimulated.

9. Intracranial pressure may be elevated, especially if there is respiratory depression.

10. The effect of narcotic analgesics on the thermoregulation center is species-variable. In some animals, hypothermia is produced; in others, hyperthermia is produced.

11. More consistent CNS depression occurs in the dog; the cat may show varying degrees of excitation following narcotic administration.

D. Cardiovascular effects
   1. At therapeutic doses the narcotics have minimal effects on the cardiovascular system.
   2. They produce little or no change in blood pressure.
   3. They produce no change in cardiac contractility.
   4. They can produce sinus bradycardia as a result of stimulation of the vagal center. The sinus bradycardia produced can be counteracted by an anticholinergic.
   5. They can affect the ability of the vascular system to compensate for positional changes and blood volume changes in the patient, resulting in hypotension.

E. Respiratory effects
   1. Narcotic analgesics are potentially potent respiratory depressants.
   2. The depression is drug- and dose-dependent and may occur at dosages that do not produce marked CNS depression or analgesia.
   3. These drugs directly depress the pontine and medullary respiratory centers.
   4. A decrease in respiratory rate and tidal volume is produced by most narcotics.
   5. They produce a delayed response (altered threshold) and a decreased response (altered sensitivity) to arterial carbon dioxide.
   6. The panting seen in the dog following the administration of some narcotic analgesics (morphine, oxymorphone, fentanyl) may be due to initial stimulation of the respiratory centers or alteration of the thermoregulation center.

F. Other physiologic effects
   1. Some narcotics can cause histamine release, which may produce vasodilation and cause a fall in blood pressure.

2. Usually an initial stimulation of the gastrointestinal tract is followed by a decrease in motility.

3. Some patients may be extremely responsive to noise or sensory stimuli following narcotic administration.

4. Most narcotics cause release of antidiuretic hormone (ADH).

G. Opioids are classified as agonists, agonist-antagonists, or antagonists.

1. Agonists

a. Opioid agonists occupy the opioid receptor sites. Depending on the specific drug, the dose, and the species of animal patient, they produce the full range of physiologic responses associated with opioid drugs.

b. Pure opioid agonists include morphine, meperidine, oxymorphone, fentanyl, sufentanil, alfentanil, carfentanil, codeine, and heroin.

2. Agonist-antagonists

a. Opioid agonist-antagonists are opioids that are agonists or partial agonists at one or more of the opioid receptors and are antagonistic or partially antagonistic at other opioid receptor sites.

b. Opioid agonist-antagonists can partially antagonize the effects of pure opioid agonists.

c. The opioid agonist-antagonists include pentazocine, nalbuphine, nalorphine, butorphanol, and buprenorphine.

3. Antagonists

a. Opioid antagonists are drugs that occupy the opioid receptors and exert none of the opioid physiologic effects.

b. Opioid antagonists will reverse the effects of opioid agonists and agonist-antagonists.

c. Opioid antagonists include naloxone, naltrexone, and nalmefene.

H. Morphine sulfate

1. Morphine is the prototype narcotic agonist.

2. Its primary effect is to produce analgesia with some degree of sedation.

3. The use of morphine as a preanesthetic agent has generally been limited to the dog.

4. In large doses (>1.0 mg/lb), morphine will produce mania and tonic convulsions in the cat. Small doses (0.05 mg/lb SC) can produce analgesia lasting more than 4 hours in the cat.

5. It depresses respiration as previously outlined.

6. It does not significantly depress myocardial contractility or cardiac output.

7. It causes histamine release, producing vasodilation and potential hypotension, especially when administered intravenously.

8. It can produce significant sinus bradycardia as a result of increased vagal tone.

9. It stimulates release of ADH and may decrease renal output by as much as 90%.

10. It directly stimulates the vomition center.

11. It is metabolized by the liver to morphine 3-0-glucuronide, which is excreted by the kidney.

12. Its duration of action is 1–4 hours in the dog.

I. Meperidine hydrochloride (Demerol)

1. Meperidine is a synthetic narcotic agonist that has one tenth to one fifth the analgesic potency of morphine.
2. Meperidine has been used in both the dog and cat.
   a. It has not been proven whether significant analgesia is produced by meperidine in the cat.
   b. It allows a dog or cat to be more easily handled; however, no marked CNS depression or sedation occurs.
3. At therapeutic doses it usually produces less cardiovascular depression than morphine.
4. At therapeutic doses, it usually causes less respiratory depression than morphine.
5. The dog and cat metabolize meperidine very rapidly in the liver.
6. Its duration of action is 1–2 hours.

J. Oxymorphone hydrochloride (Numorphan)
1. Oxymorphone is a semisynthetic narcotic agonist that has 10 times more analgesic potency than morphine.
2. It can be used in both the dog and cat.
3. It produces more sedation and less hypnosis than morphine.
4. It can be combined with a tranquilizer to produce neuroleptanalgesia.
5. It may produce less respiratory depression than morphine.
6. Its effects on the cardiovascular system are similar to those of morphine.
7. Its duration of action is 1–3 hours.

K. Fentanyl citrate (Sublimaze)
1. Fentanyl is a synthetic narcotic agonist that is 100 to 150 times more potent than morphine.
2. Fentanyl is not recommended for use in the cat.
3. It has a rapid onset of action following intramuscular or intravenous administration (3–8 minutes) and has a short duration of action, with peak effects lasting for 30 minutes in the dog.
4. Fentanyl has minimal effects on blood pressure and cardiac output but can produce profound sinus bradycardia (counteracted by atropine).
5. Its respiratory effects are not consistent and may range from hyperventilation to respiratory depression and occasional apnea. Even though peak effects last approximately 30 minutes, respiratory depression has occurred for several hours following its use.
6. It rarely produces histamine release.
7. It rarely stimulates vomition, although defecation is often produced because of relaxation of the anal sphincter.
8. Fentanyl is used in combination with droperidol under the trade name of Innovar-Vet.

L. Pentazocine lactate (Talwin)
1. Pentazocine is a benzomorphan narcotic analgesic with both agonist and antagonist properties. It has one third the potency of morphine.
2. It has been used in dogs as an analgesic.
3. It produces minimal CNS depression.
4. It has minimal cardiovascular depressant effects and only mild respiratory depressant effects.
5. Intramuscular doses of pentazocine will produce effects in 15 minutes, and they will last for approximately 2 hours.

M. Butorphanol tartrate (Stadol, Torbutrol, Torbugesic)

1. Butorphanol is a synthetic opioid agonist-antagonist.

   a. It has a strong affinity for opioid receptors.

   b. Butorphanol's analgesic potency is three to five times that of morphine.

   c. Butorphanol's antagonistic potency is about equal to nalorphine and is about 50 times less potent than naloxone.

2. Butorphanol can produce significant decreases in heart rate as a result of increased vagal tone.

   a. The bradycardia is responsive to anticholinergics.

   b. Butorphanol can produce decreases in cardiac output and blood pressure, but its effect is less strong than that of morphine.

3. The respiratory depressant effects of butorphanol are similar to those of morphine except that the respiratory depression produced seems to reach a "ceiling" beyond which higher doses do not cause significantly more respiratory depression.

4. It is rapidly absorbed after intramuscular injection, with peak blood levels occurring in 15–30 minutes. Its duration of effect is 1–4 hours at the usually administered doses.

5. It is rapidly and completely absorbed from the gastrointestinal tract; however, because of significant first-pass hepatic metabolism, only 17% of the dose is available systemically.

6. It has good analgesic and fair sedative properties.

7. It is extensively metabolized by the liver.

   a. The metabolites do not appear to have analgesic properties.

   b. Approximately 70% of the metabolites are excreted in the urine. Biliary excretion also occurs.

8. When butorphanol is combined with acepromazine, a benzodiazepine tranquilizer, or an alpha-2 agonist, a very good neuroleptanalgesic is produced.

N. Buprenorphine (Buprenex, Temgesic)

1. Buprenorphine is a partial mu-opioid agonist-antagonist derived from thebaine.

2. Its agonistic properties are approximately 30 times that of morphine.

3. Following intravenous or intramuscular administration, it requires 20–30 minutes to reach full effect.

   a. Buprenorphine's duration of action is 6–8 hours after intravenous or intramuscular use.

   b. In some patients, the effect of buprenorphine may last up to 12 hours.

4. Its cardiopulmonary effects are similar to those of butorphanol. It may produce slightly more respiratory depression.

5. It has been combined with acepromazine or an alpha-2 agonist to produce a neuroleptanalgesic.

O. Advantages

1. Narcotic analgesics sedate and calm patients prior to local or general anesthesia.

2. They provide pre- and postoperative analgesia.

3. They allow for a decrease in the amount of general anesthetic needed.

4. They have minimal depressant effects on the cardiovascular system.

5. Their physiologic effects are reversible with narcotic antagonists.
P. Disadvantages, precautions, and contraindications
  1. Narcotic analgesics can cause marked depression of the respiratory system. They should be used with caution in patients with preexisting respiratory distress.
  2. They can cause hypotension in some patients.
  3. They can produce sinus bradycardia, sometimes severe. This reaction can readily be counteracted by an anticholinergic.
  4. They can cause excitement in some patients, depending on the specific agent, the dose, and the species of animal patient.
  5. They should be used with caution in patients with head trauma as they can cause an increase in intracranial pressure. This increase is due to respiratory depression and the subsequent increase in PA_{CO_2}, which causes cerebral vasodilation.
  6. These are controlled substances; therefore, they must be kept in a secured area, and accurate records need to be kept.
Q. Narcotic antagonists
  1. Nalorphine hydrochloride (Nalline) and levallorphan tartrate (Lorfan)
    a. These drugs are synthetic congeners of morphine. They produce both agonistic and antagonistic activity.
    b. They tend to produce more antagonistic than agonistic activity.
    c. They act by competitive inhibition at the opioid receptor sites.
    d. Nalorphine and levallorphan are specific for narcotics and will not antagonize other CNS depressants.
    e. They should not be used in the absence of narcotics or as general analeptics (respiratory stimulants) as they can cause mild to moderate respiratory depression resulting from their agonistic effects.
    f. Both drugs will enhance CNS depression caused by other CNS depressants of non-narcotic types.
    g. Refer to Table 2–2 for dose and duration of action.
  2. Naloxone hydrochloride (Narcan)
    a. Naloxone is the N-allyl derivative of oxymorphone.
    b. It is a pure narcotic antagonist, having no agonistic activity.
    c. It does not produce CNS or respiratory depression when used alone.
    d. It is three times more potent than levallorphan and 13 times more potent than nalorphine in antagonizing the physiologic effects of narcotic analgesics.
    e. Naloxone will not antagonize the CNS depressant effects of non-narcotic agents.
    f. Naloxone's half-life is much shorter than that of levallorphan or nalorphine. Its antagonism lasts only 15–45 minutes. Therefore, additional doses may be needed to maintain narcotic antagonism.
    g. Naloxone will antagonize the effects of butorphanol and buprenorphine. Higher doses may be needed to antagonize butorphanol because of its high affinity for opioid receptors.
X. Neuroleptanalgesics
  A. A neuroleptanalgesic is a combination of a neuroleptic (tranquilizer) and an analgesic (narcotic).
  B. Virtually any tranquilizer and narcotic can be used in combination with each other to enhance the CNS depressant effects of each.
  C. For other neuroleptanalgesic combinations, refer to Table 2–3.

Table 2–3. Neuroleptanalgesic Combinations for the Dog and Cat

Neuroleptic (Tranquilizer)	Analgesic (Narcotic)
Acetylpromazine 0.05 mg/lb IM or IV to a maximum total dose of 1.0 mg	Oxymorphone 0.1 mg/lb IM or IV to a maximum total dose of 3 mg
Diazepam 0.1 to 0.2 mg/lb IM or IV to a maximum total dose of 10 mg*	Oxymorphone—same as above
Acetylpromazine—same as above	Meperidine 1 to 2 mg/lb IM or IV
Acetylpromazine—same as above	Butorphanol 0.1–0.2 mg/lb IM or IV to a maximum dose of 20 mg
Diazepam—same as above*	Butorphanol—same as above

*Diazepam cannot be mixed in the same syringe with the opioid as it will cause precipitation. When administering the opioid and diazepam IV, give the opioid first, and then give diazepam 2 to 3 minutes later to prevent diazepam-induced behavioral changes.

Suggested Readings

Benson GJ, Tranquilli WJ: Advantages and guidelines for using opioid agonist-antagonist analgesics. Vet Clin North Am Small Anim Pract Opin Small Anim Anesth 22(2):363–365, 1992.

Chang KJ, Cooper BR, Hazum E, Cuatrecasas P: Multiple opiate receptors: Different regional distribution in the brain and differential binding of opiates and opioid peptides. Mol Pharmacol 16:91, 1979.

Clark KW, England GCW: Medetomidine, a new sedative-analgesic for use in the dog and its reversal with atipamezole. J Small Anim Pract 30:343–348, 1989.

Gilman AG, Rall TW, Niles AS, Taylor P: The Pharmacological Basis of Therapeutics, 8th ed. New York: Pergamon Press, 1990.

Green SA, Thurmon JC: Xylazine—A review of its pharmacology and use in veterinary medicine. J Vet Pharmacol Ther 11:295–313, 1988.

Haskins SC, Lkide AM (eds): Veterinary Clinics of North America: Small Animal Practice, Opinions in Small Animal Anesthesia. Philadelphia: WB Saunders, 1992.

Moye RJ, Pailet A, Smith MW Jr: Clinical use of xylazine in dogs and cats. Vet Med Small Anim Clin 68(3):236–239, 1973.

Pert A: Neuropharmacology of analgesics. Surg Pract News 10:10, 1981.

Scheinin M, MacDonald E: An introduction to the pharmacology of alpha-2 adrenoceptors in the central nervous system. Acta Vet Scand 85:11–19, 1989.

Short CE: Effects of anticholinergic treatment on the cardiac and respiratory systems in dogs sedated with medetomidine. Vet Rec 129(4):310–313, 1991.

Stoelting RK: Pharmacology and Physiology in Anesthetic Practice, 2nd ed. Philadelphia: JB Lippincott, 1991.

Thurmon JC, Tranquilli WJ, Benson GJ: Preanesthetic and anesthetic adjuncts. In Lumb and Jones' Veterinary Anesthesia, 3rd ed. Baltimore: Williams & Wilkins, 1996.

Tranquilli WJ, Benson GJ: Advantages and guidelines for using alpha-2 agonists as anesthetic adjuvants. Vet Clin North Am Small Anim Pract 22(2):289–293, 1992.

Tranquilli WJ, Maze M: Clinical pharmacology and use of alpha-2 agonists in veterinary anesthesia. Anaesth Pharmacol Rev 1(3):297–309, 1993.

Virtanen R: Pharmacologic profiles of medetomidine and its antagonist atipamezole. Acta Vet Scand 85:29–37, 1989.

Anesthetic Agents

Robert R. Paddleford

Section 1: Injectable General Anesthetics

I. Barbiturates

  A. Historical perspective

    1. The parent compound for all barbiturates is barbituric acid, which was first prepared in 1867 by combining urea and malonic acid.

    2. Barbital (diethyl barbituric acid) was first prepared in 1903 and was the first barbiturate to be used clinically.

    3. Pentobarbital sodium was the first barbiturate to be used as a general anesthetic in 1930, followed by thiopental sodium in 1934 and thiamylal sodium in 1948.

    4. Depending on the dose administered, the barbiturates can be used as sedatives, hypnotics, or general anesthetics.

    5. In veterinary medicine, the primary use of barbiturates is to induce or maintain general anesthesia and to control seizures.

  B. Classifications of barbiturates

    1. Barbiturates are classified according to the following:

      a. Chemical substitutions on the barbituric acid molecule

      b. Duration of action

    2. Classification of barbiturates based on chemical structure

      a. The barbituric acid molecule itself does not possess CNS depressant activity.

      b. Substitutions are made at one or more of the four radicals (Fig. 3–1) in order to provide CNS depressant activity.

        (1) Thousands of barbiturates are theoretically possible.

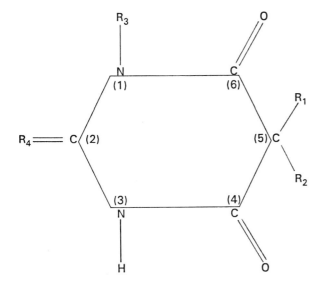

Figure 3–1. Barbituric acid molecule. R_1–R_4 indicate the sites for substitution of radicals.

Table 3–1. Structural Formulas for Some Commonly Used Barbiturates

Drug	R_1	R_2	R_3	R_4
		Oxybarbiturates		
Barbital	—CH$_2$—CH$_3$	—CH$_2$—CH$_3$	H	O
Phenobarbital	—CH$_2$—CH$_3$		H	O
Pentobarbital	—CH$_2$—CH$_3$	—CH—CH$_2$—CH$_2$—CH$_3$ CH$_3$	H	O
		Methylated oxybarbiturate		
Methohexital (Brevital)	—CH$_2$=CH=CH$_2$	—CH—C=C—CH$_2$—CH$_3$ CH$_3$	CH$_3$	O
		Thiobarbiturate		
Thiopental (Pentothal)	—CH$_2$—CH$_3$	—CH—CH$_2$—CH$_2$—CH$_3$ CH$_3$	H	S

    (2) Approximately 20 have been used clinically, and only 10 have
been used as general anesthetics.

  c. Chemical classifications (see Table 3–1 for chemical structures)

    (1) Oxybarbiturates—pentobarbital, phenobarbital, barbital, seco-
barbital

    (2) Methylated oxybarbiturates—methohexital (Brevital), hexobar-
bital

    (3) Thiobarbiturates—thiopental (Pentothal), thialbarbital

  d. If the side chain is lengthened beyond two carbons at radical 2 but
made no longer than five carbons, the onset of action and the
duration of action of the barbiturate are both decreased.

  e. As the side chain at radical 2 increases beyond five carbons, the
CNS depressant properties of the barbiturate decrease and the
convulsive or excitatory properties increase.

  f. Lipid solubility of the barbiturate is increased by substituting a
sulfur molecule for the oxygen molecule at radical 4. The sulfur
molecule decreases the onset of action and the duration of action
(Table 3–2).

3. Classification of barbiturates based on duration of action

  a. Long-acting barbiturates

    (1) Included in this group are barbital and phenobarbital.

    (2) These barbiturates have a slow onset of action after intravenous
administration (see Table 3–2).

Table 3–2. Onset and Duration of Anesthesia as Related to Substitutions at Radicals 1, 2, and 4 of the Barbituric Acid Molecule

Drug	Substitutions			Lipid Solubility (Barbital = 1)	Onset of General Anesthesia Following IV Injection	Duration of General Anesthesia
	R_1	R_2	R_4			
Barbital	Ethyl	Ethyl	Oxygen	1	22 minutes	6–12 hours
Phenobarbital	Ethyl	Phenyl	Oxygen	3	12 minutes	6–12 hours
Pentobarbital	Ethyl	1-Methylbutyl	Oxygen	40	30–60 seconds	1–3 hours
Thiopental	Ethyl	1-Methylbutyl	Sulfur	600	15–30 seconds	10–20 minutes

    (3) Their duration of anesthesia ranges from 6 to 12 hours after intravenous injection.

    (4) They are not utilized as general anesthetics because of their slow onset of action and their long duration of action.

    (5) They are used mainly as sedatives and hypnotics and to control seizures.

  b. Short-acting barbiturates

    (1) Included in this group are pentobarbital, hexobarbital, and secobarbital.

    (2) Their onset of action is fairly rapid (30–60 seconds) after intravenous injection, and their duration of action is 1–3 hours.

    (3) Pentobarbital is the primary drug of this group used in veterinary anesthesia. It has been used as a sedative and as a general anesthetic, although its use as a general anesthetic has declined in recent years.

  c. Ultra-short-acting barbiturates

    (1) Included in this group are thiopental and methohexital.

    (2) Their onset of action is very rapid (15–30 seconds) following intravenous administration, and their duration of action is very short (5–20 minutes).

    (3) These agents are used in veterinary anesthesia as induction agents and as the primary anesthetic for short procedures.

C. Physiologic effects

  1. CNS effects

    a. All of the barbiturates depress the CNS; however, they differ in the effective dosage, onset of action, and duration of action.

    b. The degree of CNS depression varies from mild sedation to surgical plane anesthesia.

    c. Barbiturates depress the cortex, thalamus, and motor areas of the brain.

    d. Part of their CNS depressant activity is related to prolongation of central inhibitory transmission processes thought to be mediated by gamma-aminobutyric acid (GABA).

    e. The reticular activating system in the mesencephalon seems very sensitive to the depressant effects of the barbiturates.

    (1) The reticular activating system controls the overall degree of CNS activity, including wakefulness and sleep.

    (2) The reticular activating system also controls a patient's ability to direct attention toward specific areas of the conscious mind.

    f. Barbiturates depress cellular activity of the CNS, but the exact mechanism is not clear.

    (1) Barbiturates are potent depressants of CNS oxygen consumption.

    (2) They can decrease oxygen consumption by as much as 55%.

    g. Barbiturates raise the threshold of spinal reflexes.

    h. Barbiturates *do not* produce analgesia.

    i. The medullary centers, thermoregulating center, vagus center, respiratory center, and vasomotor center are all depressed at anesthetic doses of barbiturates.

  2. Cardiovascular effects

    a. Barbiturates produce variable responses in the cardiovascular sys-

tem depending on the species of animal patient and the specific barbiturate, dose, and route of administration.
   b. Heart rate usually increases as a result of depression of the cardiac portion of the vagal center or arterial pressoreceptor reflexes.
   c. Stroke volume and myocardial contractility usually decrease.
      (1) The decrease in myocardial contractility may be related to calcium-dependent mechanisms.
      (2) Pentobarbital appears to decrease binding availability of calcium at superficial membrane sites in cardiac cells.
   d. An initial increase in cardiac output is followed by a decrease. The initial increase is probably due to the increased heart rate.
   e. Barbiturates cause an initial decrease in total peripheral resistance followed by a return to normal.
   f. Usually an initial fall in blood pressure occurs, followed by a return toward normal.
      (1) The fall in blood pressure is due to the decreased peripheral resistance and depression of the vasomotor center.
      (2) The vasomotor center appears to be affected by the concentration of the barbiturate administered.
      (3) Significant peripheral vasodilation can occur when relatively safe doses of barbiturate are given very rapidly or when large doses are given rapidly.
   g. Cardiac dysrhythmias may occur following barbiturate administration.
      (1) They seem to occur more with the thiobarbiturates.
      (2) The dysrhythmias produced are usually premature ventricular contractions and of a bigeminal nature.
      (3) The dysrhythmias are usually transitory.
3. Respiratory effects
   a. Barbiturates are potent respiratory depressants.
   b. At anesthetizing doses, they depress the respiratory centers of the brain.
   c. Barbiturates can depress respiratory rate and tidal volume and therefore minute ventilation.
   d. Both the threshold and sensitivity of the respiratory center to carbon dioxide is altered.
   e. The carotid-aortic chemoreceptors are also depressed.
4. Other physiologic effects
   a. Barbiturates have no direct effect on the gastrointestinal tract or liver, although they may reduce hepatic blood flow.
   b. Barbiturates have no direct effect on the kidneys, although they may reduce renal blood flow by as much as 40%. Uremia enhances the effects of barbiturates in a patient.
   c. Anesthetic doses of barbiturates depress basal metabolism.
   d. Body temperature may drop as a result of decreased basal metabolism, peripheral vasodilation, and depression of the thermoregulation center.
   e. Barbiturates readily cross the placenta and will affect in utero young.
D. Factors determining the plasma levels of the barbiturates and therefore the depth and duration of anesthesia

1. Dose
   a. Factors determining plasma levels of a barbiturate include the dose given, the route of administration, and, if given intravenously, the rate of administration.
   b. Once the barbiturate is injected into the patient, the effect of the drug and the time course depend on hemodynamic and physiochemical factors.
2. Ionization
   a. Barbiturates are weak acids and therefore have an ionized and nonionized form.
   b. The ionized form interacts strongly with the water dipoles in the cell walls and does not readily penetrate the cell.
   c. The nonionized form is pharmacologically active and readily diffuses into cells and produces the effects.
   d. The arterial pH determines the proportion of the ionized to the nonionized form of the barbiturate.
   e. At a pH of 7.4, 61% of thiopental and 83% of pentobarbital are in the nonionized (active) form.
   f. As the arterial pH decreases (acidosis), the amount of nonionized barbiturate increases; therefore, more active drug is available to enter the cell and cause anesthesia.
   g. As the arterial pH increases (alkalosis), the amount of nonionized barbiturate decreases; therefore, less active drug is available to enter the cell and cause anesthesia.
3. Plasma protein binding
   a. Barbiturates reversibly bind to plasma proteins.
   b. When barbiturates bind to plasma proteins, primarily albumins, they cannot cross the cell membrane and thus are not pharmacologically active.
   c. The barbiturates vary in their protein-binding abilities.
   d. The degree of protein binding depends on the arterial pH and reaches maximum binding at a pH of 7.6 or greater.
   e. As the pH decreases, plasma protein binding decreases; therefore, more active barbiturate is available to produce general anesthesia.
   f. Percentage of protein-bound barbiturate at an arterial pH of 7.4
      (1) Thiopental—75% protein bound
      (2) Pentobarbital—40% protein bound
      (3) Phenobarbital—20% protein bound
      (4) Barbital—5% protein bound
   g. The percent of binding is reduced as the amount of barbiturate increases in the blood, although the total amount of protein-bound barbiturate increases.
   h. It should be remembered that the thiobarbiturates, because of their greater protein affinity, can and will displace weaker protein-bound drugs on the albumin molecule.
4. Redistribution (Fig. 3–2)
   a. Induction and arousal from anesthesia produced by the thiobarbiturates (thiopental) largely depend on redistribution of these agents in body tissues.
   b. Although the thiobarbiturates are ultimately biotransformed by the

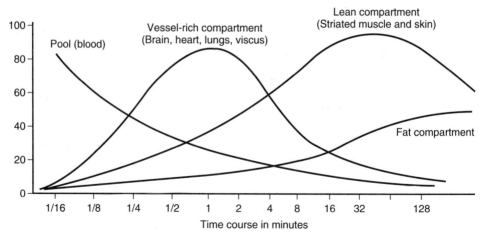

Figure 3–2. Distribution of sulfonated ultra-short-acting barbiturates. (Modified from Price H, et al: Uptake of thiopental by body tissues and its relation to duration of narcosis. Clin Pharmacol Ther 1:16, 1960.)

      liver and excreted, this is not the major reason a patient awakens from these drugs.

  c. The body organ systems can be divided into various compartments depending on what percent of the cardiac output goes to any given compartment.

    (1) Vessel-rich compartment—consists of organs such as brain, heart, lungs, liver, intestines, and kidneys. This compartment represents 6–10% of the body mass and receives 75% of the cardiac output.

    (2) Lean-organ compartment—consists of striated muscle and skin. This compartment represents 50% of the body mass and receives only 20% of the cardiac output.

    (3) Fat compartment—consists of the adipose tissue of the body. In a normally fleshed patient this compartment represents 20% of the body mass and receives 5% of the cardiac output.

    (4) Vessel-poor compartment—consists of bone, cartilage, and tendons. This compartment represents 20% of the body mass and receives less than 5% of the cardiac output. This compartment does not play a significant role in thiobarbiturate redistribution.

  d. When a dose of a thiobarbiturate is injected into the bloodstream, it reaches maximum concentration within the brain and other organs in the vessel-rich compartment in only 30–45 seconds because of the large amount of cardiac output going to that compartment.

  e. Uptake of the thiobarbiturate is slower in the lean compartment. Although the uptake by muscle and skin is slower (because of a lower percentage of cardiac output going to these tissues), it is important.

    (1) Maximum uptake by the lean compartment occurs 10–15 minutes after the thiobarbiturate injection and corresponds with arousal from the ultra-short-acting thiobarbiturates.

    (2) The ultra-short action of the thiobarbiturates is due to their redistribution into the non-nervous tissue (except fat) of the body.

   f. Finally, the thiobarbiturates redistribute into the fat compartment.
      (1) In the dog, maximum redistribution into the fat compartment occurs within 4 hours, with final equilibration of the fat/plasma ratio in 6 hours.
      (2) The thiobarbiturates are extremely lipid-soluble and tend to stay in the body fat.
      (3) As they are gradually released from the fat, they are metabolized by the liver, and the by-products are excreted by the kidneys.
      (4) In the dog, fat concentrations of thiopental at 24 and 36 hours are 22% and 5%, respectively.
   g. When final redistribution to the fat occurs, elimination of the thiobarbiturate from the body depends on liver, brain, and kidney metabolism.
   h. Redistribution is less of a factor in arousal from methylated oxybarbiturate methohexital (Brevital), although it does play some role.
   i. Redistribution plays no significant role in arousal from the short-acting oxybarbiturates (pentobarbital) or the long-acting oxybarbiturates (phenobarbital).
5. Metabolism
   a. Hepatic metabolism is the major factor in determining plasma clearance and ultimate arousal from anesthesia from the short-acting oxybarbiturate pentobarbital.
      (1) How rapidly metabolism occurs is species-dependent.
      (2) In the dog, approximately 15% of the total dose of pentobarbital is detoxified per hour.
      (3) When approximately 30–45% of the dose is detoxified, arousal occurs in the dog.
      (4) Metabolic by-products are eliminated in the urine.
   b. The ultra-short-acting thiobarbiturates are primarily detoxified in the liver; however, some metabolism also occurs in the brain and kidney. In the dog only 5% of the total dose of thiobarbiturate is metabolized per hour.
   c. Hepatic metabolism is the major factor in determining plasma clearance and ultimate arousal from anesthesia from the ultra-short-acting methyloxybarbiturate methohexital.
   d. The long-acting oxybarbiturates undergo minimal hepatic detoxification.
   e. Barbiturate metabolism occurs by the following:
      (1) Oxidation of radicals at carbon 5 (most important)
      (2) Dealkylation of the alkyl group
      (3) Desulfonation of the thiobarbiturates
      (4) Destruction of the barbituric acid ring (least important)
6. Renal excretion
   a. Plasma clearance and ultimate arousal from the long-acting oxybarbiturates (phenobarbital) are primarily dependent on renal excretion. Very little hepatic metabolism of these barbiturates occurs unless hepatic enzyme induction has occurred.
   b. The metabolites of the short-acting oxybarbiturates are excreted in the urine.
   c. The kidneys play a minor role in thiobarbiturate metabolism.

E. Clinical uses of specific barbiturates
   1. Phenobarbital
       a. Phenobarbital is primarily used as a sedative/hypnotic and anticonvulsant drug.
       b. It is not recommended for use as a general anesthetic for surgery because of its slow onset of action.
       c. It is generally given orally although it has been used intravenously "to effect" to control seizures of varying etiologies.
   2. Pentobarbital sodium (Nembutal)
       a. Pentobarbital is the most commonly used short-acting oxybarbiturate in veterinary anesthesia.
       b. It has been used as a preanesthetic sedative in the dog and cat at a dose of 1–2 mg/lb (2.2–4.4 mg/kg) intramuscularly.
       c. Its primary use in the small animal patient has been as the sole general anesthetic for surgical and diagnostic procedures. Extreme variations can exist among patients in regard to total dose needed for anesthesia as well as duration of anesthesia from a given dose.
       d. Pentobarbital is supplied in concentrations of 50 mg/ml, 60 mg/ml, and 65 mg/ml.
       e. The total calculated dose for a dog or cat that has not been premedicated with a CNS depressant (tranquilizer, sedative, narcotic) is 8–12 mg/lb (17.6–26.4 mg/kg) intravenously.
           (1) Approximately one half of this dose is given moderately rapidly to get the patient past the initial excitement stage (stage II) of anesthesia.
           (2) One should wait 30–60 seconds for the maximum effects of the initial dose to be produced in the patient before giving additional pentobarbital.
           (3) Additional barbiturate is then given to effect in small increments until the desired depth of anesthesia is reached. Allow at least 1 minute for the maximum effect for each additional dose of pentobarbital given.
       f. The total calculated dose of pentobarbital for a dog or cat that has been premedicated with a CNS depressant is 4–6 mg/lb (8.8–13.2 mg/kg) intravenously.
           (1) Depending on the degree of CNS depression achieved with the preanesthetic medication, anywhere from 10–50% of the total calculated dose is initially given intravenously.
           (2) Again wait 30–60 seconds for maximum effects of the initial dose of pentobarbital, and titrate the remainder to effect. Allow at least 1 minute for the maximum effect for each additional dose of pentobarbital.
       g. The total dose of pentobarbital needed for anesthesia for an individual patient will depend on a number of factors (see section F).
       h. Pentobarbital will provide 1–3 hours of anesthesia. For longer periods, additional pentobarbital may need to be administered.
       i. It is recommended that a preanesthetic CNS depressant be given to patients prior to pentobarbital anesthesia in order to do the following:
           (1) Decrease the amount of pentobarbital needed
           (2) Provide for a smoother induction (less chance of excitement)
           (3) Provide for a smoother recovery

Table 3–3. Pharmacokinetics of Intravenous General Anesthetic Agents

Drug Group	Drug Name	Distribution Half-Life (minutes)	Elimination Half-Life (hours)
Barbiturates	Thiopental	2–4	10–12
	Methohexital	5–6	3–5
Imidazoles	Etomidate	2–4	2–5
Arylcyclohexylamines	Telazol	11–17	2–3
Alkylphenols	Propofol	2–4	1–3

3. Thiobarbiturates (Thiopental)

   a. Thiobarbiturates are used in the small animal patient as the sole anesthetic agent for short diagnostic or surgical procedures or as inducing agents prior to inhalation anesthesia (Tables 3–3 and 3–4).

   b. The only thiobarbiturate currently available is thiopental sodium (Pentothal).

   c. The duration of surgical anesthesia from a single dose is approximately 10–15 minutes.

   d. Thiopental is supplied as a powder to which diluent is added to produce the desired concentration. A 1–5% solution is usually used.

   e. The same dosages used for pentobarbital apply to thiopental as well.

      (1) In contrast to pentobarbitol, maximum effects from a dose of thiopental are seen within 15–30 seconds.

      (2) It is very unlikely that a patient will develop excitement or delirium during ultra-short-acting barbiturate induction in view of the rapid onset of its effects.

      (3) Because of the preceding two reasons, an initial dose of 35–40% is usually given to an unpremedicated patient, with the remainder titrated to effect as needed; wait approximately 30 seconds between each dose of the drug.

      (4) In premedicated patients, depending on the degree of CNS depression, only 10–30% of the total calculated dose is given

Table 3–4. Summary of Comparative Pharmacologic Properties of IV Induction Agents

Properties	Thiopental	Etomidate	Tiletamine (Telazol)	Propofol
Solubility	Water	Propylene glycol	Water	Egg lecithin
Dose (mg/lb)	4–6 IV	0.7–1.5 IV	2 IM 1–2 IV	1–3 IV
Onset	Rapid	Rapid	Rapid	Rapid
Induction	Smooth	Pain/myoclonus	Excitatory/smooth	Smooth/pain
Cardiovascular effect	Depression	Minimal	Stimulation	Depression
Respiratory effect	Depression	Minimal	Minimal/moderate depression	Depression
Analgesia	None	None	Superficial—yes Deep visceral (?)	None
Amnesia	Minimal	Minimal	Minimal	Minimal
Recovery	Rapid	Rapid	Intermediate	Rapid

IM = intramuscular.
IV = intravenous.

initially. Additional thiopental is given to effect until the desired level of anesthesia is reached.

4. Methohexital (Brevane, Brevital)

   a. This methyloxybarbiturate is approximately twice as potent as thiopental (see Table 3–3).

   b. It is used in the same way as the thiobarbiturates.

   c. The total calculated dose for an unpremedicated dog or cat is 5 mg/lb (11.0 mg/kg) IV. Approximately one half the dose is given rapidly. The remainder is titrated to effect.

   d. The total calculated dose of methohexital in a dog or cat premedicated with a CNS depressant is 2.5–3 mg/lb (5.5–6.6 mg/kg) intravenously. Approximately 10–30% of the dose is given rapidly intravenously, with the remainder of the dose titrated to effect.

   e. Surgical anesthesia is maintained for 5–15 minutes following a single dose of methohexital.

   f. Recovery is rapid but can be accompanied by muscle tremors and violent excitement. For this reason it is recommended that a patient receiving methohexital receive a preanesthetic CNS depressant such as a tranquilizer, sedative, or narcotic.

   g. Unlike the thiobarbiturates, methohexital is rapidly detoxified by the liver. This rapid detoxification along with rapid tissue redistribution account for its very short duration of action.

   h. Methohexital has been advocated for use in the coursing (sight) hound breeds (such as Greyhound, Whippet, Borzoi) in place of the thiobarbiturates because it does not depend on redistribution for the reversal of its effects.

F. Factors that cause variations in the response to barbiturates

   1. All general anesthetics, injectable or inhalant, must be administrated to effect on an individual basis to each patient. Various factors, especially in regard to the barbiturates, will cause variations in response among individuals.

   2. Body weight

      a. The barbiturates are administered on a mg/lb (mg/kg) basis; therefore, body weight will determine total calculated dose.

      b. Even more important than body weight is percentage of body fat.

      c. In the obese patient it is quite possible to produce an initial relative barbiturate overdose when recommended doses are used.

         (1) Remember that body fat receives a very small percentage of the cardiac output (less than 5%) as compared with the vessel-rich and lean-organ compartments.

         (2) Therefore, if a patient is obese, and the dose of barbiturate is calculated on total body weight, an overdose can occur because a higher percentage of body mass is receiving a small percentage of cardiac output and therefore of barbiturate.

         (3) In turn, the vessel-rich compartment—including the brain, heart, and viscera—will be exposed to a relatively higher dose of barbiturate because this compartment now constitutes a lower total percentage of body mass but is still receiving the majority of the cardiac output. The vessel-rich group of organs receives approximately 70–75% of the cardiac output.

         (4) This factor will be important regardless of which type of barbiturate is used.

(5) Obesity also specifically affects the action of the thiobarbiturates. Because they are ultimately absorbed by the fat, an obese patient can in theory absorb more thiobarbiturate than the thin patient.

d. Lack of body fat can greatly prolong recovery from thiobarbiturates.

(1) The thiobarbiturates are extremely lipid-soluble.

(2) Rapid recovery from the effects of the thiobarbiturates is determined by redistribution from the CNS to other body organs, including adipose tissue.

(3) If a patient lacks body fat for thiobarbiturate storage, the detoxification of these drugs by the liver, brain, and kidneys becomes important in the reversal of their effects.

(4) Since detoxification is slow, recovery from these drugs can be very prolonged (6–24 hours or longer).

(5) Therefore, the use of thiobarbiturates in very lean or thin patients should be used with caution.

(6) Lack of body fat is not as major a concern with methohexital or pentobarbital as redistribution to fat is not a major factor in their reversal.

3. Age and sex of patient

a. The age of a patient may affect barbiturate response in two ways.

(1) Very young patients may not have fully developed hepatic enzyme systems; therefore, barbiturate detoxification may be delayed.

(2) Very old patients may have impaired liver function; therefore, barbiturate detoxification may be delayed.

b. The sex of a patient appears not to have a major influence on recovery from barbiturates.

4. Shock or hypovolemia

a. Shock or reduced blood volume will intensify the responses of a patient following barbiturate administration.

b. Any condition that decreases the central pool of blood into which the barbiturate is injected results in a greater percentage of the blood volume—and therefore of the barbiturate—being delivered to the vessel-rich group of organs (the CNS, heart, lungs, kidneys, and viscera).

c. In addition, shock is usually accompanied by metabolic acidosis. Therefore, less barbiturate will be protein bound and more will be in the nonionized, or active, form, further intensifying its effects.

d. Liver perfusion may decrease, slowing barbiturate detoxification.

e. Barbiturates must be used with extreme caution in patients suffering from shock or hypovolemia.

5. Liver dysfunction

a. Liver dysfunction can delay barbiturate detoxification and ultimately clearance from the body.

b. Liver dysfunction is more of a problem with the short-acting oxybarbiturates and the ultra-short-acting methyloxybarbiturates because arousal from these barbiturates depends on liver metabolism.

c. Liver dysfunction is less of a problem with the thiobarbiturates because arousal is due to redistribution, although ultimately these drugs are metabolized in the liver. But if for some reason (lack of body fat, excessive amount of thiopental given) liver metabolism becomes the primary route for arousal from anesthesia, liver dysfunction may *greatly* prolong the effects of thiopental.

6. Hypothermia
   a. Hypothermia may cause a decrease in the metabolic rate of the liver, thereby delaying barbiturate metabolism.
   b. Both shock and general anesthesia can produce hypothermia.

7. Acid-base imbalance
   a. Acidosis increases the amount of nonionized barbiturate as well as decreasing the amount of protein-bound barbiturate. Therefore, more barbiturate is available to produce effects in the patient.
   b. Many disease processes can produce metabolic or respiratory acidosis. In these patients, barbiturates must be used with care.

8. Uremia
   a. Uremia seems to prolong the sleep time of barbiturates.
   b. The prolonged sleep time may be due to acid-base or electrolyte imbalance.

9. Hypoproteinemia
   a. Hypoproteinemia will enhance the effects of the barbiturates because there is less protein for them to bind with.
   b. The protein-bound fraction of the barbiturate is pharmacologically inactive.
   c. Hypoproteinemia is very important when considering the use of thiobarbiturates because up to 75% of the injected dose is protein bound.

10. Potentiating drugs
    a. Any CNS depressant—that is, any tranquilizers, sedatives, narcotics, or other general anesthetics—can enhance the patient's response to barbiturate anesthesia as the effects are additive.
    b. Drugs that competitively bind with plasma proteins may prevent the barbiturates from binding and thus enhance the barbiturates' effect.
    c. Drugs that are detoxified by the same hepatic metabolic pathways may prolong the effect of barbiturate anesthesia.
    d. Atropine has been shown to prolong the effect of barbiturate anesthesia.

11. Repeated doses of barbiturates
    a. Repeated doses of barbiturates will obviously prolong their effects; however, sometimes the additional anesthesia time is excessive.
    b. Repeated doses of thiopental can result in very prolonged recovery periods.
       (1) Primary recovery is due to tissue redistribution.
       (2) When repeated doses of thiopental are given, the tissue compartments may become saturated, and thus redistribution cannot occur.
       (3) When redistribution cannot occur, metabolism becomes the major reason for recovery and arousal.
       (4) Because thiopental metabolism is very slow in the dog and cat, recovery and arousal may take a very long time—up to 12 hours or more.

    c. Repeated doses of the short-acting barbiturates may cause prolonged recoveries because the hepatic enzyme systems are able to metabolize the barbiturates at a certain rate and no faster. Thus, large or excessive doses will take longer to metabolize.

12. Chronic tolerance

    a. Barbiturates can cause enzyme induction in the liver.

    b. Therefore, repeated administrations of anesthesia with short-acting or ultra-short-acting barbiturates can increase the liver's ability to detoxify these drugs.

    c. When the liver is thus affected, patients will often require more barbiturate to produce the same degree of anesthesia, and the sleep time will be decreased.

13. Acute tolerance

    a. Some patients receiving a barbiturate for the first time seem to develop an acute tolerance in that their recovery times from the barbiturate are much shorter than normal.

    b. The reason for this acute tolerance is unknown.

14. Excited or apprehensive patients

    a. Excited or apprehensive patients often require larger doses of barbiturate to produce anesthesia.

    b. This need for larger doses is in part due to heightened CNS activity.

    c. Another part of the reason that larger doses are required may be that anxious patients have an increased blood flow going to the striated muscles ("fight or flight" phenomenon) because of beta-2 receptor stimulation. Therefore, less of the cardiac output is going to the CNS.

    d. One reason for the use of preanesthetic medications is to prevent this problem.

G. Precautions and contraindications for barbiturates

1. Thiobarbiturates should be used with care in thin patients. Recovery in thin patients may be prolonged because of the diminished fat compartment producing problems with redistribution.

2. Barbiturates should also be used with care in obese patients, as a relative overdose may occur.

3. Patients with hepatic dysfunction may have longer recovery times from pentobarbital anesthesia.

4. Renal dysfunction may prolong the effects of barbiturates.

5. Because barbiturates are potent respiratory depressants, respiratory function should be monitored closely.

6. Preexisting hypoproteinemia or acidosis will enhance a patient's response to barbiturates.

II. Dissociative anesthetics

A. Dissociative anesthetics are cyclohexamine derivatives that produce a cataleptic state characterized by CNS excitement (rather than depression), analgesia, immobility, dissociation from one's environment, and amnesia.

B. Included in this group of drugs are phencyclidine HCl, ketamine HCl, and tiletamine HCl.

C. Phencyclidine HCl (Sernylan, Sernyl)

1. Phencyclidine HCl is the parent compound for the other drugs in this group.

    2. It is not available for use as it is a Schedule I controlled substance.

    3. It was never approved for use in dogs or cats, although it has been used in subhuman primates, large exotic cats, and swine.

D. Ketamine HCl (Ketalar, Ketaset, Vetalar)

    1. Ketamine is a congener of phencyclidine. It was first used in human anesthesia in 1965 and in veterinary anesthesia in 1970.

    2. Ketamine has been used in humans, subhuman primates, cats, dogs, horses, pigs, ruminants, birds, reptiles, laboratory rodents, and numerous exotic species.

    3. The ketamine molecule exists as two optical isomers.

        a. This racemic mixture is used clinically.

        b. The positive isomer produces hypnosis lasting twice as long as the negative isomer.

        c. The positive isomer produces more profound analgesia.

        d. The mixture is intermediate in effect.

    4. Ketamine can be administered either intramuscularly or intravenously in the cat and dog (Table 3–5).

    5. CNS effects

        a. Ketamine appears to selectively depress the thalamocortical system (association region of the cerebral cortex) while stimulating the reticular activating and limbic systems.

        b. It produces anesthesia by functional disruption of the CNS.

        c. It appears to be a potent inhibitor of GABA binding in the CNS and seems to enhance CNS inhibitory mechanisms through the action of the GABA systems.

        d. It appears to block neuronal transport processes for the monoamine transmitters such as 5-hydroxytryptamine (serotonin), dopamine, and norepinephrine.

        e. It increases cerebral spinal fluid pressure and intracranial pressure.

        f. It can increase CNS stimulation to the point of causing seizures

Table 3–5. Suggested Dosages of Some Ketamine–Tranquilizer/ Sedative/Narcotic Combinations

Type of Patient	Tranquilizer/Sedative/Narcotic (mg/lb)	Ketamine (mg/lb)	Duration of Action (minutes)
Cat	Acepromazine 0.1 IM*	1–2 IV	3–10
	Acepromazine 0.1 IM†	5–15 IM†	15–60
	Diazepam 0.1–0.2 IV†	1–2 IV†	5–10
	Xylazine 0.25–0.5 IM†	5–10 IM†	30–45
	Medetomidine 0.04 IM†	2–3 IM†	30–60
	Butorphanol 0.1–0.2 IM† *plus* acepromazine 0.25 mg total dose IM†	2–10 IM†	20–40
Dog	Acepromazine 0.1 IM (3 mg maximum)†	5–10 IM†	20–40
	Diazepam 0.1–0.2 IV (10 mg maximum)†	1–2 IV†	10
	Xylazine 0.25–0.5 IM†	5 IM†	20–40
	Medetomidine 0.02 IM†	2.5 IM†	20–35
	Butorphanol 0.1–0.2 IM (20 mg maximum)† *plus* acepromazine 0.25–1.0 mg total dose IM†	5–10 IM†	20–40

*Administered 15–20 minutes prior to ketamine.
†Mixed together in one syringe and given as an injection.
Note: Numerous combinations, or "cocktails," of tranquilizers, alpha-2 agonists, and narcotics have been used with ketamine.

in dogs and cats. Ketamine should be used with caution in patients with a history of seizures.

   g. It increases cerebral blood flow and oxygen consumption.

   h. It may provide better analgesia for somatic pain than for visceral pain.

   i. It may provide analgesia by the following actions:

     (1) Blocking the spinal reticular tracts

     (2) Depressing the nuclei of the medial medullary reticular formation

     (3) Suppressing the lamina of the spinal cord

     (4) Interacting with CNS and spinal cord opiate receptors

     (5) Antagonizing N-methyl-D-aspartate receptors

   j. It is not recommended for use alone in patients undergoing abdominal or thoracic procedures.

   k. It seems to be more effective in patients undergoing surgery of the skeletal/integumentary systems and extremities than in patients undergoing other types of surgery.

   l. Hallucinations and/or delirium may occur during ketamine recovery.

     (1) Emergence delirium may be accompanied by ataxia, increased motor activity, avoidance behavior, sensitivity to touch, hyperreflexia, or violent recovery reactions.

     (2) Premedication with tranquilizers, sedatives, or opioids can decrease the incidence of adverse emergence reactions.

6. Cardiovascular effects

   a. Ketamine tends to indirectly stimulate the cardiovascular system. The mechanisms by which this occurs are not completely understood, and controversy exists about them.

   b. Ketamine exerts a selective positive inotropic effect on heart muscle.

     (1) It is independent of heart rate and of the autonomic nervous system.

     (2) This effect may be due to alteration of intracellular cyclic adenosine monophosphate (cAMP).

   c. Ketamine causes an increase in heart rate, cardiac output, mean arterial blood pressure, pulmonary arterial blood pressure, and central venous pressure.

     (1) The adrenergic system must be intact for these effects to occur.

     (2) Therefore, ketamine acts either directly by stimulating the central adrenergic centers or indirectly by preventing the uptake of the catecholamines.

   d. Ketamine's effect on peripheral vascular resistance is variable.

   e. It seems to have antidysrhythmic activity.

   f. It can markedly increase myocardial oxygen demands and consumption.

   g. Large doses of ketamine, especially when administered intravenously, can have a marked depressant effect on the cardiovascular system.

   h. The cardiovascular stimulating effect of ketamine can be decreased or prevented by the prior administration of benzodiazepines, phenothiazines, or alpha-2 agonists or the concomitant administration of inhalation anesthetics.

7. Respiratory effects

   a. Ketamine produces apneustic ventilation—that is, ventilatory pattern characterized by a prolonged pause after inspiration. In patients receiving high doses, respirations may be irregular and shallow.

   b. In general, ketamine does not affect blood gases; however, in some patients it can produce marked hypoxia and hypercarbia—especially when additional CNS depressant drugs are used in combination with it.

   c. It often decreases the respiratory rate and may decrease minute volume.

   d. It does not decrease ventilatory responses to hypoxia.

   e. Pharyngeal and laryngeal reflexes are not depressed by ketamine, although they may be activated only with stimulation. As a result, a patient may be more prone to laryngospasm, bronchospasm, and coughing.

   f. Ketamine increases salivation and respiratory secretions.

      (1) Salivation may increase to the point of aspiration and respiratory obstruction.

      (2) For this reason, the use of an anticholinergic in combination with ketamine is recommended.

8. Other physiologic effects

   a. Ketamine produces muscle tonus and increased limb rigidity.

   b. It may produce spontaneous, random limb movements unassociated with pain.

   c. Eyelid and corneal reflexes remain intact and the eyes remain open; therefore, eye ointment should be used to prevent corneal drying.

   d. Both hypothermia and hyperthermia have been observed following ketamine administration.

      (1) Hypothermia is due to depression of the thermoregulation center.

      (2) Hyperthermia is most likely due to increased muscle activity or hyperactive recoveries.

   e. Ketamine can produce transient increases in liver enzymes.

9. Metabolism and elimination

   a. Ketamine undergoes extensive hepatic metabolism in the dog, horse, and human.

      (1) Biodegradation occurs by N-demethylation and hydroxylation of the cyclohexanone ring.

      (2) The metabolites formed are water-soluble and are excreted in the urine.

   b. In the cat, the majority of the injected ketamine is eliminated intact via the kidneys. Very little hepatic metabolism appears to occur.

   c. The physiologic effects of ketamine may be partially antagonized by yohimbine.

      (1) Yohimbine is an alpha-2-adrenergic blocker.

(2) It may antagonize ketamine by means of a release of central neuronal dopamine and norepinephrine.

10. Doses, routes of administration, and duration of effect

    a. Ketamine is used both in the dog and cat intramuscularly or intravenously.

    b. It is highly lipid-soluble and is readily distributed to all body tissues, even with an intramuscular injection.

    c. Refer to Table 3–3 for doses.

    d. Following intravenous administration the patient will lose its righting reflex in 30–90 seconds. Ketamine's duration of effect is usually 3–10 minutes following intravenous administration.

    e. It is rapidly effective when given intramuscularly, with loss of the righting reflex occurring in 3–5 minutes and maximum anesthetic effect occurring in 10–15 minutes.

    f. Following intramuscular administration, its duration of effect is 20–30 minutes in the dog and 30–60 minutes in the cat. Duration of effect depends on dose and on the concurrent use of CNS depressants (tranquilizers, sedatives, opioids, general anesthetics).

    g. Extreme variations in the duration and depth of anesthesia produced by ketamine may exist among individuals.

    h. It can be absorbed orally through the mucous membranes.

11. Adjunct medications

    a. Ketamine is often used in combination with a preanesthetic tranquilizer or narcotic in order to provide better muscle relaxation and smoother recoveries.

    b. Preanesthetic CNS depressants will also prolong the effects of ketamine.

    c. It has been used in combination with the phenothiazine tranquilizers, the narcotic analgesics, xylazine, and diazepam (see Table 3–5).

    d. Significant respiratory depression may occur when these drugs are used in combination with ketamine.

    e. An anticholinergic agent should be used to decrease the salivation caused by ketamine.

    f. An eye ointment should be used to prevent corneal drying.

12. Clinical uses

    a. Ketamine has been used both intramuscularly and intravenously in the dog and cat as an induction agent prior to the use of an inhalation anesthetic.

       (1) Even though laryngeal reflexes are not depressed, intubation can usually be accomplished following its use.

       (2) Ketamine is compatible with all the commonly used inhalant anesthetics.

    b. Intramuscular doses of ketamine, in combination with a preanesthetic CNS depressant, may be used for short surgical and anesthetic procedures lasting from 10–40 minutes.

       (1) If additional anesthesia is needed, one half of the original dose of ketamine may be given, or the ketamine can be supplemented with inhalant anesthetic agents.

       (2) The original intramuscular dose plus supplemental doses should probably not exceed 20 mg/lb (44 mg/kg).

    c. Intravenous doses of ketamine may be used for surgical or diagnostic procedures lasting less than 10 minutes.

      d. Low intramuscular doses of ketamine can be used for chemical restraint.

  13. Precautions, adverse effects, and contraindications

      a. Ketamine may cause convulsions in some patients. Convulsions are more likely to occur in dogs.

        (1) The seizures may result from dopamine release.

        (2) For this reason, ketamine is contraindicated in epileptics.

        (3) Concurrent use of benzodiazepine or phenothiazine tranquilizers can be used to prevent seizures.

      b. Myoclonic jerking of the extremities may occur.

      c. Some patients fail to reach surgical levels of anesthesia with recommended doses.

      d. Prolonged recovery times of 12–24 hours have been reported in both the dog and cat, especially with large intramuscular doses.

      e. It is contraindicated in cats with primary renal dysfunction and in dogs with hepatic dysfunction.

      f. Hypothermia or hyperthermia may occur.

      g. Significant respiratory depression may occur, especially when ketamine is combined with CNS depressants.

      h. It may not prevent visceral pain, so it should be combined with analgesics or inhalant anesthetic agents for abdominal or thoracic surgery.

      i. It is contraindicated in patients with head trauma because it may cause an increase in CSF pressure.

      j. It will cause pain at the intramuscular injection site because of its low pH.

      k. Personality changes have been reported in patients lasting from several hours to several weeks.

      l. It should be used with extreme caution in patients with myocardial disease because it increases the heart rate and the oxygen consumption and demands of the myocardium.

      m. Emergence delirium consisting of vocalization, uncoordination, agitation, or "pawing" at the mouth may occur. The administration of a tranquilizer may help decrease the severity of the emergence delirium.

  E. Tiletamine (Telazol)

    1. At present, the dissociative agent tiletamine is available only as Telazol (CI-744) (see Tables 3–3 and 3–4).

    2. Telazol is a combination of equal parts by weight of tiletamine and zolazepam (a benzodiazepine tranquilizer).

      a. It is supplied as a lyophilized powder in sterile vials containing 500 mg of active drug (250 mg of tiletamine and 250 mg of zolazepam).

      b. It is reconstituted with 5 ml of sterile diluent to produce 100 mg/ml of active drug.

      c. After reconstitution, its shelf life is 4–5 days at room temperature and 14–21 days when refrigerated.

    3. Telazol is a Class III controlled substance.

    4. Telazol has been approved for use in the dog and cat.

    5. Central nervous effects

      a. The CNS effects of Telazol are very similar to those of ketamine.

b. Tiletamine is more potent than ketamine.

6. Cardiovascular effects

  a. The cardiovascular effects of Telazol vary markedly among species and are similar to those of ketamine.

  b. In the dog and cat, it produces cardiovascular stimulation much like ketamine.

  c. It increases the heart rate, most likely because of direct CNS stimulation. It causes increased sympathetic tone and a possible decrease in vagal tone.

  d. Arterial blood pressure may initially decrease but then returns to normal or above normal.

  e. The increase in blood pressure is caused by direct CNS stimulation and increased sympathetic tone, prevention of the uptake of catecholamines, and inhibition of vagal baroreceptor reflex activity.

7. Respiratory effects

  a. The respiratory effects of Telazol are similar to those of ketamine.

  b. High doses may produce apneustic ventilation, apnea, a decreased tidal volume, a decreased respiratory rate, and a decreased minute ventilation.

  c. Low doses seem to have only minimal respiratory depressant effects.

  d. When other CNS depressants (tranquilizers, alpha-2 agonists, opioids, injectable anesthetics, inhalant anesthetics) are used in combination with Telazol, *significant* respiratory depression may occur. The respiratory depression may be observed even when low doses of Telazol are used.

8. Other physiologic effects

  a. Other physiologic effects of Telazol are similar to those of ketamine.

  b. It can cause excess salivation that can be controlled with anticholinergics.

9. Metabolism and elimination

  a. In the dog, both tiletamine and zolazepam undergo extensive biodegradation in the liver.

  b. In the dog, the plasma half-life of zolazepam is 1 hour and of tiletamine is 1.2 hours. Therefore, the effects of tiletamine may last longer than the effects of zolazepam, and one may see the characteristic emergence delirium associated with dissociative anesthesia recoveries. Premedication with opioids, tranquilizers, or alpha-2 agonists will smooth recovery.

  c. In the cat, both tiletamine and zolazepam are excreted virtually intact by the kidneys.

  d. In the cat, the plasma half-life of zolazepam is 4.5 hours and of tiletamine is 2.5 hours.

  e. Recovery for cats is longer than for dogs because of the longer plasma half-life of zolazepam and tiletamine.

10. Dose, route of administration, and duration of effect

  a. Telazol is approved for use in both the dog and the cat. It has also been used in a wide variety of domestic, exotic, and wild species.

  b. Onset of surgical anesthesia occurs within 5–8 minutes following

intramuscular injection and within 30–60 seconds following intravenous injection.

   c. The intramuscular dose range in the dog is 3–6 mg/lb (6.6–13.2 mg/kg) and in the cat is 4–7 mg/lb (8.8–15.4 mg/kg).

   d. The duration of anesthesia from an intramuscular dose is 20–40 minutes.

      (1) Supplemental doses may be given, but any supplemental dose should not exceed more than half of the initial dose, and the total dose given (initial dose plus supplemental doses) should not exceed 10 mg/lb (22 mg/kg) in the dog and 25 mg/lb (55 mg/kg) in the cat.

      (2) Supplemental doses may *greatly prolong* recovery times.

   e. An intravenous dose of 1–2 mg/lb (2.2–4.4 mg/kg) will produce surgical anesthesia in 30–60 seconds and will have a duration of effect of 10–15 minutes.

   f. The use of preanesthetic medications such as tranquilizers, alpha-2 agonists, and opioids will enhance and extend the effects of Telazol.

   g. Telazol is compatible with the commonly used inhalant anesthetics.

11. Clinical uses

   a. Intravenous Telazol has been used to induce anesthesia in the dog and cat prior to inhalant anesthesia and as the sole anesthetic for short (10–15 minutes) procedures.

   b. In the dog, intramuscular Telazol is recommended as an anesthetic for diagnostic examinations, restraint, treatment of lacerations and wounds, castrations, and any procedure requiring mild to moderate analgesia.

      (1) Telazol is *not* recommended as the sole agent for use in the dog for procedures requiring major analgesia (such as abdominal or thoracic procedures). The intramuscular doses required can produce marked respiratory depressions.

      (2) Supplemental doses may be given to prolong anesthesia, but any supplemental dose should not exceed more than half of the previous dose.

      (3) The total dose given (initial dose plus supplemental doses) should not exceed 10 mg/lb (22 mg/kg) in the dog.

   c. In the cat, intramuscular Telazol is recommended as an anesthetic for procedures ranging from diagnostic examinations and restraint to declawing and ovariohysterectomies.

      (1) As with the dog, supplemental doses may be given to the cat, but any supplemental dose should not exceed more than half of the previous dose.

      (2) The total dose given (initial dose plus supplemental doses) should not exceed 25 mg/lb (55 mg/kg) in the cat.

   d. Telazol has a wider margin of safety in cats than in dogs.

   e. Repeated doses of Telazol increase the duration of effect of the drug but may not further diminish muscle tone.

      (1) Recovery times may be *greatly* prolonged with repeated or multiple doses of Telazol.

      (2) The quality of anesthesia varies with repeated doses because the ratio between tiletamine and zolazepam within the patient

changes with each injection. These changes are due to the different plasma half-life of each drug.

(3) The practice of giving repeated doses of Telazol to prolong anesthesia should be avoided if possible.

  f. An intramuscular injection of 1–2 mg/lb (2.2–4.4 mg/kg) of Telazol, combined with 0.2 mg/lb (0.44 mg/kg) of butorphanol in the same syringe can be used to sedate fractious, mean, or vicious dogs or cats.

(1) This combination will usually produce lateral recumbency in 5–7 minutes.

(2) Anesthesia induction can then be accomplished by mask with an inhalant agent or by using an injectable agent intravenously.

(3) Ventilation must be closely watched, even with this low dose, as some patients will have respiratory depression when injectable or inhalant general anesthetics are added to the Telazol-butorphanol combination.

  12. Precautions, adverse effects, and contraindications

    a. Precautions, adverse effects, and contraindications for Telazol are similar to those for ketamine and ketamine combinations.

    b. It can markedly depress ventilation, especially when high intramuscular or intravenous doses are used or when it is used in combination with other CNS depressants.

    c. Its duration of action can vary widely among individuals and among species.

    d. Hypothermia may occur as a result of muscle relaxation.

    e. Tachycardia may occur.

    f. Repeated doses may greatly prolong recovery time.

    g. Its margin of safety appears to be greater in cats than in dogs.

III. Propofol (Diprivan, Rapinovet)

  A. Physical properties

    1. Propofol (2,6-diisopropylphenol) is a phenolic compound unrelated to any other general anesthetic

    2. It is only slightly water-soluble and is available as an emulsion containing 10 mg propofol, 100 mg of soybean oil, 22.5 mg of glycerol, and 12 mg of egg lecithin per ml.

    3. Propofol emulsion comes in sterile glass ampules and contains no preservatives.

      a. The emulsion will support bacterial growth and endotoxin production.

      b. Once the ampule is opened, the propofol emulsion should be used or discarded within 8 hours. It should not be kept overnight for use the next day.

  B. Metabolism and elimination

    1. A single bolus dose of propofol provides approximately 10 minutes of anesthesia time, with complete recovery occurring in dogs and cats within 20–30 minutes.

    2. The rapid onset of propofol is caused by rapid CNS uptake.

    3. Its short duration of action and associated rapid recovery time are due to rapid redistribution from the brain to other tissues and organs in much the same way as occurs with thiopental.

    4. In addition, propofol is rapidly metabolized.

        a. It is metabolized primarily by conjugation, with the liver playing a major role.

        b. Its plasma clearance exceeds hepatic blood flow, suggesting that other organs, e.g., the lung and kidney, are also involved in metabolism.

        c. After 30 minutes, less than 20% of the dose can be recovered as unchanged compound.

    5. Metabolites are nonreactive and are excreted by the kidneys.

C. Physiologic properties

    1. Propofol causes CNS depression by decreasing the brain's metabolic activity and by enhancing the effects of the neurotransmitter GABA.

    2. It can produce respiratory depression and apnea in much the same way as thiopental.

    3. Its cardiovascular effects are similar to those of thiopental.

        a. It will cause a transient decrease in arterial blood pressure and myocardial contractility.

        b. It can cause hypotension primarily resulting from arterial and venous vasodilation.

        c. It is not inherently arrhythmogenic, although it will enhance the arrhythmogenicity of catecholamines.

    4. Heinz body formation has been reported in cats following repeated administration of propofol over several days.

        a. Propofol can cause oxidative injury to feline red blood cells because of the cat's decreased ability to conjugate phenol.

        b. Clinical signs of diarrhea, anorexia, and malaise have been observed following experimentally administered daily doses of propofol repeated over several days.

    5. Its pharmacokinetics (see Table 3–3) in patients with renal and hepatic dysfunction is similar to that in nondiseased patients, suggesting that it would be suitable for patients with renal or hepatic impairment.

    6. It has been safely used in sighthound dog breeds.

D. Clinical uses

    1. Propofol has been approved for use only in the dog at this time.

    2. It can be given as a single bolus for short surgical procedures and for induction of general anesthesia to allow intubation and the use of inhalant anesthesia (see Table 3–4).

        a. The dose for induction of anesthesia in unpremedicated dogs and cats is 3–4 mg/lb (6.6–8.8 mg/kg) given to effect.

        b. The dose for induction of anesthesia in dogs and cats premedicated with tranquilizers, sedatives, or opioids is 1–2 mg/lb (2.2–4.4 mg/kg).

        c. The calculated dose of propofol is given slowly over approximately 60–90 seconds to effect until the desired level of anesthesia is reached. Approximately one third of the dose is given every 30 seconds.

        d. Apnea of short duration may occur following propofol induction. The incidence and duration of apnea may be decreased by giving the dose of propofol over 60–90 seconds (slower than thiopental would be given).

    3. Propofol can be used for maintenance of anesthesia by giving a continuous infusion or by giving intermittent boluses.

   a. The amount of propofol needed for maintenance of general anesthesia will depend on the preanesthetic medications administered
and the type of surgery being done.

   b. The continuous infusion rate is 0.1–0.2 mg/lb per minute (0.22–
0.44 mg/kg per minute) given to effect.

   c. If the intermittent bolus technique is used, the dose is administered
when needed to effect. The dose may range from 0.2 mg/lb to 1
mg/lb (0.44–2.2 mg/kg). It should be given over 30–60 seconds to
decrease the incidence of respiratory depression and apnea.

   d. Recovery from the propofol usually occurs within 20–30 minutes
following the last bolus dose or discontinuation of the infusion.

   e. It seems ideally suited for use as a continuous infusion for anesthesia maintenance.

     (1) Recovery is rapid, with minimal to no "drug hangover."

     (2) No problem of drug buildup appears to exist with repeated
doses of propofol, in contrast to barbiturates or dissociative
agents.

   f. Pulmonary and cardiovascular function need to be closely monitored because of propofol's ability to depress ventilation and decrease blood pressure.

   g. Cats have a decreased ability to conjugate phenols. Therefore,
although the reported recovery times after single or repeated doses
of propofol are similar in dogs and cats, continuous infusion may
produce more prolonged recoveries in cats.

4. Pain has been reported in human patients during propofol injection.
The incidence seems much lower in animals.

5. Myoclonic twitching, muscle tremors, and muscle movement have
been reported in humans and dogs during induction and maintenance
of propofol anesthesia.

   a. This muscle reaction may be due to the carrier agents used for
propofol.

   b. The use of preanesthetic tranquilizers, sedatives, or opioids seems
to decrease the incidence of myoclonic twitching, muscle tremors,
and muscle movement.

6. Propofol does not cause tissue damage when accidentally injected
perivascularly.

7. Advantages

   a. Propofol is ideally suited for short anesthetic procedures, especially
when the patient is premedicated with a tranquilizer, sedative,
or opioid.

   b. It is associated with rapid inductions and rapid and smooth recoveries.

   c. Repeated doses or continuous infusions can be given because there
is minimal to no "drug hangover," even with repeated doses.

   d. Neither hepatic nor renal dysfunction seem to prolong propofol's
duration of effect or the recovery period associated with it.

   e. It might be useful for anesthetic inductions for cesarean sections
because puppies have good conjugation enzyme activity, and there
appears to be less fetal depression in neonates delivered from
bitches anesthetized with propofol.

8. Disadvantages

   a. Propofol can produce hypotension and can be a potent respiratory depressant. Cardiopulmonary depression is dose-dependent. Respiratory depression depends on both dose and rate of administration.

    b. It has a limited shelf life once the ampule is opened.

    c. A risk of iatrogenic sepsis exists.

    d. At the present time, it is costly.

    e. It may produce pain on injection and myoclonic twitching and muscle movements. The incidence can be decreased by using preanesthetic tranquilizers, sedatives, or hypnotics.

IV. Etomidate (Amidate)

  A. Physical properties

    1. Etomidate is a carboxylated imidazole derivative first used as an induction agent in human anesthesia in 1975 (see Tables 3–3 and 3–4).

    2. It is structurally unrelated to any other anesthetic.

    3. It is a congener of metomidate and is not water-soluble.

    4. Etomidate comes as a concentration of 2 mg/ml dissolved in 35% propylene glycol.

    5. It should be refrigerated and should not be frozen or exposed to extreme heat.

  B. Physiologic effects

    1. Etomidate is a sedative-hypnotic agent that has a rapid onset of action and is associated with a rapid recovery.

    2. It is a weak base dissolved in propylene glycol; therefore, intravenous infusion can be associated with pain and venous irritation.

    3. At clinically used doses, it does not depress cardiopulmonary function.

       a. It does not produce a change in heart rate, blood pressure, or myocardial contractility.

       b. Cardiovascular stability may be better with etomidate because it maintains baroreceptor-mediated responses.

       c. It does not cause histamine release.

       d. It can produce a mild to moderate dose-dependent respiratory depression.

    4. It has been demonstrated to temporarily inhibit adrenal steroidogenesis in humans and dogs, but whether this inhibition is significant to the patient is a point of controversy. A single dose may depress adrenal function for up to 3 hours.

    5. Retching, myoclonus, and apnea have been reported in humans and dogs during induction.

    6. Etomidate injection can produce acute hemolysis. This is most likely due to the propylene glycol, which causes a rapid increase in osmolality and subsequent red blood cell rupture.

    7. It depresses the reticular system of the brain stem and will decrease CNS oxygen consumption.

    8. Neonates born to mothers anesthetized with etomidate have minimal respiratory depression.

  C. Metabolism and elimination

    1. A single dose of etomidate will produce 10–20 minutes of anesthesia depending on the dose administered.

    2. Recovery is rapid.

    3. Etomidate undergoes rapid hepatic hydrolysis to inactive metabolites.

This rapid hydrolysis results in rapid recovery for the patient and lack of accumulation of the drug when used in repeated boluses or as an infusion.

    4. The metabolites are excreted via the urine.

D. Clinical uses

    1. The induction dose of etomidate is 0.7–1.5 mg/lb (1.5–3.0 mg/kg) intravenously.

      a. The dose is given to effect intravenously and will depend on the preanesthetic medications administered to the patient and the physical status of the patient.

      b. Etomidate produces a rapid loss of consciousness.

    2. Etomidate is primarily used as an induction agent in human patients.

    3. Venous pain and myoclonus can occur during injection; however, use of preanesthetic tranquilizers, sedatives, or opioids will help decrease the incidence.

    4. Nausea and vomiting have been reported in human patients during induction and recovery.

      a. Nausea and vomiting are more likely to occur following multiple doses.

      b. Preanesthetic sedation can help prevent nausea and vomiting.

    5. Etomidate's minimal cardiopulmonary depressant effects and its rapid metabolism and recovery make it seem ideally suited as an induction agent for high-risk patients.

      a. In human patients, it has been used as an induction agent in patients suffering trauma, cardiovascular instability and myocardial disease, and liver disease, and in patients undergoing cesarean section.

      b. The high cost of etomidate may limit its use in veterinary anesthesia at the present time.

Section 2: Inhalant General Anesthetics

I. Factors influencing absorption and elimination of inhalant anesthetics

  A. Inspired anesthetic concentration

    1. The greater the inhaled concentration, the greater the alveolar anesthetic tension, and therefore the pressure gradient, will be. Consequently, the greater the inhaled concentration, the more rapidly the inhalant anesthetic will diffuse across the alveoli.

    2. Rate of diffusion is directly proportional to the pressure differences at the oral cavity and the alveoli (Fick's law).

    3. Rate of diffusion is inversely proportional to molecular size (Graham's law).

    4. The upper limit of the inspired concentration of an inhalant agent is determined by the vapor pressure of that agent, which in turn depends on temperature.

    5. The patient delivery circuit of the anesthetic machine is a major factor in determining the inspired anesthetic concentration. Characteristics of the breathing circuit that are important follow:

      a. Volume of the system

      b. Amount of rubber or plastic components of the system

      c. Amount of fresh gas inflow into the circuit

      d. Vaporizer position relative to the circuit (in circuit versus out of circuit)

B. Minute ventilation

   1. Minute ventilation directly affects movement of anesthetic vapor into the alveoli.

   2. Increased rate and depth of ventilation will aid in moving more anesthetic vapor to the alveoli.

C. Alveolar partial pressures or anesthetic tension

   1. Inhalation of volatile anesthetics does not alter the carbon dioxide and water tension in the alveoli, but the volatile anesthetics will displace nitrogen and oxygen in the alveoli.

   2. The alveolar tension of an anesthetic gas will vary with the following:

      a. Uptake of gas by blood and tissue

      b. Warming effect of cool gases within the alveoli

      c. Presence of other gases or vapors

   3. Factors causing an increased alveolar delivery

      a. Increased inspired anesthetic concentration

         (1) Increased vaporization of the inhalant agent

         (2) Increased vaporizer dial setting

         (3) Increased fresh gas flow

         (4) Decreased gas volume of patient's breathing circuit

      b. Increased alveolar ventilation

         (1) Increased minute ventilation

         (2) Decreased dead space (mechanical and physiologic)

   4. Factors causing a decreased removal from the alveoli

      a. Decreased blood solubility of anesthetic

      b. Decreased cardiac output

      c. Decreased alveolar-venous anesthetic gradient

D. Diffusion surface and diffusion velocity

   1. Diffusion of an anesthetic gas into the blood is directly proportional to the size of the alveolar surface exposed to the gas.

   2. Diffusion is indirectly proportional to the thickness of the alveolar membrane.

   3. Diffusion through the alveolar membrane is a physical process and is determined by the following:

      a. Solubility coefficient of the gases

      b. Molecular weight of the gases

      c. Pressure gradient from the alveolus and plasma

E. Partition coefficient

   1. The partition coefficient is the ratio between the number of molecules of an anesthetic gas existing in two phases. It indicates the solubility of an anesthetic gas in a particular tissue or in blood.

   2. An inhalant anesthetic with a low numeric partition coefficient will quickly saturate the blood and tissues; thus the induction and recovery times will be rapid.

   3. An inhalant anesthetic with a high numeric partition coefficient will

be slow to saturate blood and tissues; thus the induction and recovery times will be slow.

F. Pulmonary blood flow

1. The amount of blood flowing through the lungs will help determine the amount of anesthetic gas uptake from the alveoli.

2. The more blood exposed to the anesthetic gas, the more molecules will move into the blood.

G. Tissue absorption

1. The amount of anesthetic gas passing into the tissues depends on the following:

a. The degree of perfusion of the tissue

b. The solubility of the anesthetic gas (solubility coefficient) in the tissue

2. Highly perfused tissues receive and absorb the majority of the anesthetic gas taken up from the alveoli.

a. Approximately 75% of the cardiac output perfuses the brain, heart, lungs, liver, kidneys, intestine, and endocrine glands (6–10% of the body mass). These tissues are the first to reach equilibrium during uptake of an anesthetic gas and the first to desaturate.

b. Approximately 20% of the cardiac output perfuses the muscles and skin (50% of the body mass). These tissues are the next to reach equilibrium.

c. Approximately 5% of the cardiac output perfuses the adipose tissue (20% of the body mass). Adipose tissue is slow to reach equilibrium.

H. Lipid content of tissues

1. Lipid-rich cells take up more of an anesthetic gas than do lipid-poor cells.

2. The brain is very lipid-rich.

3. If a lipid-rich cell and a lipid-poor cell are equally perfused, the anesthetic gas will reach equilibrium in the lipid-rich cell first.

I. Perfusion of the brain

1. Anesthetic uptake by the brain is directly proportional to the amount of perfusion of the brain cells.

2. Anesthetic uptake of the brain depends on the following:

a. Cerebral blood flow

b. Blood-brain barrier (all anesthetics rapidly pass this barrier because of their lipophilic characteristics)

c. Lipid content of the brain

II. Methoxyflurane (Metofane, Penthrane)

A. Methoxyflurane was synthesized in 1958 and first used clinically in human anesthesia in 1959.

B. Physical properties (refer to Table 3–6).

1. Methoxyflurane is a methyl-ethyl-ether that is nonflammable and nonexplosive at commonly used anesthetic concentrations.

2. It is very soluble in blood, body tissues, and conductive rubber components of the anesthetic circuit (Table 3–7).

a. This solubility accounts for its slow induction time (10–15 minutes) and the associated slow recovery time (30 minutes to several hours, depending on the length of anesthesia).

b. Because it is very soluble in blood, the blood will absorb many

Table 3-6. Physical Properties of Currently Used Inhalation Anesthetics

Property	Sevoflurane	Desflurane	Isoflurane	Halothane	Methoxyflurane	Nitrous Oxide
Formula	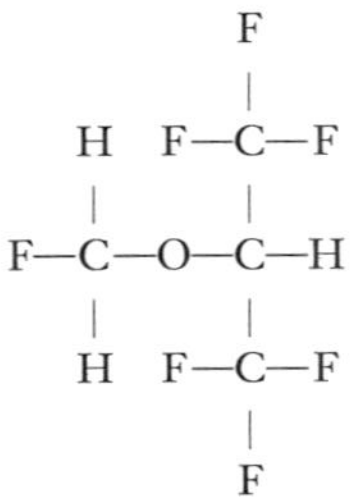 (see structure below)	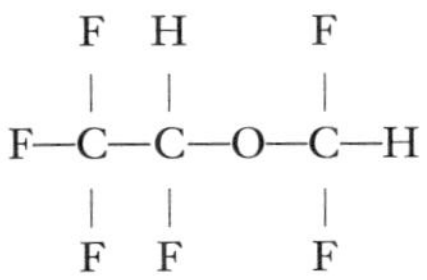 (see structure below)	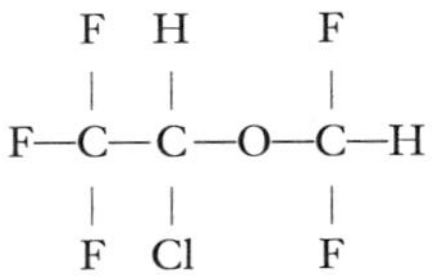 (see structure below)	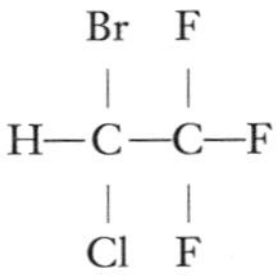 (see structure below)	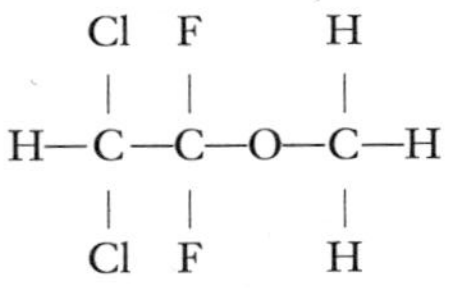 (see structure below)	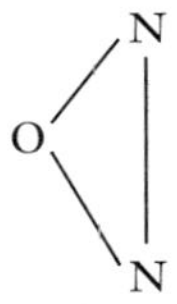 (see structure below)
Molecular weight	200	168	184.5	197.4	165.3	44
Specific gravity (20°C)	1.52	1.47	1.49	1.86	1.41	—
Boiling point (°C)	59	23.5	48.5	50.2	104.7	—
Vapor pressure at 20°C (mm Hg)	160	664	239.5	244.1	22.8	—
mL Vapor/mL liquid at 20°C	182.7	209.7	194.7	227	207	—
Preservative	None	None	None	0.01% thymol	0.01% butyl hydroxytoluene	None
Stability Soda lime	No?	Stable	Stable	Decomposes	Decomposes	Stable
UV light	—	—	Stable	Decomposes	Decomposes	—

Structural formulas:

Sevoflurane:
```
            F
            |
    H   F-C-F
    |       |
F-C-O-C-H
    |       |
    H   F-C-F
            |
            F
```

Desflurane:
```
 F  H   F
 |  |   |
F-C-C-O-C-H
 |  |   |
 F  F   F
```

Isoflurane:
```
 F  H   F
 |  |   |
F-C-C-O-C-H
 |  |   |
 F  Cl  F
```

Halothane:
```
 Br F
 |  |
H-C-C-F
 |  |
 Cl F
```

Methoxyflurane:
```
 Cl F   H
 |  |   |
H-C-C-O-C-H
 |  |   |
 Cl F   H
```

Nitrous Oxide:
```
 N       N
  \     /
     O
```

Table 3–7. Solvent/Gas Partition Coefficients at 37°C

Solvent	Nitrous Oxide	Desflurane	Sevoflurane	Isoflurane	Halothane	Methoxyflurane
Blood	0.47	0.42	0.68	1.46	2.54	15.00
Brain	0.50	1.30	1.70	1.60	1.90	20.00
Liver	0.38	1.30	1.80	1.80	2.10	29.00
Kidney	0.40	1.00	1.20	1.20	1.00	11.00
Muscle	0.54	2.00	3.10	2.90	3.40	16.00
Fat	1.08	27.00	48.00	45.00	51.00	902.00
Conductive rubber*	1.2	—	—	62	120	630

*Rubber/gas partition coefficient at room temperature.
Note: Tissue samples derived from human sources.

molecules of methoxyflurane before they start to saturate the body tissues, hence the slow induction.

   c. When it is discontinued, the opposite effect occurs: recovery is slow because the methoxyflurane is so soluble in body tissues that it takes a longer period of time for it to diffuse back into the blood and from the blood back into the alveoli.

   d. It is very soluble in the rubber components of the anesthetic delivery circuit. Therefore, induction and recovery times can be prolonged because of uptake and release of methoxyflurane from the rubber.

   e. Because of its solubility characteristics, the depth of anesthesia cannot be changed rapidly.

3. The minimum alveolar concentration (MAC) for methoxyflurane is 0.23% in the dog and 0.27% in the cat (Table 3–8).

   a. The lower the MAC value is, the lower the anesthetic concentration needed to maintain anesthesia, and thus the more potent the inhalant anesthetic.

   b. Methoxyflurane is the most potent of the modern inhalant anesthetic agents.

4. Methoxyflurane reactivity

   a. It decomposes when exposed to soda lime or to ultraviolet light.

   b. Butylated hydroxytoluene is added to the methoxyflurane as a preservative to prevent acid formation.

Table 3–8. Minimum Alveolar Concentration (MAC) Values of Modern Inhalant Anesthetics

Anesthetic Gas	MAC (%)*		
	Dog	Cat	Human
Methoxyflurane	0.21	0.2–0.3	0.16
Halothane	0.9	0.8–1.2	0.7–0.8
Isoflurane	1.3–1.4	1.68	1.27
Sevoflurane	2.1–2.4	2.6	1.7–2.0
Desflurane	7.2	9.8	6.0–7.2
Nitrous oxide	188–297	250	104

*MAC is the concentration that will render 50% of patients unresponsive to a painful stimulus. MAC is the ED_{50} of the inhalant anesthetics. The anesthetic concentration that corresponds to the ED_{95} (95% of the individuals are anesthetized) is 1.2–1.4 MAC. Two times MAC (2.0 MAC) usually represents a deep plane of anesthesia.

      c. Methoxyflurane changes from a clear color to a yellowish amber color in the vaporizer; however, this color change does not affect its potency.

      d. It is highly reactive with most metals.

C. Vaporization and administration

   1. The vapor pressure of methoxyflurane at 20°C is 22.8 mm Hg.

   2. The lower the vapor pressure of a liquid, the harder it is to vaporize; therefore, methoxyflurane is difficult to vaporize.

   3. At room temperature, the maximum amount of anesthetic vapor that can be produced by methoxyflurane is approximately 3%.

   4. The low vaporization pressure allows methoxyflurane to be used in either nonprecision in-circuit vaporizers (Ohio Heidbrink #8 vaporizer) or precision out-of-circuit vaporizers (Pentec, Pentomatic, the Vapor Penthrane vaporizer, Copper Kettle, etc.).

   5. Induction is usually achieved with 1.5–2.5%. Once induction has been achieved, a patient can usually be maintained at 0.5–1.25% for surgical procedures.

D. CNS effects

   1. Methoxyflurane is a general CNS depressant.

   2. It produces very good analgesia, even at subanesthetic doses. This may partially account for the prolonged recovery times associated with it; the patient is not stimulated by postoperative pain.

   3. The classic signs of determining anesthetic depth are not of value with methoxyflurane.

      a. The pedal and palpebral reflexes are lost early in the dog and cat under methoxyflurane.

      b. The eye tends to centrally fix early under low concentrations.

      c. The pupils do not dilate until anesthesia is very deep.

      d. One should closely monitor the cardiopulmonary parameters during methoxyflurane anesthesia and depend less on monitoring the classic signs of Guedal.

E. Cardiovascular effects

   1. As with all inhalant anesthetics, severe cardiovascular depression can occur when excessive doses of methoxyflurane are administered.

   2. It decreases myocardial contractility.

      a. Of the modern inhalant agents, it is the third most potent in its ability to depress contractility.

      b. The cardiodepressant effects of methoxyflurane—and the other inhalant agents—may be due to alterations in calcium-accumulating abilities of microsomal and mitochondrial membranes.

   3. Cardiac output may be reduced as much as 25–40% during methoxyflurane anesthesia.

   4. Both heart rate and stroke volume decrease as more methoxyflurane is administered.

   5. Spontaneous cardiac dysrhythmias are not common during methoxyflurane anesthesia.

      a. Methoxyflurane sensitizes the myocardium to catecholamines but to a much lesser degree than does halothane.

      b. Exogenous use of epinephrine and norephinephrine seems to be well tolerated in patients receiving methoxyflurane.

   6. Arterial blood pressure decreases during methoxyflurane anesthesia.

  a. The degree of hypotension is dose-related and is due primarily to a decreased cardiac output.

  b. At normal anesthetic concentrations, peripheral vascular resistance is usually maintained; therefore, large falls in arterial blood pressure may not be observed even though cardiac output decreases.

  c. As methoxyflurane overdose occurs, significant falls in blood pressure may occur because of a decrease in the peripheral resistance as well as a decrease in cardiac output.

F. Respiratory effects

  1. Methoxyflurane is a respiratory depressant.

     a. It depresses both respiratory rate and tidal volume.

     b. The amount of respiratory depression is dose-dependent.

     c. Increasing concentrations of methoxyflurane will eventually lead to respiratory arrest.

  2. It is nonirritating to the respiratory tract and does not increase salivary or respiratory secretions.

G. Hepatic effects

  1. Methoxyflurane does not appear to be directly hepatotoxic to animals, although isolated cases of hepatic toxicity have been reported in humans and dogs.

  2. It appears to depress hepatic function, but this effect is transitory.

H. Renal effects

  1. Methoxyflurane may alter renal function because of decreased renal blood flow and vasoconstriction.

  2. It has been shown to produce direct renal toxicity in human patients.

     a. The toxicity is related to the metabolic by-products of methoxyflurane, not the methoxyflurane molecule itself.

     b. The toxicity is characterized by proximal renal tubule necrosis with a high renal output, hypernatremia, elevated BUN, and dehydration.

     c. The most likely cause is the inorganic fluoride ion and oxalic acid released during methoxyflurane metabolism.

     d. The degree of toxicity is directly related to the concentration of methoxyflurane delivered, the length of anesthesia, and the obesity of the patient.

  3. Urine fluoride and serum fluoride increase in the dog during and after methoxyflurane anesthesia; however, nephrotoxicity is very rare if it occurs at all.

I. Other physiologic effects

  1. Methoxyflurane produces good skeletal-muscle relaxation.

  2. It readily crosses the placenta.

  3. It decreases smooth-muscle tone, motility, and peristalsis in the gastrointestinal tract.

J. Excretion and metabolism

  1. The majority of the methoxyflurane is exhaled from the lungs unchanged following anesthesia.

  2. As much as 50% of the inspired concentration can be metabolized by the liver.

     a. Longer procedures allow more time for metabolism and fat saturation.

       b. A patient with a high percentage of body fat will absorb more methoxyflurane.

       c. High levels of methoxyflurane are found in fat up to 30 hours following its administration.

       d. The methoxyflurane is slowly released from the fat, allowing more time for hepatic metabolism to occur.

    3. The metabolites of methoxyflurane consist of carbon dioxide, inorganic fluoride ion, dichloroacetic acid, and oxalic acid. They are excreted in the urine.

  K. Contraindications and precautions

    1. No specific contraindications exist to the use of methoxyflurane.

    2. It should be used with caution in the presence of renal or hepatic dysfunction.

III. Halothane (Fluothane, Halocarbon)

  A. Halothane was synthesized in 1951 and first used clinically in human patients in 1956.

  B. Physical properties (see Table 3–6)

    1. Halothane is a halogenated hydrocarbon that is nonflammable and nonexplosive at commonly used anesthetic concentrations.

    2. Halothane is much less soluble in blood, body tissues, and conductive rubber components of the anesthetic circuit than is methoxyflurane (see Table 3–7).

       a. This lesser solubility accounts for its rapid induction time (3–5 minutes) and the associated rapid recovery time (5–20 minutes).

       b. Since halothane is less soluble in blood than methoxyflurane, fewer molecules are absorbed into the blood before they are released into the tissues.

       c. Halothane is less soluble in the body tissues, including the brain, and it therefore diffuses from the body more quickly when it is discontinued.

       d. Because of halothane's solubility characteristics, the depth of anesthesia can be changed fairly rapidly.

    3. The MAC for halothane in the dog and cat is 0.87% and 0.82%, respectively (see Table 3–8).

    4. Halothane reactivity

       a. Halothane decomposes when exposed to ultraviolet light; therefore, 0.01% thymol is added to it as an antioxidant.

       b. The thymol is preferentially oxidized by ultraviolet light, thus preserving the halothane.

       c. Halothane will decompose when exposed to soda lime, but no toxins are formed.

       d. It is highly reactive with metal.

  C. Vaporization and administration

    1. The vapor pressure of halothane at 20°C is 244.1 mm Hg.

    2. This high vapor pressure means that halothane is very easy to vaporize.

    3. At 20°C the maximum amount of halothane vapor that can be produced is approximately 32%.

    4. Its high vapor pressure prevents halothane from being safely used in nonprecision in-circuit vaporizers.

    5. Only out-of-circuit precision vaporizers (Fluotec, Fluomatic, the Va-

por Fluothane Vaporizer, Copper Kettle, Vernitrol, etc.) should be used to administer halothane.

   a. With the exception of the Copper Kettle and Vernitrol, these vaporizers are designed to deliver a maximum concentration of 5% halothane to the patient.

   b. The maximum concentration is only 5% because this volatile anesthetic is very potent, and concentrations in the patient can be quickly changed. Therefore, anesthetic overdose may occur when concentrations in excess of 2–2.5% are maintained for extended periods of time.

6. Generally mask induction with halothane can be achieved with a concentration of 3.5–5%. Once induction of anesthesia has been accomplished, the patient can usually be maintained at 1–1.5% of halothane.

   a. As with all inhalant anesthetics, ultimate induction and maintenance concentrations are given to effect with halothane and will depend on the physical status of the patient and the type and dose of other CNS depressant drugs administered.

   b. Remember, because of halothane's solubility characteristics, one can rapidly increase or decrease the depth of anesthesia.

D. CNS effects

1. Halothane is a general CNS depressant.

2. It does not provide analgesia during recovery the way methoxyflurane does. In fact, halothane has an almost antianalgesic effect during recovery, and emergence delirium may occur in the presence of pain.

3. The vomiting center, cough center, respiratory center, vasomotor center, temperature-regulating center, and reticular activating system are all depressed by halothane.

4. Recovery from halothane is generally rapid, with little or no depression of the sensorium evident soon after recovery.

E. Cardiovascular effects

1. Halothane produces cardiovascular depression directly related to the administered concentration. A sustained concentration of 2% can produce marked cardiovascular depression.

2. It is a direct myocardial depressant, decreasing myocardial contractility.

   a. It affects myocardial contractility by decreasing the binding and availability of calcium at superficial membrane sites in myocardial cells.

   b. It may also affect intracellular calcium inotropic processes.

3. Cardiac output and heart rate are also decreased in a dose-dependent manner.

4. It may produce severe arterial hypotension.

   a. The hypotension is dose-dependent.

   b. The hypotension occurs because of direct myocardial depression, decreased peripheral resistance, and direct depression of the vasomotor center.

5. Spontaneous cardiac dysrhythmias are more common with halothane than with methoxyflurane.

   a. Halothane sensitizes the myocardium to catecholamines.

   b. This sensitization seems to be most pronounced during the first 30 minutes of halothane anesthesia.

    c. Because of this sensitization, exogenous catecholamines should be used with caution during halothane anesthesia.

    d. Halothane slows the conduction of impulses through the His-Purkinje system, which tends to facilitate the reentry of impulses and thus leads to dysrhythmias.

6. It increases the baroreceptor discharge at any given arterial pressure.

7. It decreases or prevents digitalis-induced cardiac dysrhythmias.

8. Like most inhalant and injectable anesthetics, halothane has an additive effect on sinoatrial or atrioventricular conduction disturbances.

F. Respiratory effects

1. Halothane is a respiratory depressant.

2. It decreases tidal volume.

3. Initially the respiratory rate may increase to compensate for the decreased tidal volume. As anesthesia deepens, the respiratory rate will also decrease.

4. As with all general anesthetics, increasing doses of halothane will eventually produce respiratory arrest.

5. It can depress chemoreceptor function to a significant degree.

6. It is nonirritating to the respiratory mucous membranes and does not increase salivary or respiratory secretions.

G. Hepatic effects

1. Halothane is an inert molecule and is not directly hepatotoxic.

2. It can produce transitory depression of hepatic function.

3. "Halothane hepatitis"

    a. Halothane has been implicated as a possible cause of post-anesthetic hepatitis in human patients.

    b. The phenomenon is extremely rare, occurring in 1:7000–10,000 of cases of halothane anesthesia.

    c. The hepatitis is most likely related to the metabolites of halothane biodegradation.

    d. Halothane can be metabolized via an oxidative hepatic microsomal enzyme pathway (major pathway) that produces relatively harmless metabolites, or it can occur via a reductive pathway (non-oxygen-dependent, minor pathway) that produces potentially harmful metabolites.

    e. The reactive intermediate metabolites produced by the reductive pathway could covalently bind to hepatic proteins, lipoproteins, and lipids, altering their function and resulting in hepatic necrosis.

    f. Certain factors seem to increase the risk of halothane hepatitis in human patients.

        (1) Intraoperative hepatic hypoxemia seems to be very important.

        (2) Reductive metabolism of halothane by the liver seems to be very important.

        (3) Repeated exposure to halothane seems to be less important.

        (4) Genetics may play a major role.

    g. The rarity of halothane hepatitis in human surgical patients is probably due to its multifactorial etiology, with genetic predisposition playing a major role.

    h. If halothane hepatitis ever occurs clinically in animal patients, its incidence is probably rare.

(1) It has been experimentally produced in guinea pigs and rats.

(2) Its etiology in animal patients would most likely be similar to its etiology in human patients.

H. Renal effects

1. Halothane does not have a direct nephrotoxic effect.

2. It can indirectly decrease renal function by decreasing renal blood flow.

I. Other physiologic effects

1. Halothane provides adequate muscle relaxation.

2. It can cause hypothermia as a result of peripheral vasodilation and depression of the thermoregulation center.

3. It readily crosses the placenta.

J. Excretion and metabolism

1. The majority of halothane is exhaled from the lungs unchanged following anesthesia.

2. Up to 20% of the inspired concentration can be biodegraded by the liver.

3. The normal metabolic by-products include trifluoroacetic acid, bromide ion, and chloride ion.

4. It is not defluorinated by the liver the way methoxyflurane is.

5. When it is reduced instead of oxidized, reactive metabolites may be formed.

K. Precautions and contraindications

1. Halothane should be used with extreme caution in patients with cardiac conduction problems or other dysrhythmias.

2. It should be used with caution in patients with myocardial disease.

3. It is contraindicated in patients with a history of an unexplained postanesthetic hepatitis developing following its use and in patients with active hepatitis.

4. Chronic hepatitis or chronic liver dysfunction may be a contraindication for the use of halothane.

IV. Isoflurane (Forane, AErrane)

A. Isoflurane was synthesized in 1968 and first used clinically in human patients in 1970.

B. Physical properties (see Table 3–6)

1. Isoflurane is a halogenated ether that is nonflammable and nonexplosive at commonly used anesthetic concentrations.

2. It is a structural isomer of enflurane (Ethrane). Enflurane is no longer routinely used in clinical practice.

3. It is one of the least soluble of the volatile inhalation anesthetic agents in blood, body tissues, and conductive rubber components of the anesthetic circuit.

4. This low solubility accounts for its very rapid induction time (3–5 minutes) and the associated very rapid recovery time (less than 5 minutes).

5. The MAC for isoflurane in the dog and cat is 1.28 and 1.63, respectively.

6. Isoflurane reactivity

a. It is a very stable compound and does not require a preservative.

b. It does not react with metals.

      c. It does not decompose when exposed to ultraviolet light.

C. Vaporization and administration

  1. The vapor pressure of isoflurane at 20°C is 239.5.

  2. This high vapor pressure means it is easily vaporized, so only precision, out-of-circuit vaporizers should be used to administer it.

  3. At 20°C, the maximum amount of isoflurane vapor that can be produced is approximately 31.5%.

  4. Since isoflurane and halothane have almost identical vapor pressures, isoflurane can be used in precision, out-of-circuit vaporizers that are calibrated for halothane.

    a. Studies have shown that the percent of anesthetic vapor output from these vaporizers is the same whether halothane or isoflurane is used.

    b. If one is going to use isoflurane in a vaporizer intended for halothane, the vaporizer should be serviced and thoroughly cleaned before isoflurane is placed in it.

  5. Generally 3.5–5% isoflurane is needed for mask induction. Once induction has been achieved, the patient can usually be maintained at 1.5–2%.

    a. As with all inhalant anesthetics, ultimate induction and maintenance concentrations are given to effect and will depend on the physical status of the patient and the type and dose of other CNS depressant drugs administered to the patient.

    b. Because isoflurane is so insoluble, increases and decreases in the depth of anesthesia can be achieved very rapidly.

D. CNS effects

  1. Isoflurane is a general CNS depressant.

  2. Unlike its isomer, enflurane, isoflurane does not produce convulsive or seizure activity even in the presence of hypercapnia or at deep levels of anesthesia.

  3. Deep levels of anesthesia do not produce muscle twitching.

E. Cardiovascular effects

  1. In normal patients, the isoflurane concentrations used to provide clinical surgical anesthesia have minimal to moderate effects on the cardiovascular system.

  2. In vivo, isoflurane administered at 1 and 2 MAC produces little or no myocardial depression; however, when concentrations above 2 MAC are administered, cardiovascular depression does occur.

  3. The cardiovascular margin of safety may be greater with isoflurane than with halothane, enflurane, or methoxyflurane.

    a. Isoflurane has the highest cardiac index of the inhalant anesthetics. (The cardiac index is obtained by dividing the myocardial anesthetic concentration at cardiac collapse by the concentration in the heart at MAC.)

    b. A high cardiac index equates to less myocardial depression.

    c. Cardiac index of the inhalant agents.

      (1) Isoflurane = 5.7.

      (2) Methoxyflurane = 3.7.

      (3) Halothane = 3.0.

  4. Cardiac output does not decrease significantly with clinically used concentrations of isoflurane.

  a. Isoflurane decreases stroke volume.

  b. The heart rate stays the same or increases slightly and compensates for the decreased stroke volume; therefore, cardiac output does not fall.

 5. The heart rate is not depressed with isoflurane and may increase slightly. This occurs because of the following reasons:

  a. Isoflurane depresses both vagal and preganglionic sympathetic activity; however, the vagal depression is more than the sympathetic depression.

  b. Isoflurane may also have mild beta-sympathetic stimulating properties.

 6. Isoflurane decreases arterial blood pressure in a dose-related fashion.

  a. The decrease in blood pressure is due to a decreased vascular resistance (vasodilation) and not to a decreased cardiac output.

  b. Part of the vasodilation may also be due to a direct effect of isoflurane on the blood vessels.

 7. Isoflurane decreases myocardial oxygen consumption and coronary vascular resistance without decreasing coronary blood flow.

 8. Peripheral perfusion is usually adequately maintained with isoflurane.

 9. Isoflurane produces a very stable heart rhythm.

  a. It does not sensitize the myocardium to exogenous epinephrine.

  b. The lack of dysrhythmias with isoflurane is also due to the fact that it does not slow the conduction of impulses through the His-Purkinje system.

F. Respiratory effects

 1. Isoflurane depresses respiration in a dose-related fashion.

 2. It may be slightly more depressant than halothane but is less depressant than enflurane.

 3. Lung compliance is slightly decreased and pulmonary resistance slightly increased by isoflurane.

G. Hepatic and renal effects

 1. Isoflurane does not appear to produce any direct liver damage even when used for long procedures or administered during hypoxia.

 2. Like other inhalant anesthetics, isoflurane decreases renal blood flow, glomerular filtration rate, and urine flow.

  a. This depression is transitory.

  b. No direct renal injury has been reported.

H. Other physiologic effects

 1. Isoflurane produces adequate muscle relaxation for most procedures.

 2. It readily crosses the placenta.

I. Excretion and metabolism

 1. Essentially all of the isoflurane is exhaled from the lungs unchanged.

 2. Only about 0.2% of the inhaled isoflurane undergoes biodegradation in the liver.

J. Precautions and contraindications

 1. No major precautions or contraindications exist for isoflurane.

 2. As with any inhalant anesthetic, excessive concentrations of isoflurane can lead to cardiopulmonary collapse.

 3. Evidence is emerging that exposure of carbon dioxide absorbants

(soda lime and barium hydroxide lime) to isoflurane, desflurane, and enflurane can lead to carbon monoxide production.

   a. Carbon monoxide production is most likely caused by letting oxygen flow through an unused rebreathing circuit (circle system) for a prolonged period.

   b. Some human patients have been known to inhale significant amounts of carbon monoxide.

   c. Most of these cases occurred after the anesthetic machine had not been used for several days.

   d. One study suggests that barium hydroxide lime is the absorbant with the greatest potential for carbon monoxide production when exposed to isoflurane, desflurane, or enflurane. Carbon monoxide can also be formed if these inhalants are passed across dried soda lime.

   e. It is critical to use fresh carbon dioxide absorbants and not let them dry out in order to prevent carbon monoxide formation.

   f. Pulse oximetry is not a reliable method for detecting this problem.

   g. If a patient is suspected to have inhaled carbon monoxide during anesthesia, remove the carbon dioxide absorbant immediately, and provide 100% oxygen to the patient.

V. Desflurane (Suprane)

  A. Desflurane was first used clinically in human anesthesia in the early 1990s.

  B. Physical properties (see Table 3–6)

    1. Desflurane is a halogenated ether that is nonflammable and nonexplosive at commonly used anesthetic concentration.

    2. It is the least soluble of the volatile inhalation anesthetic agents in blood and body tissues.

    3. This low solubility accounts for its very rapid induction and associated rapid recovery times. It is the most rapid-acting volatile anesthetic agent.

    4. The MAC for desflurane in the dog and cat is 7.20% and 9.79%, respectively. Desflurane is the least potent of the modern volatile inhalant anesthetics.

    5. Reactivity

      a. Desflurane is a very stable compound and does not require a preservative.

      b. It does not react with metals.

    6. Desflurane has fluorine molecules substituted for chloride and bromide molecules.

      a. These fluorine molecules improve stability.

      b. These fluorine molecules decrease potency (MAC).

  C. Vaporization and administration

    1. The vapor pressure of desflurane at 20°C is 664.

    2. Desflurane's boiling point is 23.5°C, which is close to room temperature.

      a. Because of its low boiling point, even evaporative cooling of desflurane will greatly influence vapor pressure and thus anesthetic vapor concentration delivered to the circuit.

      b. A special vaporizer had to be developed to administer desflurane.

      c. The cost of the vaporizer is extremely high, which limits the routine use of desflurane in most veterinary settings.

  3. Because desflurane is so insoluble in blood and tissues, changes in anesthetic depth can be achieved extremely quickly.

D. CNS effects

  1. Desflurane produces a dose-dependent CNS depression.

  2. It is the least potent of the modern volatile anesthetic agents.

E. Cardiovascular effects

  1. Desflurane produces a dose-dependent depression of the cardiovascular system.

  2. The cardiovascular effects of desflurane are similar to those of isoflurane.

  3. All volatile anesthetic agents can decrease cardiac output.

     a. Desflurane, like isoflurane and sevoflurane, tends to maintain cardiac output at clinically used concentrations.

     b. The decreases in cardiac output are primarily due to a decrease in myocardial contractility, producing a decrease in stroke volume.

  4. Desflurane will cause a dose-dependent decrease in blood pressure, primarily because of a decrease in stroke volume. A decrease in peripheral vascular resistance also plays a role in decreasing blood pressure.

  5. Desflurane, like isoflurane, does not sensitize the myocardium to the catecholamines and thus is not considered arrhythmogenic.

F. Respiratory effects

  1. Desflurane produces a dose-dependent decrease in pulmonary function.

  2. It will produce a decrease in both rate and tidal volume.

  3. Desflurane, like the other volatile anesthetics, depresses the patient's ability to respond to increases in arterial carbon dioxide levels and to decreases in arterial oxygen levels.

G. Hepatic effects

  1. Desflurane has not been associated with direct hepatocellular damage.

  2. Desflurane, like all the volatile anesthetics, may indirectly produce hepatocellular damage by decreasing hepatic blood flow and oxygen delivery.

H. Renal effects

  1. Desflurane, like all the volatile anesthetics, can decrease renal blood and glomerular filtration rate in a dose-related manner.

  2. It has not been shown to produce direct nephrotoxicity.

 I. Excretion and metabolism

  1. Desflurane is excreted into the alveoli and exhaled during recovery.

  2. Only 0.02% of the inspired anesthetic concentration can be recovered as metabolites.

J. The expense of desflurane and the added expense of a special vaporizer for its administration will probably limit the use of this drug in veterinary anesthesia.

VI. Sevoflurane (Ultane)

A. Sevoflurane is the newest of the volatile anesthetics to be approved for human use in the United States.

B. Physical properties (see Table 3–6)

  1. Sevoflurane is a halogenated ether that is nonflammable and nonexplosive at commonly used anesthetic concentrations.

2. Its blood solubility is similar to desflurane, which accounts for its very rapid induction and associated rapid recovery times.

3. Sevoflurane is nonpungent and has a nonirritating odor, making mask inductions easier.

4. The MAC for sevoflurane is 2.1–2.4% in the dog and 2.6% in the cat. It is less potent than isoflurane but more potent than desflurane.

5. Reactivity

    a. Sevoflurane will react with soda lime or Baralyme to produce olefin, a nephrotoxic compound. The concentration threshold for nephrotoxicity in the rat model is within the clinically used concentration ranges.

    b. Sevoflurane does not require a preservative.

C. Vaporization and administration

1. The vapor pressure of sevoflurane at 20°C is 160, making it a highly volatile agent.

2. It should be used only in precision, agent-specific, out-of-circuit vaporizers.

3. Changes in anesthetic depth can be rapidly achieved with sevoflurane because of its decreased solubility in blood.

D. CNS effects

1. Sevoflurane produces a dose-dependent CNS depression.

2. It is similar to isoflurane and desflurane in its CNS effects.

E. Cardiovascular effects

1. The cardiovascular effects of sevoflurane are similar to those of isoflurane and desflurane.

2. It will produce a dose-dependent decrease in cardiac output and blood pressure.

3. It does not sensitize the myocardium to catecholamines.

F. Respiratory effects

1. Sevoflurane produces a dose-dependent decrease in pulmonary function similar to that of the other volatile inhalant anesthetics.

2. It will produce a decrease in both rate and tidal volume.

3. Sevoflurane, like the other volatile anesthetics, depresses the patient's ability to respond to increases in arterial carbon dioxide levels and to decreases in arterial oxygen levels.

G. Hepatic effects

1. Sevoflurane has not been associated with direct hepatocellular damage.

2. It can produce indirect hepatocellular damage by decreasing hepatic blood flow and oxygen delivery.

H. Renal effects

1. Sevoflurane has not been associated with direct nephrotoxicity.

2. It can indirectly affect renal function by decreasing renal blood flow and the glomerular filtration rate.

I. Excretion and metabolism

1. Almost all of the inspired sevoflurane is excreted into the alveoli and exhaled during recovery.

2. Only 3% of sevoflurane is metabolized.

J. The expense of sevoflurane may limit its use in veterinary anesthesia.

VII. Nitrous oxide

A. Nitrous oxide was first prepared in 1776, and its anesthetic properties were first noted in 1799.

B. Physical properties (see Table 3–6)
   1. Nitrous oxide is a colorless, nonirritating, sweet-smelling, inorganic gas.
   2. It is nonflammable but will support combustion in the absence of oxygen.
   3. It is compressed to form a liquid and is supplied in cylinders.
   4. It is very insoluble in blood, body tissues, and rubber components of the anesthetic delivery circuit.
      a. It has the lowest solubility coefficients of any of the inhalant anesthetics.
      b. Because of its low solubility, nitrous oxide rapidly diffuses into the blood from the alveoli and from the blood into the tissues.
      c. When it is discontinued, the opposite result occurs, and most of the nitrous oxide is eliminated from the body within 5 minutes.
   5. It is 30 times more soluble than nitrogen.
      a. It displaces nitrogen from the alveoli, blood, and gas-filled pockets of the body.
      b. It therefore diffuses into the gas-filled cavities, intestines, and cerebral ventricles, where it may cause distension or increased pressure.
   6. The MAC of nitrous oxide in the dog is 188–297% and in the cat 250%.
      a. This means nitrous oxide is a very weak CNS depressant and is not capable of producing general anesthesia by itself.
      b. Additional CNS depressant drugs must be used in combination with nitrous oxide.
   7. It is very stable and does not react with the soda lime or metal components of the anesthetic machine.

C. Administration
   1. Like oxygen, nitrous oxide is metered to the patient via a flowmeter.
   2. It must always be used in combination with oxygen to prevent hypoxia.
   3. Although it is a very weak, or mild, anesthetic, the CNS depression it produces in a patient occurs very rapidly.

D. CNS effects
   1. Nitrous oxide is a mild anesthetic agent that rarely produces anesthesia below very light levels of anesthesia.
   2. Some cortical depression occurs, but nitrous oxide is unable to produce general anesthesia alone.
   3. To obtain surgical anesthesia, hypnotics, narcotics, or other inhalation anesthetics must be used in combination with nitrous oxide.

E. Cardiovascular effects
   1. The heart rate is unaffected by nitrous oxide unless hypoxia occurs.
   2. Cardiac output and arterial blood pressure are unchanged.
   3. Spontaneous cardiac dysrhythmias are uncommon with nitrous oxide unless hypoxia is produced with it.

F. Respiratory effects
   1. Nitrous oxide is nonirritating to the respiratory tract and does not increase salivary or respiratory secretions.

2. It has no significant effect on the respiratory rate, tidal volume, or minute volume.

G. Other physiologic effects

   1. Nitrous oxide has no appreciable effects on other organ systems in the body.

   2. It does cross the placenta.

   3. It does not produce good muscle relaxation.

H. Excretion and metabolism

   1. Biologically, nitrous oxide is not inert; however, if any metabolism of nitrous oxide occurs, it is of no significance.

   2. The majority of the nitrous oxide is eliminated through the lungs, unchanged, within 2–3 minutes after administration is discontinued.

      a. This rapid elimination of nitrous oxide from the blood will dilute the air in the alveoli and will displace oxygen, causing diffusion hypoxia.

      b. Therefore, 100% oxygen should be continued to the patient for 3–5 minutes after the nitrous oxide is turned off to prevent diffusion hypoxia.

   3. Minute traces of nitrous oxide may be present in the blood for several hours.

I. Clinical uses

   1. Induction

      a. Nitrous oxide can be used with the more potent inhalant anesthetics during mask induction to more rapidly induce anesthesia in the patient.

      b. The more rapid induction occurs as the result of a concentrating, or "second gas effect," of the nitrous oxide.

   2. Maintenance

      a. Nitrous oxide must be combined with other CNS depressant drugs or anesthetics for maintenance of anesthesia.

      b. For maintenance it is recommended that 50–66% nitrous oxide be used in combination with 33–50% oxygen.

      c. At least 30% oxygen should always be administered with the nitrous oxide.

      d. The concentration of the other more potent inhalation anesthetic agents can be decreased by one third to one half when nitrous oxide is used in combination with them.

   3. Nitrous oxide and oxygen can be used in combination with hypnotics, narcotics, or local anesthetics for minor procedures or in sick and debilitated patients.

J. Advantages

   1. Nitrous oxide is nonflammable and nonexplosive.

   2. It has no significant physiologic effects on the cardiovascular, respiratory, hepatic, or renal systems.

   3. Induction and recovery are rapid.

   4. It is compatible with all hypnotics, narcotics, muscle relaxants, and general anesthetics commonly used.

   5. It possesses fair to good analgesic properties, depending on the species of animal patient.

   6. It gives added safety to anesthesia by allowing a decrease in the amount of other more potent anesthetic agents.

K. Disadvantages
   1. General anesthesia cannot be produced with nitrous oxide alone.
   2. It produces inadequate muscle relaxation.
   3. It may cause increased tension in the gas pockets of the body. Therefore, it may compound problems when used in the presence of a pneumothorax or intestinal obstruction.
   4. Diffusion hypoxia may occur when nitrous oxide is discontinued and the patient is allowed to breathe room air immediately.
   5. Hypoxia is always a danger with nitrous oxide unless at least 30% oxygen is administered with it.

VIII. Health hazard of exposure to anesthetic waste gases
   A. Strong evidence exists that exposure to waste anesthetic gases can be a health hazard.
   B. The National Institute for Occupational Safety and Health (NIOSH) has recommended that the environmental concentration of halogenated anesthetic agents (halothane, methoxyflurane, enflurane, isoflurane) not exceed 2 ppm when used alone, or 0.5 ppm when used with nitrous oxide, and that the nitrous oxide concentration not exceed 25 ppm.
   C. Cellular mechanism of anesthetic toxicity
      1. Long-term organ toxicity of the inhalant agents is most likely caused by the metabolic by-products of their biodegradation.
      2. Biotransformation may produce toxicity by means of the following:
         a. The accumulation of metabolites in excess of the organ toxicity threshold
         b. The production of reactive intermediates that covalently bond to tissue macromolecules
         c. The formation of metabolites that act as haptens, which can produce hypersensitivity or immune responses
      3. All modern volatile anesthetic agents are capable of biodegradation by the body.
      4. Percentage of the inspired anesthetic concentration that can be metabolized
         a. Methoxyflurane (50%)
         b. Halothane (20–25%)
         c. Sevoflurane (3%)
         d. Isoflurane (<0.2%)
         e. Desflurane (0.02%)
         f. Nitrous oxide (0.0004%)
      5. Potentially toxic metabolites produced by biodegradation of the inhalant anesthetics
         a. Inorganic fluoride ion
         b. Oxalic acid
         c. Inorganic bromide ion
         d. Free radicals
   D. Reproductive problems
      1. Strong evidence exists that chronic exposure to waste anesthetic gases may lead to reproductive problems.
      2. In retrospective studies conducted with physician anesthesiologists and nurse anesthetists, there was a statistically significant increase in the

relative risk of spontaneous abortion among the females in the groups. The relative increased risk was 1.3-fold.

3. The increased risk for congenital abnormalities was of borderline statistical significance.

E. Mutagenicity and carcinogenicity

1. Evidence does not support mutagenicity of inhalant anesthetic agents.

2. Experimental evidence using animal models and cell cultures has not demonstrated carcinogenicity of halothane, methoxyflurane, enflurane, isoflurane, or nitrous oxide.

3. Epidemiologic studies likewise do not support the carcinogenicity of these agents.

F. Hepatic dysfunction

1. Mounting evidence exists that halothane and possibly methoxyflurane are potential hepatotoxins and that chronic exposure to these waste anesthetic gases may increase the risk of liver disease in operating room personnel.

2. The hepatotoxicity is probably due to the formation of reactive intermediates during the metabolism of these agents, which in turn covalently bind to liver macromolecules.

3. The increased risk of liver disease in operating room personnel exposed to waste anesthetic gases is 1.6-fold in men and 1.5-fold in women.

4. Evidence does not support hepatotoxicity of enflurane, isoflurane, or nitrous oxide.

G. Renal dysfunction

1. Methoxyflurane can produce primary renal dysfunction in clinical patients. Proximal renal tubular necrosis is produced by the inorganic fluoride ion released during methoxyflurane biodegradation.

2. Direct nephrotoxicity from halothane, enflurane, isoflurane, or nitrous oxide has not been reported.

3. A statistically significant increase in renal disease is reported only among female operating room personnel.

H. CNS dysfunction

1. Several reports have described an increased incidence of headaches, nausea, fatigue, and irritability in physician anesthesiologists and nurse anesthetists exposed to waste anesthetic gases.

2. In addition, chronic exposure to nitrous oxide has been associated with myeloneuropathies.

3. Exposure to waste anesthetic gases may produce not only short-term neurologic effects (headache, nausea, depression, lethargy, ataxia), but also long-term effects (myoneuropathies, muscle weakness, neuron destruction, learning disabilities).

I. Methods to reduce operating room contamination

1. Scavenging

a. Scavenging is the single most important factor in reducing operating room contamination.

b. A scavenging system consists of the following:

(1) Gas-capturing system

(2) Interface

(3) Disposal system

c. Gas-capturing system

(1) A gas-capturing system is incorporated into the pop-off valve of the anesthetic machine.

(2) A gas-capturing system is also available for non-rebreathing delivery circuits.

d. Interface

(1) The interface joins the gas-capturing mechanism of the breathing circuit with the disposal system.

(2) The interface is designed to (i) relieve positive pressure if the scavenging system occludes and (ii) prevent vacuum, or negative, pressures from reaching the breathing circuit when central suction or a blower is used to eliminate the waste anesthetic gases.

e. Disposal system

(1) The disposal system ultimately removes the waste gases from the operating room.

(2) Several options are available:

(i) A system for exhausting the waste gases into a non-recirculating air conditioning system

(ii) A central vacuum system

(iii) A passive through-wall system

(iv) Charcoal absorbers

2. Equipment leaks

a. Continuous in-house maintenance by veterinary personnel is necessary to identify and correct leaks in the anesthetic machine.

b. High-pressure leaks

(1) The high-pressure system of an anesthetic machine extends from the nitrous oxide tanks or central nitrous oxide supply to the anesthetic flowmeters.

(2) The most likely leak sites in the high-pressure system are as follows:

(i) "Quick connects" on the central inflow lines (crimp joints, screw joint seals, spring ooals, and O-rings)

(ii) Nitrous oxide tank yolk connector

(iii) Nitrous oxide regulator

(3) A 10% detergent solution can be placed on the joints to check for leaks. Bubbles will form wherever there are leaks.

c. Low-pressure leaks

(1) The low-pressure system extends from the flowmeters of the anesthetic machine to the patient.

(2) The most likely leak sites in the low-pressure system are as follows:

(i) At the connection between the flowmeters and vaporizer

(ii) At the unidirectional valves

(iii) At the soda lime canister

(iv) Around the endotracheal tube

(v) From holes in the rebreathing bag and delivery hoses

(vi) From the pop-off valve

3. Altering anesthetic techniques

a. Always make sure the waste anesthetic disposal system is attached and functional.

    b. Do not turn on the vaporizer or nitrous oxide until the patient is attached to the delivery system.

    c. Use cuffed endotracheal tubes of the proper size.

    d. Empty the rebreathing bag into the scavenging system—not the room.

    e. Scavenge all non-rebreathing systems.

    f. Use a chamber or mask induction only when indicated, and make sure the mask is a tight fit.

    g. Avoid spilling anesthetic when filling the vaporizer, and, if possible, fill vaporizers just before the staff leaves for the day.

    h. Keep the patient on 100% oxygen as long as possible at the end of the procedure.

    i. When possible, personnel should stay at least 3 feet away from the anesthetic machine exhaust, the head of the recovering animal, and any anesthetic spills.

J. Monitoring waste anesthetic gases

    1. The only way to determine waste anesthetic gas concentrations in the environment is to (a) send air samples to a laboratory or (b) monitor rooms "in-house" by using portable infrared analysis equipment.

    2. Nitrous oxide dosimeters are available that can be worn by an individual. At the end of a specified period of time these are sent to a laboratory for analysis of total nitrous oxide exposure.

References and Suggested Readings

Booth NH: Intravenous and other parenteral anesthetics. In Booth NH, McDonald LE (eds): Veterinary Pharmacology and Therapeutics. Ames, IA: Iowa State University Press, 1988, p. 212.

Branson KE, Gross ME: Propofol in veterinary medicine. J Am Vet Med Assoc 204(12):1888–1890, 1994.

Corssen G, Reves JG, Stanley TH: Dissociative anesthesia. In Intravenous Anesthesia and Analgesia. Philadelphia: Lea & Febiger, 1988, p. 99.

Dreesen DW, Jones GL, Brown J, Rawlings CA: Monitoring for trace anesthetic gases in a veterinary teaching hospital. J Am Vet Med Assoc 179:797–799, 1981.

Eger EI, II: New inhaled anesthetics. Anesthesiology 80:906–922, 1994.

Fragen RJ, Avram MJ: Nonopioid intravenous anesthetics. In Barash PG, Cullen BF, Stoelting RK, (eds): Clinical Anesthesia. Philadelphia: JB Lippincott, 1989, pp. 227–253.

Hartsfield SM: Advantages and guidelines for using ketamine for induction of anesthesia. Vet Clin North Am Small Anim Pract Opin Small Anim Anesth 22(2):268, 1992.

Haskins SC, Farver TB, Patz JD: Ketamine in dogs. Am J Vet Res 46:1855, 1985.

Ilkin JE: Other potentially useful new injectable anesthetic agents. Vet Clin North Am Small Anim Pract Opin Small Anim Anesth 22(2):281–288, 1992.

Kruse-Elliott KT, Swanson CR, Aucion DP: Effects of etomidate function on canine surgical patients. Am J Vet Res 48:1098–1100, 1987.

Lin HC: Dissociative anesthetics. In Thurmon JC, Tranquilli WJ, Benson GJ (eds): Lumb and Jones' Veterinary Anesthesia, 3rd Ed. Baltimore: Williams & Wilkins, 1996, pp. 241–296.

Manley SV, McDonell WF: Recommendations for reduction of anesthetic gas pollution. J Am Vet Med Assoc 176:519–524, 1980.

Morgan DWT, Legge K: Clinical evaluation of propofol as an intravenous anesthetic agent in cats and dogs. Vet Rec 124:31–33, 1989.

Muir WW, Mason DE: Side effects of etomidate in dogs. J Am Vet Med Assoc 1994:1430–1434, 1989.

Robertson S: Advantages of etomidate as an anesthetic agent. Vet Clin North Am Small Anim Pract Opin Small Anim Anesth 22(2):277–280, 1992.

Short CE: Dissociative anesthetics. In Principles and Practice of Veterinary Anesthesia. Baltimore: Williams & Wilkins, 1987, p. 158.

Short CE: Inhalant anesthetics. In Principles and Practice of Veterinary Anesthesia. Baltimore: Williams & Wilkins, 1987, pp. 70–90.

Smith I, White PF, Nathanson M, Goldson R: Propofol, an update on its clinical use. Anesthesiology 81(4):1005–1043, 1994.

Steffey EP: Inhalation anesthetics. In Thurmon JC, Tranquilli WJ, Benson GJ (eds): Lumb and Jones' Veterinary Anesthesia, 3rd Ed. Baltimore: Williams & Wilkins, 1996, pp 297–329.

Steffey EP, Howland D Jr: Isoflurane potency in the dog and cat. Am J Vet Res 38:1833–1836, 1977.

Stoelting RK: Nonbarbiturate induction drugs. In Pharmacology and Physiology in Anesthetic Practice, Philadelphia: JB Lippincot, 1991, p. 134.

Thurmon JC, Tranquilli WJ, Benson GJ: Injectable anesthetics. In Lumb and Jones' Veterinary Anesthesia, 3rd Ed. Baltimore: Williams & Wilkins, 1996, pp. 210–240.

Wertz EM, Benson GJ, Thurmon JC, Tranquilli WJ: Pharmacokinetics of etomidate in cats. Am J Vet Res 51(2):281–285, 1990.

White PF, Way WL, Trevor AJ: Ketamine—its pharmacology and therapeutic uses. Anesthesiology 56:119, 1982.

Zoran DL, Riedesel DH, Dyer DC: Pharmacokinetics of propofol in mixed-breed dogs and greyhounds. Am J Vet Res 54:755–760, 1993.

Chapter

4

Neuromuscular Blocking Agents

Robert R. Paddleford

I. Normal nerve transmission
   A. An electrical impulse causes release of the neurotransmitter acetylcholine from vesicles located near the nerve end plate.
   B. Acetylcholine reacts with postjunctional receptors located directly opposite the acetylcholine-releasing sites.
   C. Membrane permeability to all ions is charged, and depolarization occurs.
      1. Acetylcholine receptors are composed of five protein subunits arranged parallel to each other, forming a cylinder. The central core of the cylinder forms an ion channel through the cell membrane.
         a. The junctional receptors are composed of two alpha, one beta, one gamma, and one epsilon subunit.
         b. Both alpha subunits must be stimulated by acetylcholine simultaneously for the ion channel to open.
         c. If the alpha subunits are occupied by two antagonists, or by one agonist and one antagonist, the channel remains closed.
      2. Sodium ions and calcium ions migrate into the muscle cell, and potassium ions migrate out of the muscle cell when the channel is open.
      3. The ion current produces depolarization of the cell membrane.
      4. The exterior of the muscle membrane becomes negatively charged, and the interior becomes positively charged, resulting in an action potential.
      5. The action potential proceeds to the interior of the muscle fiber, causing it to contract.
   D. Acetylcholinesterase in the end plate becomes active and hydrolyzes the acetylcholine, restoring permeability so that the muscle membrane repolarizes.
      1. Sodium ions move out of the muscle cell, and potassium ions move in.
      2. A negative resting potential is restored.
   E. A phenomenon called "channel block" may occur when certain drug molecules enter the protein channel of the acetylcholine receptor and become lodged inside without binding to the acetycholine subunit receptor sites.
      1. This phenomenon of channel block will prevent ion currents from forming and subsequent depolarization from occurring.
      2. Channel block is dose-dependent, and the mechanism appears very similar to that of local anesthetics and sodium channels.
      3. Drugs that can produce channel block include naloxone, the local anesthetics, and verapamil. Antibiotics that have been associated with channel block include polymyxin-B, lincomycin, clindamycin, and the aminoglycoside antibiotics.
      4. Drugs that cause channel block will enhance the effects of nondepolar-

78

izing neuromuscular blockers and therefore may prolong the neuromuscular block.

F. Some drugs bind to protein subunits other than their alpha subunits and thus distort the acetylcholine receptor.

1. Even if both alpha subunits are occupied by an agonist, the acetylcholine receptor cannot change to allow the channel to open. This inability to change is referred to as receptor desensitization.

2. Drugs that can cause desensitization include chlorpromazine, lidocaine, thiopental, methoxyflurane, halothane, isoflurane, verapamil, and polymyxin B.

3. Some drugs decrease postsynaptic membrane sensitivity to acetylcholine. These drugs include diazepam, midazolam, droperidol, morphine, fentanyl, the barbiturates, ketamine, procainamide, corticosteroids, and magnesium.

4. All of these drugs will potentiate the neuromuscular blocking effect of the nondepolarizing drugs in a dose-dependent manner.

G. Adverse side effects

1. When higher than normal clinical doses of neuromuscular blockers are used, they may bind to other muscarinic receptors besides the cholinergic receptors.

2. Bradycardia may result from stimulation of cardiac muscarinic receptors.

3. Tachycardia may occur if the cardiac muscarinic receptors are inhibited.

4. Hypotension may occur if receptors in the autonomic ganglia are blocked.

5. Bronchial constriction may occur.

6. Salivary secretions may increase.

7. Neuromuscular blockers cause the release of norepinephrine and histamines.

   a. Some neuromuscular blocking agents may cause the release of histamine at clinically used doses.

   b. These anaphylactoid reactions do not appear to be IgE-mediated reactions but instead involve degranulation of mast cells.

   c. Administering the nondepolarizing neuromuscular blockers slowly over 1–2 minutes helps to decrease the incidence of anaphylactoid reactions.

II. Classifications of neuromuscular blocking agents

A. Neuromuscular blocking drugs are classified as acetylcholine agonists, which are depolarizing drugs, or acetylcholine antagonists, which are nondepolarizing drugs.

1. All neuromuscular blocking drugs are polar, ionized, lipophobic, water-soluble agents that produce clinical effects by acting at the postjunctional receptors.

2. The nondepolarizing neuromuscular blockers also decrease mobilization of acetylcholine through their actions at the prejunctional receptors.

3. Neuromuscular blocking drugs are not degraded by acetylcholinesterase and thus will persist at the neuromuscular junction for longer periods of time, depending on their pharmacokinetic profile.

B. Depolarizing muscle relaxants

1. Depolarizing muscle relaxants are quaternary bases and act in a manner similar to acetylcholine.

2. They cause initial depolarization (muscle contraction) the same way acetylcholine does, but their effects persist longer than those of acetylcholine, therefore producing a persistent depolarization (muscle paralysis).

3. These drugs are broken down at the muscle sites by plasma cholinesterase (pseudocholinesterase).

4. No antagonists exist for these muscle relaxants.

5. Included in this group of muscle relaxants are succinylcholine (Anectine, Sucostrin) and decamethonium (Syncurine).

6. They produce a Phase I block.

7. Excessive or repeated doses can produce a Phase II block. Phase II block resembles a nondepolarizing block.

C. Nondepolarizing muscle relaxants

1. Nondepolarizing muscle relaxants are quaternary bases that act by competitive inhibition and preferentially bind to both the alpha subunits at the end plates, causing the ion channel to stay closed.

2. They do not act like acetylcholine but prevent acetylcholine from binding with the alpha subunit receptor sites, therefore, there is no initial muscle contraction, only flaccid paralysis.

3. They are not broken down by plasma cholinesterase (pseudocholinesterase). Instead, they are metabolized by the liver, excreted by the kidneys, or broken down by the Hofmann reaction.

4. Their effects can be antagonized by anticholinesterase drugs such as edrophonium or neostigmine.

5. Included in this group of muscle relaxants are *d*-tubocurarine, gallamine (Flaxedil), pancuronium (Pavulon), atracurium (Tracrium), vecuronium (Norcuron), and mivacurium (Mivacron).

6. They produce a Phase II block.

III. General statements regarding depolarizing and nondepolarizing neuromuscular blocking agents

A. All neuromuscular blocking agents produce striated-muscle paralysis in the following sequence:

1. The first muscles to be paralyzed are the ocular muscles, followed, in order, by the muscles of the face, pharynx, jaw and tail, extremities, abdomen, and finally the intercostal and diaphragmatic muscles.

2. The intercostal and diaphragmatic muscles are the last to be paralyzed and the first to regain function.

B. Because of their large molecular size, neuromuscular blocking agents do not readily cross the placenta or blood-brain barrier.

C. *They produce no analgesia or CNS depression.*

D. Any neuromuscular blocking agent is capable of producing complete paralysis of the respiratory muscles at any clinical dose; therefore, patients *must be ventilated* manually or mechanically when these agents are used.

IV. Clinical uses of the neuromuscular blocking agents

A. Neuromuscular blocking agents are used as adjuncts to general anesthesia to produce complete muscle relaxation to facilitate manipulations during surgery.

B. They are used as an adjunct to facilitate intubation.

C. They are used to stop spontaneous ventilation and allow for controlled ventilation, either manually or with a mechanical ventilator.

D. They are used to relieve laryngeal spasm.

V. Advantages of neuromuscular blocking agents
  A. Neuromuscular blocking agents provide excellent muscle relaxation with lighter levels of anesthesia; therefore, the amount of general anesthetic can be reduced.
  B. They have no CNS depressant effects.
  C. Relaxation can be produced rapidly without deepening anesthesia.
  D. Less potent anesthetic agents can be used to provide adequate muscle relaxation.

VI. Disadvantages of neuromuscular blocking agents
  A. Clinical doses will cause apnea.
  B. Cumulative effects and prolonged muscle paralysis and weakness can result with repeated doses.
  C. Their effects are influenced by electrolyte imbalances.
  D. *They produce no analgesia or anesthesia.*
  E. Depolarizing agents may cause postoperative muscular pain.
  F. Prolonged apnea of unknown etiology has been reported.
  G. Antagonists are either not available (depolarizing relaxants) or are not fully reliable (nondepolarizing relaxants).
  H. Complete muscle activity may not be fully recovered for many hours after apparent return of muscle tone.
  I. Hypotension may develop as a result of ganglionic blockade caused by excessive doses of neuromuscular blocking agents or histamine release.
  J. Tachycardia and decreased cardiac output may occur.

VII. Factors affecting intensity and duration of neuromuscular blockade
  A. Dose
    1. The larger the dose is, the more pronounced and the longer the duration of blockade.
    2. Repeated doses can produce a cumulative effect and a prolonged paralysis.
  B. Distribution, excretion, and metabolism
    1. Some neuromuscular blocking agents are excreted by the kidneys (gallamine, pancuronium); therefore, renal dysfunction can prolong their effects.
    2. Liver disease may cause a decreased plasma level of plasma cholinesterase and thereby prolong the effects of depolarizing neuromuscular blockers (succinylcholine, decamethonium). The effects of neuromuscular blockers that require hepatic metabolism (pancuronium) may also be prolonged in patients with liver disease.
    3. Redistribution of accumulated neuromuscular blocking agent may result in reparalyzation.
  C. Body temperature
    1. Hypothermia may potentiate neuromuscular blocking agents as a result of decreased renal and biliary excretion.
    2. Hypothermia also decreases enzyme activity, which may prolong the effects of neuromuscular blocking agents.
  D. Electrolyte imbalance/acid-base imbalance
    1. Hypokalemia prolongs the effects of neuromuscular blockers.
    2. Hypernatremia decreases the effects of neuromuscular blockers.
    3. Increased magnesium levels enhance the effects of depolarizing and nondepolarizing neuromuscular blockers.

4. Acidosis enhances the effects of nondepolarizing neuromuscular blockers.

E. Certain drugs will increase or prolong the effects of neuromuscular blockers (refer to outline items IE, IF, and IIC).

VIII. Depolarizing neuromuscular blocking agents

A. Succinylcholine (Anectine, Sucostrin)

1. Action of drug

a. It acts by persistent depolarization of the muscle membrane.

b. The area beyond the membrane also becomes inactivated.

c. Excessive or repeated doses of succinylcholine can cause a Phase II block; that is, it acts like a nondepolarizer.

2. Dose, duration of action, and route of administration

a. The effective dose and duration of action are extremely variable among species and among individuals within a species.

b. Duration of action is prolonged by organophosphates because they decrease plasma cholinesterase, which is necessary to hydrolyze succinylcholine.

c. Neostigmine and edrophonium prolong the action of succinylcholine.

d. Doses (intravenous)

(1) Dog—0.15–0.20 mg/lb (paralysis lasts 5–30 minutes)

(2) Cat—0.5 mg/lb (paralysis lasts 4–6 minutes)

e. Its latency (time until onset of maximum paralysis) is 15–60 seconds

f. Cases of prolonged apnea after repeated doses of succinylcholine have been reported.

(1) This reaction is probably due to an accumulation of succinyl monocholine (the first breakdown product of succinylcholine).

(2) Succinyl monocholine can also depolarize the muscle membrane, and after prolonged use, Phase II block occurs (the drug in the muscle fiber then acts like a nonpolarizer).

3. Physiologic effects

a. Respiratory effects

(1) Succinylcholine does not affect the respiratory center except in massive doses; then it depresses it.

(2) Apnea is due to muscle paralysis.

(3) Succinylcholine can increase bronchial and salivary secretions.

b. Cardiovascular effects

(1) Heart rate is not usually affected except following repeated doses. Then bradycardia may result from stimulation of the vagal ganglia.

(2) No significant effects on the myocardium are produced.

(3) Cardiac rhythm is unaffected.

(4) Large doses of succinylcholine cause transient blood pressure elevation.

(5) Hypotension is uncommon; however, with large doses, ganglionic blockade and histamine release can occur, resulting in a fall in blood pressure.

c. Liver and kidney effects

(1) Succinylcholine has no direct effect on renal or hepatic function.

(2) The kidney excretes 5–15% of the injected dose unchanged.

(3) Plasma cholinesterase is produced in the liver, and this enzyme rapidly destroys succinylcholine in the plasma. Therefore, liver disease may prolong paralysis.

    d. CNS effects

        (1) Succinylcholine does not depress the CNS.

        (2) *It produces no analgesia or anesthesia.*

  4. No antagonists are available for succinylcholine.

B. Decamethonium (Syncurine)

  1. Decamethonium is essentially identical to succinylcholine.

  2. It differs in the following ways:

    a. It does not produce histamine release.

    b. It is not metabolized by plasma cholinesterase.

    c. It is excreted by the kidneys unchanged.

    d. It is longer acting than succinylcholine.

IX. Nondepolarizing neuromuscular blocking agents

A. *d*-Tubocurarine (Curare)

  1. Action of drug

    a. The drug *d*-tubocurarine acts by competitive inhibition of acetylcholine.

    b. It does not inhibit cholinesterase or acetylcholine formation.

    c. It does not change the electrical activity of the muscle membrane.

    d. It elevates the threshold to acetylcholine at the myoneural junction.

  2. Dose, duration of action, and route of administration

    a. For veterinary use, the drug should be diluted from 20 units (3.0 mg/ml) to 2 units (0.3 mg/ml). Use physiologic saline.

    b. It has been used in the dog at a dose of 0.06 mg/lb IV (paralysis lasts up to 100 minutes).

    c. It has been used in the cat at a dose of 0.1 mg/lb IV (paralysis lasts approximately 20 minutes).

    d. Always premedicate the patient with 0.02 mg/lb atropine intramuscularly to prevent the following:

        (1) Bradycardia

        (2) Salivation

        (3) Bronchial secretions

    e. Administer slowly, to effect (over a 2-minute period). Rapid intravenous injection may cause bradycardia, tachycardia, or cardiovascular collapse.

    f. No cumulative effects occur with repeated administration.

  3. Physiologic effects

    a. Respiratory effects

        (1) *d*-Tubocurarine has no effect on the respiratory center.

        (2) Respiratory arrest is due to muscle paralysis.

        (3) It may increase bronchial and salivary secretions.

    b. Cardiovascular effects

        (1) *d*-Tubocurarine may produce bradycardia or tachycardia.

        (2) It has no significant effects on the myocardium.

        (3) It can produce hypotension as a result of ganglionic blockade and histamine release.

    c. Liver and kidney effects

(1) A small portion of *d*-tubocurarine is metabolized by the liver.

(2) The majority of the drug is excreted unchanged in the urine.

(3) It has no direct effect on hepatic or renal function.

d. CNS Effects

(1) It produces no CNS depression or change in the electroencephalogram.

(2) *It produces no analgesia or anesthesia.*

4. The effects of *d*-tubocurarine can be antagonized by edrophonium or neostigmine.

B. Gallamine (Flaxedil)

1. The action of gallamine is similar to that of *d*-tubocurarine.

2. Dose, duration of action, and route of administration

a. Gallamine is one fifth as potent as *d*-tubocurarine in producing neuromuscular blockade, and its duration of action is shorter.

b. Its latency period (time until onset of maximum paralysis) is 2–4 minutes.

c. Doses (intravenous)

(1) Dog—0.2–0.5 mg/lb (paralysis lasts 15–30 minutes)

(2) Cat—0.5–0.6 mg/lb (paralysis lasts 10–20 minutes)

d. Repeated doses may result in cumulative effects.

e. If repeated doses are needed, administer no more than half of the preceding dose.

3. Physiologic effects

a. Respiratory effects

(1) Gallamine has no effect on the respiratory center except in massive overdose, and then it causes depression.

(2) Respiratory arrest is due to muscle paralysis.

(3) Secretions continue but are not increased.

b. Cardiovascular effects

(1) Gallamine causes some vagal blockade and therefore bradycardia.

(2) It has no significant effects on the myocardium or electrocardiogram.

(3) It does not cause histamine release.

(4) It rarely causes a fall in arterial blood pressure in the dog.

(5) Transient decreases in blood pressure have been observed in the cat.

c. Liver and kidney effects

(1) Gallamine is excreted unchanged by the kidneys.

(2) It has no direct effect on hepatic or renal function.

d. CNS effects

(1) Gallamine's effects are similar to those of *d*-tubocurarine.

(2) It does not readily cross the blood-brain barrier.

(3) *It produces no analgesia or anesthesia.*

4. The effects of gallamine can be antagonized by edrophonium and neostigmine.

C. Pancuronium (Pavulon)

1. The action of pancuronium is similar to that of *d*-tubocurarine.

2. Dose, duration of action, and route of administration

a. Its latency period (time until onset of maximum paralysis) is 30–90 seconds.

b. The intravenous dose in the dog is 0.01–0.03 mg/lb (paralysis lasts 20–100 minutes).

c. The intravenous dose in the cat is 0.01 mg/lb (paralysis lasts 15–20 minutes).

d. If repeated doses are needed, administer no more than half of the preceding dose.

3. Physiologic effects

a. Respiratory effects

(1) Respiratory arrest occurs as a result of muscle paralysis produced by pancuronium.

(2) It does not produce bronchospasm or bronchoconstriction.

(3) Increased salivation may occur.

b. Cardiovascular effects

(1) Pancuronium may cause an increased heart rate, which is most likely due to a vagolytic affect.

(2) The cardiac output may increase as a result of the increased heart rate.

(3) Blood pressure is either unaffected or increases only slightly.

(4) Pancuronium does not cause histamine release and does not produce sympathetic ganglionic blockade.

c. Liver and kidney effects

(1) Approximately 30% of pancuronium undergoes hepatic metabolism.

(2) The remainder of the drug is excreted unchanged via the kidneys.

(3) No prolongation of the neuromuscular block appears to occur in patients with hepatic or renal dysfunction.

(4) It has no direct effect on hepatic or renal function.

d. CNS effects

(1) Pancuronium's effects are similar to those of d-tubocurarine.

(2) It does not readily cross the blood-brain barrier.

(3) *It produces no analgesia or anesthesia.*

4. The effects of pancuronium can be antagonized by edrophonium and neostigmine.

D. Atracurium (Tracrium)

1. The action of atracurium is similar to that of d-tubocurarine.

2. Dose, duration of action, and route of administration

a. Its latency period (time until onset of maximum paralysis) is 3–5 minutes.

b. The intravenous dose in the dog and cat is 0.05 to 0.1 mg/lb (paralysis lasts 20–45 minutes).

c. Because of its unique metabolism, atracurium can be administered in repeated doses or as an infusion without residual effects.

(1) Infusion of atracurium is started by giving a loading dose of 0.1 mg/lb intravenously.

(2) The constant infusion is started approximately 5–10 minutes later at a rate of 0.0015–0.004 mg/lb per minute.

(3) The infusion rate is adjusted to the individual patient.

      (4) Atracurium infusion has been used during anesthesia and in ICU patients needing long-term controlled ventilation (adequate analgesia and sedation must be provided to the patient).

  3. Atracurium metabolism

    a. Atracurium has a unique metabolism. It does not depend entirely on hepatic metabolism or renal excretion.

    b. At normal physiologic temperature and pH, atracurium is metabolized by an extrahepatic process known as the Hofmann elimination. Approximately 40% of the injected dose is eliminated by Hofmann degradation. The remainder is metabolized via other pathways.

    c. Atracurium can be given repeatedly or as an infusion because it has no cumulative effects.

    d. Hypothermia and acidemia will prolong its effects.

    e. Alkalemia will decrease its effects.

  4. Physiologic effects

    a. Respiratory effects

      (1) Respiratory arrest occurs as a result of muscle paralysis caused by atracurium.

      (2) It may cause bronchospasm or bronchoconstriction in the dog because of histamine release.

    b. Cardiovascular effects

      (1) Atracurium causes minimal to no cardiovascular effects.

      (2) Although it causes release of small quantities of histamine, the amount is probably not significant at clinically used doses.

      (3) When hypotension has been reported following atracurium use, it has been attributed to histamine release.

    c. Liver and kidney effects

      (1) Renal or hepatic dysfunction do not seem to prolong the effects of atracurium.

      (2) It has no direct effect on hepatic or renal function.

    d. CNS effects

      (1) Atracurium's effects are similar to those of *d*-tubocurarine.

      (2) Laudanosine is a metabolite of atracurium that easily crosses the blood-brain barrier and can cause CNS stimulation.

      (3) *Atracurium produces no analgesia or anesthesia.*

X. Neuromuscular blocking agent antagonists

  A. Depolarizing blocking agents *cannot* be effectively antagonized. The use of cholinesterase inhibitors will intensify and prolong the duration of block of the depolarizing blocking agents.

  B. The nondepolarizing blocking agents can be antagonized by using cholinesterase inhibitors.

  C. Neostigmine (Prostigmin)

    1. Mechanism of action

      a. Neostigmine inhibits the production of cholinesterase and thus allows acetylcholine to accumulate.

      b. Because the nondepolarizing blocking agents are competitive with acetylcholine, the increased concentrations of acetylcholine will decrease the intensity of the neuromuscular block.

      c. Neostigmine will produce a more rapid and complete antagonism if some spontaneous muscular movements are already present in the patient.

    d. It may fail to antagonize a nondepolarizing agent when there are large amounts of the nondepolarizing blocking agent still present. Conditions that may lead to this failure include the following:

      (1) Overdosage of the nondepolarizing neuromuscular blocker

      (2) Factors that delay metabolism or excretion of the nondepolarizing neuromuscular blocker, including hepatic or renal dysfunction

      (3) Hypothermia

      (4) Acid-base imbalance

      (5) Decreased plasma proteins

  2. Neostigmine is administered at a dose of 0.02 mg/lb intravenously.

    a. Antagonism should occur within 2–4 minutes.

    b. If the initial dose does not produce antagonism, additional doses of 0.02 mg/lb may be given; however, *do not* exceed a total administered dose of 0.06 mg/lb.

  3. Because neostigmine is a cholinesterase inhibitor, it will produce parasympathetic effects including the following:

    a. Bradycardia

    b. Increased salivation

    c. Increased gastrointestinal motility and secretions

    d. Miosis

  4. In order to prevent the preceding adverse side effects, always administer 0.01 mg/lb atropine intravenously 1–2 minutes prior to administering the neostigmine.

  5. Patients must be watched closely after a nondepolarizing block has been antagonized with neostigmine in the event reparalyzation should occur, requiring that additional neostigmine be given.

D. Edrophonium (Tensilon)

  1. Edrophonium is a very rapid and short-acting anticholinesterase.

  2. It has been used as a test for residual nondepolarizing neuromuscular blockade.

  3. Edrophonium's duration of action is too brief for it to be used clinically as an antagonist.

E. Doxapram (Dopram) test

  1. Doxapram is a CNS and respiratory stimulant used to test for residual neuromuscular blockade.

  2. A dose of 1–2 mg/lb is administered intravenously.

    a. If there are no respiratory movements, the patient is most likely apneic because of residual neuromuscular blockade.

    b. If there are respiratory movements, the apnea is due to a level of anesthesia that is too deep.

IX. Monitoring neuromuscular function following neuromuscular block

A. Whenever possible, neuromuscular function should be monitored following the use of neuromuscular blockers.

B. Neuromuscular function is monitored to determine the following:

  1. The quantity of neuromuscular blocker required to produce the desired muscle relaxation

  2. When and if an antagonist should be administered

3. When adequate muscle function has returned for spontaneous breathing and recovery
C. The simplest method for determining neuromuscular function is to electrically stimulate a peripheral nerve and evaluate the evoked muscle contraction.
1. Many small, hand-held nerve stimulators are available for monitoring neuromuscular blockade.
2. A nerve stimulator should be able to deliver various patterns of nerve stimulation, including a single stimulus, a tetanic stimulus, a train-of-four stimulus and a double-burst stimulus.
3. The ulnar, peroneal, and tibial nerves have been used in the dog and cat to monitor neuromuscular function.

Suggested Readings

Bowman WC: Neuromuscular block and its antagonism: Basic concepts. In JF Nung, JE Utting, BR Brown (eds): General Anesthesia, 5th ed. London: Butterworth, 1989.
Cullen LK: Muscle relaxants and neuromuscular block. In JC Thurmon, WJ Tranquilli, GJ Benson (eds): Lumb and Jones' Veterinary Anesthesia, 3rd ed. Baltimore: Williams & Wilkins, 1996.
Hughes R, Chapple DJ: The pharmacology of atracurium: A new competitive neuromuscular blocking agent. Br J Anaesth 53:31, 1981.
Hunter JM: Adverse effects of neuromuscular blocking drugs. Br J Anaesth 59:46, 1987.
Jones RS: New skeletal muscle relaxants in dogs and cats. J Am Vet Med Assoc 187:281, 1985.
Klein LV: Neuromuscular blocking agents. In Short CE (ed): Principles and Practice of Veterinary Anesthesia. Baltimore: Williams & Wilkins, 1987.
Klein L, Beck E, Hopkins J, Burton B: Characteristics of neuromuscular blockade by gallamine, pancuronium and vecuronium (Org N C 45) and antagonism with neostigmine in anesthetized horses. Proc Assoc Vet Anaesth Gr Br Jr 10:173, 1982.
Miller RD, Savarese JJ: Pharmacology of muscle relaxants and their antagonists. In RD Miller (ed): Anesthesia, 3rd ed. New York: Churchill Livingstone, 1990.
Standaert FG: Neuromuscular physiology. In RD Miller (ed): Anesthesia, 3rd ed. New York: Churchill Livingstone, 1990.

Anesthetic Equipment

Chapter

5

Sandee M. Hartsfield

I. Introduction

   A. Inhalant anesthetics are delivered to patients via the respiratory system. Various techniques and equipment have facilitated the delivery of inhalant anesthesia since the introduction of ether and nitrous oxide (N_2O) in the mid nineteenth century, but this discussion will focus on current equipment and procedures that are generally accepted as safe both for patients and anesthesia personnel.

   B. Most inhalant anesthetics (desflurane, enflurane, halothane, isoflurane, methoxyflurane, sevoflurane) are liquids and are vaporized for delivery. Oxygen (O_2) and N_2O are gases at normal temperatures and pressures. Modern anesthesia machines and breathing systems control the delivery of inhalant anesthetics and O_2 and eliminate waste gases from the environment of the operating room.

II. The anesthesia machine

   A. An anesthesia machine is designed to deliver a precise yet variable mixture of inhalant anesthetic and O_2 to the breathing system and to the patient. Anesthesia machines for human and veterinary patients have been described in detail.[1-5]

   B. Components of an anesthesia machine include sources, regulators, and flowmeters for medical gases, plus one or more vaporizers for volatile liquid anesthetics (Fig. 5–1). Although most anesthesia machines incorporate a circle breathing system, other breathing systems can be substituted.

   C. Medical gases

      1. An anesthesia machine is typically fitted for two sources of O_2, with a small cylinder attached at the hanger yoke and a pipeline inlet for the hospital's central O_2 system. Machines may have similar fittings for N_2O.

      2. Compressed-gas cylinders, rather than bulk sources of medical gases, supply O_2 and N_2O for most veterinary practices.

         a. Cylinders are made of steel, steel alloy, or aluminum and are strictly regulated by the Department of Transportation. Gas passes from the cylinder, through a brass valve body, to the regulator (Fig. 5–1). Cylinder sizes are designated alphabetically; "A" is the smallest. Cylinders are color-coded (green = O_2; blue = N_2O). A color-coded label displaying the name of the gas, the principal hazards associated with the cylinder and its contents, and the name and address of the manufacturer or distributor is required.[2]

         b. "H" and "E" cylinders contain 6900 L and 660 L of gaseous O_2, respectively. Similarly, "H" and "E" cylinders of N_2O contain 15,800 L and 1590 L, respectively. Service pressures for "H" cylinders of O_2 and N_2O are 2200 psi and 745 psi, respectively; for "E" cylinders, service pressures are 745 psi for N_2O and 1900 psi for O_2. The service pressure is the maximum filling pressure at 70°F.[1] Generally, on the basis of cost per liter, medical gases are more economically supplied in larger cylinders.

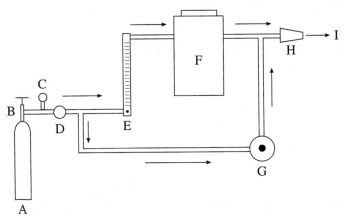

Figure 5–1. Diagram of the basic parts of a simple anesthesia machine. Upstream from D is the high-pressure (200–2200 psi) part of the machine. Downstream from D and upstream from E and G is an area of intermediate pressure ($\approx$ 50 psi). Downstream from E and G is the low-pressure area (minimal but variable pressure). Arrows show the direction of gas flow.
A = oxygen cylinder
B = oxygen cylinder valve
C = pressure gauge (indicates the pressure in the O_2 cylinder)
D = regulator
E = oxygen flowmeter (flow is continuous from A through D, E, and F to H as long is the flowmeter control valve is open and the source of O_2 has not been depleted)
F = VOC vaporizer
G = oxygen flush valve (gas flow from D through G to H occurs only when the flush valve is activated)
H = common gas outlet
I = to the breathing system

    c. The pressure in an O_2 cylinder is proportional to its contents, and the O_2 in a cylinder can be estimated by assessing the pressure in the cylinder. For example, 500 psi in an "E" cylinder indicates that about 25% of the original contents remain, $\approx$ 175 L.

    d. Full N_2O cylinders contain both liquid and gas. The content can be determined accurately only by weighing the cylinder.[2] When the pressure in the cylinder drops just below the service pressure (<745 psi), the content has been depleted by about 75%.

    e. Gases in cylinders are under high pressure and support combustion; explosion and fire are potential hazards. Therefore, cylinders should be handled carefully, secured properly (attached to machines, placed in storage racks, or secured to a wall by chains), and stored in a moderate ambient temperature. The cylinder valve should be turned "on" completely when the cylinder is in use. Hazards, precautions, and care and use of medical gas cylinders have been discussed in detail.[1, 2]

3. Bulk and bank sources of medical gases

    a. Bulk sources of O_2 and N_2O are delivered to various locations (station outlets) within a hospital through pipeline systems. Color-coded station outlets are fitted with noninterchangeable gas-specific connectors that accept only the appropriate high-pressure hose connectors from the pipeline inlet of an anesthesia machine. Diameter-indexed safety system (DISS) connectors or proprietary "quick connectors" may be used.[2]

    b. Bulk tanks of liquid O_2 are located outside a medical facility and are conveniently filled without movement of heavy cylinders.

A. Oral mucous membranes are blue or white.

B. Respiratory movements may or may not increase; the animal may begin to gasp.

C. The cardiovascular system is initially stimulated, resulting in tachycardia and hypertension. Prolonged or severe hypoxemia produces bradycardia and hypotension. EKG changes include reversed polarity of T waves with ST segment depression and slur.

IV. Causes

A. Low inspired oxygen concentration

1. Anesthesia machine malfunction: oxygen supply failure, broken or sticking flowmeter, disconnects, empty rebreathing bag, incorrect attachment of hoses

2. Nitrous oxide: accumulation in rebreathing circuit when low gas flows are used, decreased alveolar oxygen concentration during the first few minutes after nitrous oxide is discontinued (diffusion hypoxia phenomenon)

B. Hypoventilation

1. CNS depression: trauma, uremia, acidosis, opioids, anesthetic drugs

2. Mechanical impairment of ventilation: airway obstruction, external pressure on ribs, increased intra-abdominal pressure, increased pressure within the thorax from air or abdominal organs

C. Diffusion impairment: thickened alveolar blood gas barrier (interstitial pneumonia)

D. Ventilation-perfusion inequality

1. Alveolar collapse: general anesthesia, pneumothorax, pulmonary edema

2. Decreased cardiac output or excessive vasodilation: anesthetic drugs, other causes of hypotension

E. Shunt (blood perfusing nonventilated areas of lung): large areas of lung collapse, insertion of endotracheal tube beyond the carina into one bronchus, bronchial obstruction by secretions, severe pneumothorax, ruptured diaphragm

F. Hypotension.

G. Any combination of the preceding causes.

V. Treatment

A. Treat cardiac arrest (cardiopulmonary resuscitation).

B. Supply 100% oxygen by endotracheal tube. Check anesthesia machine for oxygen source, empty rebreathing bag, or closed pop-off valve.

C. Treat hypoventilation. Check for airway obstruction. Pneumothorax may develop unexpectedly during surgery of the neck, especially ventral decompression or tracheal surgery, or during exploratory laparotomy, especially during surgery around the liver.

D. Treat hypotension.

E. Use oxygen flow of at least 30 ml/kg per minute when including nitrous oxide.

F. Remove cause of hypoxemia.

Irregular Breathing

I. General considerations

A. Irregular breathing is an indication that respiratory control is impaired and that (1) large fluctuations in arterial carbon dioxide and oxygen concentrations, (2) increased carbon dioxide concentration, or (3) decreased oxygen concentration is probably occurring.

II. Clinical signs

A. Cheyne-Stokes breathing

1. Depth of breathing is at first shallow but becomes progressively deeper until definite hyperpnea is present. Breathing then gradually decreases and may cease before the pattern begins again. The cycle repeats every 45 seconds to 3 minutes.

B. Apneustic breathing

1. Prolonged end-inspiratory pauses of several seconds' duration (lungs remain inflated longer than usual) are evident.

C. Cluster breathing

1. A disorderly breathing pattern is interrupted by non-regular pauses.

D. Biot breathing

1. An alternating pattern of several gasps and apnea is observed.

E. Ataxic breathing

1. Both rhythm and depth of breathing are irregular.

F. Kussmaul breathing

1. Regular deep breaths without a pause are observed.

III. Causes

A. Diseases altering respiratory control

1. Cheyne-Stokes breathing is attributed to asphyxia of the CNS and has been associated with congestive heart failure, uremia, and head injury.

2. Kussmaul breathing may be caused by severe respiratory acidosis.

B. Anesthetic drugs

1. Irregular breathing may occur in the otherwise normal animal from CNS depression caused by anesthetic drugs.

2. Barbiturate anesthesia decreases the sensitivity of the respiratory centers to carbon dioxide, resulting in apnea before sufficient carbon dioxide accumulates to stimulate several breaths. Irregular breathing may persist until blood barbiturate concentration decreases.

3. Ketamine anesthesia frequently causes apneustic breathing.

4. A deep plane of anesthesia (overdose) may be accompanied by irregular or labored breathing.

C. Increased intracranial pressure caused by trauma or cerebellar herniation can produce irregular breathing.

IV. Treatment

A. Increase inspired oxygen concentration.

B. Institute controlled ventilation if minute volume is moderately or severely decreased.

C. Improve cardiovascular function.

D. Decrease anesthetic drug administration.

E. See following section on labored breathing.

Labored Breathing

I. Clinical signs

A. Jerky breathing with excessively large thoracic excursions may result in either hypoventilation or hyperventilation and may immediately precede cardiac arrest.

II. Causes

  A. Increased work of breathing

    1. Resistance to flow of air in anesthesia machine, trachea, or bronchi

    2. Increased stiffness of lungs or chest wall

  B. Inadequate tissue oxygenation

    1. Decreased oxygen uptake (decreased pulmonary function, low cardiac output or blood pressure)

    2. Decreased blood oxygen content (insufficient hemoglobin to carry oxygen)

    3. Decreased oxygen delivery (decreased cardiovascular function, peripheral vasoconstriction)

  C. Stimulation of central respiratory center: pain, hypercarbia, metabolic acidosis, drugs (doxapram)

III. Differential diagnosis

  A. Airway obstruction: kinked anesthesia hose or endotracheal tube, tracheal foreign body, endobronchial intubation, endotracheal tube too small

  B. Bronchospasm: reflex, allergic, or caused by aspiration of gastric fluid

  C. Pneumothorax, pleural effusion

  D. Pulmonary edema, pulmonary embolism

  E. Partial curarization: neuromuscular blocking drugs

  F. Hypoxia: decreased cardiovascular function from deep anesthesia, gasping

  G. Hypercarbia: exhausted soda lime; malfunction of one-way valves of circle system, resulting in rebreathing; inner tube of Bain system disconnected, resulting in rebreathing

  H. Pain

  I. Hypotension

IV. Treatment

  A. Use endotracheal intubation.

  B. Use controlled ventilation with 100% oxygen.

  C. Check depth of anesthesia and adjust administration.

  D. Check that equipment is functioning correctly.

  E. Treat initiating cause.

Pneumothorax

I. General considerations

  A. The thorax of traumatized patients should be radiographed before anesthesia to identify preexisting pneumothorax and subpleural bullae or blebs. Nitrous oxide should not be used in these patients. During controlled ventilation, the peak inspiratory pressure should be kept below 25 cm H_2O if possible.

  B. Pneumothorax occurring during artificial ventilation may be the result of incorrect application or of rupture of diseased alveolae (pneumonia or pulmonary contusions).

    1. A *tension pneumothorax* develops when the site of air entry into the thorax acts as a one-way valve. Air enters the pleural cavity or mediastinum on inspiration but is trapped and does not leave during expiration. The size of the air pocket increases with time, progressively restricting

lung inflation. Hypercapnia and, ultimately, hypoxemia together with decreased stroke volume result in hypotension. In some animals with lung rupture, air embolism of the systemic arterial or venous system occurs.

II. Clinical signs
- A. Hypotension may be the first indication in an anesthetized patient.
- B. Increased amplitude of breathing may be seen in the spontaneously breathing animal.
- C. Greater resistance than normal may be seen when the rebreathing bag is manually compressed.
- D. Cyanosis of oral mucous membranes occurs if pneumothorax is severe.
- E. Thoracic cage does not collapse on expiration.
- F. Unilateral or bilateral loss of lung sounds is evident on auscultation.
- G. Subcutaneous emphysema occurs.
- H. Shift in cardiac apex beat occurs if pneumothorax is unilateral.

III. Causes
- A. Intrapulmonary alveolar rupture
  1. High airway pressure: overexpansion or too rapid expansion of lungs during controlled ventilation, use of the emergency oxygen flush with a non-rebreathing system
  2. Weakened alveolar wall: pulmonary contusions, pneumonia
- B. Visceral pleura rupture
  1. Rupture of subpleural bleb or bulla, penetration by end of a fractured rib, lung biopsy
  2. Esophageal damage: esophageal foreign body, esophagoscopy
- C. Parietal pleura injury
  1. Chest wall injury: penetrating dog-fight wounds, surgical excision of tumors or fistulous tracts, insertion of chest tubes
  2. Neck surgery: cervical fenestration, repair of collapsing trachea, tumor excision, tracheostomy
  3. Rupture of esophagus: esophagoscopy, passage of stomach tube
  4. Tearing of diaphragm during laparotomy: surgery in cranial abdomen, nephrectomy, lumbar fenestration
- D. Nitrous oxide expansion of an existing pneumothorax or pulmonary bulla
  1. Seeking equilibrium, nitrous oxide diffuses into air pockets, and nitrogen diffuses into blood. Nitrous oxide leaves the blood and enters the air space much faster than nitrogen leaves the air space and enters the blood, resulting in an increase in volume of the air space. A minimal pneumothorax will then become significant, and a bulla may rupture, creating a pneumothorax.

IV. Differential diagnosis
- A. Pneumothorax: suggested by clinical signs and confirmed by sound of gas escaping through a needle inserted into the pleural space, smell of halothane or isoflurane in escaping gas, or view on thoracic radiography
- B. Airway obstruction: deflate endotracheal tube cuff and change tube position to eliminate bronchial intubation or kinked tube as causes of clinical signs.
- C. Cardiovascular depression from anesthetic drugs: assess depth of anesthesia.

    D. Pulmonary edema: frothy fluid should be visible in the endotracheal tube when the condition is this severe, and fluid sounds should be audible via esophageal stethoscope or stethoscope.

    E. Bronchospasm: produces similar clinical signs and may be caused by anaphylaxis, aspiration of gastric fluid, pulmonary embolism

    F. Anesthetic circle malfunction (stuck one-way valves in circle system, disconnected tubing in Bain system) resulting in carbon dioxide present in inhaled gas and causing increased amplitude of breathing

V. Treatment

    A. Discontinue use of nitrous oxide, and supply 100% oxygen.

    B. Controlled ventilation is indicated in most cases.

    C. When pneumothorax develops during laparotomy, start controlled ventilation, suture diaphragm, then aspirate air from pleural cavity using a needle inserted through the diaphragm and attached to a three-way stopcock and large syringe.

    D. Immediate treatment of severe or tension pneumothorax is to insert wide-bore needle or catheter into pleural space.

    E. Insert chest tube drain if air leak continues.

VI. Chest tube placement

    A. The degree of preparation and the technique of tube placement will depend on the urgency of the patient's condition. The decision to place one or more tubes, dorsal or ventral, in the thoracic wall will be determined by the location of the largest volume of air and by whether fluid accumulation is also a problem.

    B. A variety of types of tubes are acceptable for use as chest tubes, and some commercially available thoracostomy tubes have a trocar for easier insertion.[1]

    C. Following is a description of one acceptable method of chest tube placement.

        1. Sterile technique should be used. The hair should be clipped from just caudal to the shoulder to the last rib and from the dorsal midline to the ventral midline. The skin should be prepared as for surgery. With the skin pulled cranially by an assistant, the seventh intercostal space should be identified by counting from the thirteenth rib (Fig. 8–5 A). A 2 cm skin incision should be made between the ribs at the point where the diameter of the chest is widest (point "x" in Fig. 8–5 A), avoiding the intercostal artery, vein, and nerve that lie on the caudal border of rib (Fig. 8–5 B, C). Metzenbaum scissors should be used for blunt dissection through intercostal muscle (Fig. 8–5 C, D) until the tips of the scissors penetrate the pleura (Fig. 8–5 E). Holding the scissors with two hands will provide greater control of the instrument so that it penetrates only a short distance into the pleural cavity (Fig. 8–5 E).

        2. The tip of the chest tube (Argyle) (with stopcock or valve attached to the opposite end) should be grasped with a curved Kelly forceps, and, as the Metzenbaum scissors are gradually withdrawn, the tube should be introduced through the previously made thoracostomy hole (Fig. 8–5 F). The Kelly forceps should then be withdrawn and the tube advanced into the chest in a cranial and slightly ventral direction. The skin should be allowed to return to its normal position (Fig. 8–5 G). The tube should be secured by a suture passed through the skin and deep into fascia and muscle and then tied around the tube using a

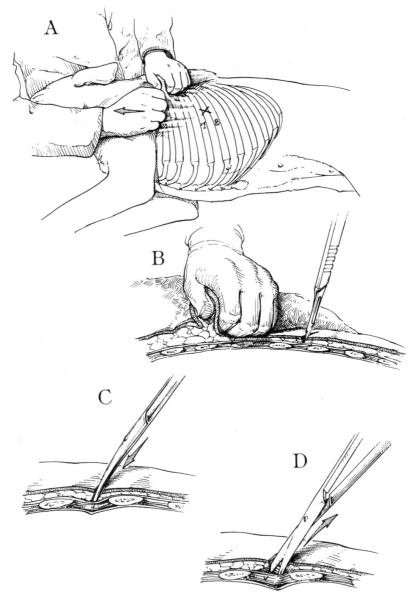

Figure 8–5. Placement of a chest tube: see text for description of technique. (From Crowe DT: The Surgical Laboratory, University of Georgia, 1986.)

friction suture pattern. Air may then be aspirated with a 60 ml syringe, or the tube may be attached to other equipment used for thoracic drainage.

Pulmonary Edema

I. Clinical signs
   A. Increased respiratory rate
   B. Labored breathing
   C. Hypoxemia

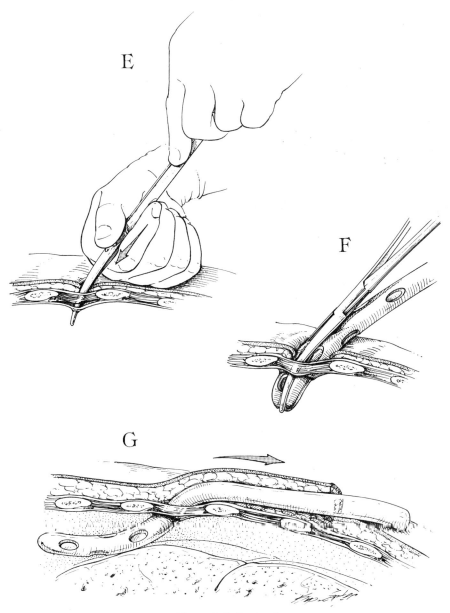

Figure 8–5 *Continued*

   D. Fluid sounds audible on auscultation of the lungs

   E. Froth in the endotracheal tube

II. Causes

   A. Increased pulmonary venous pressure

      1. Excessive intravenous infusion of fluid: lactated Ringer's solution, saline

      2. Infusion of more than 1 blood volume per hour to an anesthetized animal, unless severe fluid loss is continuing

      3. Ligation of a patent ductus arteriosus

      4. Cardiac failure

      5. Arterial hypertension

     6. Ketamine anesthesia, especially in cats

     7. Mannitol administration with renal failure

   B. Increased capillary-alveolar permeability

     1. Sepsis or endotoxemia

     2. Pancreatitis

     3. Aspiration of gastric fluid

     4. Prolonged hypotension

     5. Fat embolism

     6. Head trauma

   C. Decreased serum osmotic pressure: hypoproteinemia

   D. Lymphatic obstruction: neoplasia

III. Diagnosis

   A. Obvious associated temporal event, such as surgery for patent ductus arteriosus, manipulation of ischemic intestine, regurgitation and aspiration

   B. History of preexisting cardiac disease

   C. Evaluation of the cardiovascular system: arterial pressure, central venous pressure, EKG

   D. Measurement of plasma protein or albumin concentration

IV. Treatment

   A. Intubate trachea, and supply 100% oxygen.

   B. Institute controlled ventilation if necessary.

   C. Apply positive end-expiratory pressure (PEEP) of 5–10 cm H_2O as needed to keep the arterial P_{O_2} above 60 mm Hg. In the absence of a specific PEEP valve, take the following steps:

     1. If the patient is on a non-rebreathing anesthetic circuit, the expiratory limb of the circuit should be positioned 5–10 cm below the surface of water in a container.

     2. If the patient is on a circle circuit, the pop-off valve can be partially closed until the pressure required to open it (as observed on the circle pressure gauge) is 5 cm H_2O (3.8 mm Hg).

   D. Determine cause and treat appropriately.

   E. Treat cardiac dysrhythmias.

   F. Decrease pulmonary pressure by administering furosemide (Lasix) 2.5 mg/kg intravenously.

   G. If the cardiac output is assessed to be low, infuse dobutamine or dopamine 3–7 μg/kg per minute.

   H. If hypotension is present, expand intravascular volume with crystalloid solution, and treat patient with dobutamine or dopamine.

   I. Administer antibiotics if sepsis or endotoxin release is suspected.

   J. Administer corticosteroids if the cause is suspected to be fat embolism.

     1. The use of corticosteroids in other forms of pulmonary edema is controversial.

Tachypnea

I. General considerations

   A. Panting in dogs is a common side effect of administration of opioids and is frequently seen with the use of oxymorphone and meperidine, less frequently with butorphanol. The panting is the result of CNS stimulation;

arterial P_{O_2} may remain normal. When the opioid is administered by intravenous injection, panting is less likely to occur if the drug is injected slowly over several minutes. Deep halothane anesthesia is often accompanied by a high respiratory rate, especially in cats and small dogs.

II. Clinical signs

    A. Rapid, shallow breathing occurs.

    B. Plane of anesthesia may remain light during inhalation anesthesia if panting produces hypoventilation.

III. Causes

    A. Anesthetic drugs: opioids, halothane

    B. High inspired carbon dioxide: exhausted soda lime, one-way valves in a circle system absent or malfunctioning

    C. Hyperthermia: excessive application of external heat, anesthetic drug-induced impairment of thermoregulation, septicemia, malignant hyperthermia

IV. Diagnostic approach

    A. History

        1. Panting caused by opioids usually begins soon after their administration.

        2. Hypercarbia from exhausted soda lime or malfunctioning one-way valves may not develop until anesthesia has progressed for 1 or more hours.

        3. Hyperthermia may occur rapidly, or it may not develop until 1–2 hours of anesthesia have elapsed.

    B. Monitoring

        1. Tachypnea can occur at both light and deep planes of anesthesia.

        2. It can be difficult to assess adequacy of ventilation without measurement of end-tidal C_{O_2} or blood gas analysis. Hypoventilation should be suspected when a dog appears to be inadequately anesthetized despite administration of a usually adequate concentration of halothane or isoflurane. In this case, controlled ventilation should be instituted.

        3. Hypoventilation should be suspected and controlled ventilation instituted when a dog is at risk for inadequate ventilation (overweight, prone position, geriatric) and appears deeply anesthetized.

        4. Although cardiovascular parameters may be normal when tachypnea is caused by anesthetic drugs, nonspecific signs of hypercarbia are bright-red mucous membranes, high heart rate or blood pressure, and premature ventricular contractions.

        5. Check movement of one-way valves in circle circuit.

        6. Hyperthermia is confirmed by an increased rectal temperature of more than 39.2°C (102.5°F). Malignant hyperthermia should be suspected when the color indicator in the carbon dioxide absorber changes rapidly to an intense color and the canister is very hot to touch.

    C. Treatment

        1. Drug-induced hyperpnea is usually controlled by artificial ventilation. In some cases, reversal of an opioid with naloxone may be appropriate.

        2. Anesthesia equipment should be checked. Any soda lime canister in which the indicator has changed color to half its capacity should have the exhausted soda lime replaced.

        3. Hyperthermia should be treated as described elsewhere.

CARDIOVASCULAR EMERGENCIES AND COMPLICATIONS

Air Embolism

I. General considerations

   A. Air embolism of the systemic *arterial* system usually occurs during cardiopulmonary bypass procedures or thoracic trauma. It may result in embolism of the coronary circulation, which may be fatal, or of the cerebral circulation, which may cause neurologic deficit.

   B. Air embolism of the *venous* and pulmonary circulation is more common, and the clinical signs depend on the volume and rate of embolization and the composition of inhaled gases.

      1. Bubbles collect in the ventricle and obstruct flow into the pulmonary artery. Hypotension and dysrhythmias may follow. Bubbles leaving the heart enter and obstruct the pulmonary arterioles. The bubbles last for up to 15 minutes and gradually diffuse into solution.

      2. Usually small amounts of air have no clinical significance, but that cannot be guaranteed, as intravenous injection of only 5 ml of air has caused cardiac arrest in a 15 kg dog. In an experimental investigation of venous air embolism in dogs, injection of 0.5 ml air/kg resulted in decreased mean arterial pressure when the dogs were breathing 50% nitrous oxide.

II. Clinical signs

   A. Hypotension

   B. Dysrhythmias

   C. Tachypnea

   D. Hypoxemia

   E. EKG changes

   F. Cardiac arrest

III. Causes

   A. Intravenous injection: air bubbles in a syringe, failure to eliminate air from an infusion set, pressurized fluid or blood transfusions

   B. Incision in a vein above the level of the heart: any surgical site above heart level, especially when made during neurosurgery (craniotomy, laminectomy, fenestration); incision of the brachial vein before ligation during forelimb amputation; central venous catheterization

   C. Thoracic trauma: open chest wounds, thoracentesis

   D. Gas insufflation: pneumoperitoneoscopy (laparoscopy), pneumocystoscopy

IV. Diagnosis

   A. Air embolism in dogs may present as abrupt cessation of peripheral pulse in the presence of a normal EKG. A hand placed on the chest can feel the heart beating.

   B. Other causes of absent pulse should be ruled out, such as pressure by the surgeon on the caudal vena cava during laparotomy or increased intrathoracic pressure due to a closed pop-off valve. The diagnosis of air embolism should not be arrived at until other possible causes have been ruled out.

   C. Postmortem diagnosis of cardiac arrest from massive air embolism is confirmed by radiography of the thorax and cranial abdomen.

   D. Monitoring end-expired carbon dioxide concentration (capnography)

      1. An abrupt decrease in end-expired carbon dioxide concentration will occur when air enters the pulmonary circulation and obstructs the

capillaries. This decrease can be differentiated from decreased cardiac output in that the latter is a more gradual change. This method of monitoring will detect air embolism before major cardiovascular changes are produced.

E. Auscultation of a change in heart sounds
  1. Introduction of a small volume of air produces a tympanic quality. With increasing volumes of air, a soft but coarse systolic murmur develops, followed by a progressively louder murmur that eventually can be heard during both systole and diastole. This method of monitoring may be useful for diagnosis but will give little warning of cardiovascular collapse.

F. Monitoring reflected ultrasound by placing a Doppler flowmeter on the chest wall directly over the right heart
  1. Small volumes of air produce a change in sound, provided that the probe is correctly placed. Correct placement of the Doppler probe can be assisted by introduction of a catheter via the jugular vein into the right atrium. An audible swishing sound on the Doppler monitor when saline is forcefully injected through the catheter confirms correct placement.

G. Aspiration of air from a catheter with the tip in the right atrium

H. Observation of bubbles entering the circulation from an infusion set, followed closely by decreased cardiovascular function

V. Treatment
  A. Prevent further aspiration of air by rapidly increasing venous pressure with positive pressure ventilation, digital occlusion of the jugular veins, or rapid infusion of intravenous fluids.
  B. Discontinue nitrous oxide administration to prevent expansion of the air bubbles.
  C. A catheter may be inserted into the right atrium from the jugular vein (under fluoroscopy or by measuring venous pressures if time allows) and used to aspirate air trapped in the heart.
  D. Administer symptomatic treatment of the cardiovascular system. Administration of vasopressors will also encourage air to move out of the heart

Bradycardia (Sinus Bradycardia)

I. Clinical signs
  A. Heart rate of less than 65 beats per minute in dogs
  B. Heart rate of less than 80 beats per minute in cats
  C. Hypotension may or may not be present.

I. Causes
  A. CNS depression
    1. Anesthetic drugs, especially opioids, xylazine, medetomidine
    2. Increased intracranial pressure
    3. Hypothermia
  B. Cardiovascular failure: hypoxemia, decreased venous return, bacterial endocarditis, cardiomyopathy, hyperkalemia, congenital heart disease
  C. Vagal reflex: traction on viscera, pressure on eye, stimulation of the pharynx or larynx

II. Treatment
  A. Determine and treat cause of bradycardia.

B. Expand blood volume by intravenous infusion of balanced electrolyte solution.

C. Drugs can be used specifically to increase heart rate.

  1. Atropine 0.02 mg/kg intravenously or glycopyrrolate 0.005 mg/kg intravenously; repeat in 5 minutes if necessary

  2. Dopamine infusion (50 mg in 500 ml 0.9% saline produces 100 μg/ml solution) infused intravenously at 5–7 μg/kg per minute

  3. Isoproterenol drip (0.2 mg in 500 ml 5% dextrose in water) given intravenously to effective dose

D. External cardiac massage may be necessary when the heart rate decreases below 20 beats per minute.

E. Treat hyperkalemia.

F. Transvenous pacing is used for "sick sinus syndrome" (severe sinus bradycardia).

Cardiac Arrest: Asystole, Ventricular Fibrillation, Pulseless Electrical Activity

I. General considerations

  A. Mistakes sometimes occur during use of anesthesia. Surveys of human anesthesia records have shown that when deaths from mistakes occur, they are usually the result of not one but multiple errors. Factors quoted as frequently associated with preventable anesthetic mishaps follow:

    1. Failure to take proper history

    2. Inadequate anesthesia experience or ignorance of anesthetic pharmacology and drug interactions

    3. Inadequate familiarity with equipment

    4. Haste, fatigue, or inattentiveness to the patient

  B. It was also observed that many problems occurred during the middle of surgical procedures, and it was suggested that devices be used to improve monitoring. In veterinary practice, if an EKG or blood pressure monitor is available, it should be attached to all anesthetized patients, not just those considered to be a high risk. Equipment to monitor arterial pressure is inexpensive and frequently provides an early warning of a problem, before changes in heart rate and respiratory rate occur.

  C. With increased monitoring of the anesthetized patient, the incidence of cardiac arrest during anesthesia is small. Nonetheless, every member of the operating room staff must be familiar with the treatment plan, because delays will result in failure to resuscitate the patient.

II. Clinical signs of impending cardiac arrest

  A. Progressive and persistent tachycardia or bradycardia

  B. A decrease in systolic blood pressure below 70 mm Hg (blood pressure as low as 50 mm Hg can be palpated) or decrease in sound intensity from a Doppler probe placed over a metacarpal or metatarsal artery

  C. Capillary refill time of 2 seconds or longer

  D. Change in spontaneous breathing pattern to an irregular rhythm, sometimes labored

  E. Pale mucous membranes, cyanosis

  F. Darkening of blood oozing at the incision

  G. Cardiac arrest occurring abruptly, without warning

  H. Eye central, cornea dry, pupils dilated; note that corneal reflex may not disappear and pupils may not dilate maximally until some time after the cardiac arrest

III. Causes

    A. Direct myocardial depression

        1. Anesthetic drugs

        2. Hypoxemia

        3. Hypercarbia

        4. Metabolic acidosis

        5. Endotoxin

        6. Vasoactive substances released from an inflamed pancreas

    B. Decreased venous return

        1. Hemorrhage

        2. Hypovolemia

        3. Postural change (lateral to lateral or lateral to dorsal)

        4. Vasodilation (release of vasoactive substances by manipulation of a carcinoma of the gastrointestinal tract or bronchi, anaphylactic shock from injection of anesthetic agent or antibiotic, progressive hypotension induced by injection of an antibiotic)

    C. Cardiac dysrhythmias

        1. Bradycardia (traction on viscera or manipulation of the eye)

        2. Tachyarrhythmias (myocardial contusions, preanesthetic excitement)

IV. Diagnosis

    A. Pulse or blood pressure is absent. "False arrest" may occur if an EKG lead slips or blood pressure probe moves. These events should be identified quickly. If the abdomen or thorax is open, palpation of the aorta or a large artery will confirm or exclude cardiac arrest.

    B. Respiratory arrest usually precedes cardiac arrest. Before respiratory arrest, the breathing pattern may alter. Cyanosis may not be present at the time of cardiac arrest. If the patient is connected to an anesthesia machine, the equipment should be quickly checked for disconnections, obstructions, and adequate oxygen flow. The anesthesia circuit should be smelled for excessive concentration of anesthetic. The rebreathing bag should be compressed to check that the lungs inflate easily.

    C. The EKG recording of asystole or ventricular fibrillation should be checked. No electrical activity in the heart during asystole will result in a flat line on the EKG. Ventricular fibrillation is asynchronous depolarization of ventricular myofibrils and is identified by a coarse or fine wavy line on the EKG (Fig. 8–6). The presence of a relatively normal EKG complex when the systolic blood pressure is below 40 mm Hg is termed *pulseless electrical activity* (previously known as *electromechanical dissociation*).

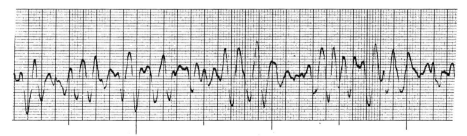

Figure 8–6. Ventricular fibrillation.

V. Treatment: cardiopulmonary resuscitation
  A. Call for help, and note the time.
  B. Intubate trachea, or discontinue anesthetic administration. Flush anesthesia circuit with oxygen.
  C. Institute artificial ventilation, 10–12 breaths per minute, 15–20 cm H_2O inspiratory pressure, using 100% oxygen and an anesthesia machine or a resuscitator bag. Ventilation can be effective for a short time by blowing down an endotracheal tube.
  D. Provide external cardiac massage, 100 compressions per minute.
    1. Insert a catheter or needle into a vein, and expand blood volume by rapid infusion of lactated Ringer's (or similar) solution, initially 10–20 ml/kg infused as rapidly as possible.
    2. Have an assistant feel for the femoral pulse. Alternatively, a Doppler probe can be placed over the lingual artery or inserted under the third eyelid to give an audible monitor of peripheral blood flow. If the pulse is absent, change site of compression for more effective massage. Presence of a pulse does not guarantee cerebral perfusion. Administration of epinephrine or dopamine is usually necessary to cause peripheral vasoconstriction and redirect blood flow to brain.
  E. Internal cardiac massage should be performed if external massage cannot be accomplished effectively, which may be the case in dogs of more than 20 kg body weight, in patients with chest wall injury or intrathoracic pathologic condition, and in patients who have undergone a thoracotomy. Decision to perform internal cardiac massage should be made within 15 minutes of cardiac arrest—earlier in large dogs.
  F. Examine electrocardiogram.
    1. *Flat line (asystole)*
      a. Dose of epinephrine is controversial. Author's preference is to use a low dose for the first injection, but to follow with a high dose if the heart does not resume beating in 2 minutes. Low-dose epinephrine is 10 μg/kg—that is, 0.1 ml/10 kg of undiluted 1:1,000 (1 mg/ml) solution of epinephrine or 1 ml of epinephrine diluted with 9 ml of saline and injected as 1 ml/10 kg intravenously or intratracheally.
      b. Intratracheal injection of epinephrine should be washed down the endotracheal tube with a few milliliters of saline.
      c. Increase the dose of epinephrine to 0.5–1.0 ml/10 kg (undiluted 1 mg/ml) if the first dose is unsuccessful.
      d. Thereafter, repeat low-dose epinephrine (10–20 μg/kg) every 4–5 minutes as necessary.
      e. An alternative recommendation for maintenance dose of epinephrine is to use 0.1 μg/kg per minute, given as an infusion by adding 1 ml undiluted epinephrine to 1 liter of lactated Ringer's solution and infusing the mixture at 1 ml/10 kg per minute.[2] Inject atropine 0.02 mg/kg.
      f. When cardiac arrest has resulted from a body position change, cardiac rhythm can be restored satisfactorily by substituting dopamine infusion of 7–10 μg/kg per minute for injection of epinephrine. Renal failure is less likely to result from dopamine than epinephrine administration.
      g. Epinephrine, atropine, dopamine, lactated Ringer's solution, sodium bicarbonate, and other drugs can be given through an interosseous needle and will be absorbed within seconds. Do not give drugs by intracardiac injection, except as a last resort, as it may stimulate the

myocardium to change asystole to fibrillation, cause myocardial or coronary vessel damage, or damage the conduction system.

   2. *Asynchronous activity (ventricular fibrillation)*

      a. Small animals may spontaneously defibrillate with ventilation and cardiac massage. Cardioversion (DC electrical defibrillation) should be attempted immediately in medium to large dogs (see section VIII). Start external cardiac massage immediately if time must elapse before the defibrillator can be brought to the patient. Chemical defibrillation with acetylcholine chloride 6 mg/kg or acetylcholine 6 mg/kg and potassium citrate or chloride 1 mg/kg can be tried if cardioversion is not an option.

   3. *EKG normal but no pulse*

      a. Start an infusion of dopamine 7–10 µg/kg per minute. Continue cardiac massage. Inject atropine 0.02–.04 mg/kg intravenously if heart rate is slow.

G. Continue cardiac massage for several minutes after the heart resumes beating. Continue artificial ventilation and circulatory support with dopamine or dobutamine at 5 µg/kg per minute. After 10 minutes, infuse sodium bicarbonate 1.5 mEq/kg. If pH and blood gas analysis is available, collect an arterial or venous blood sample for measurement of base deficit. Administer further sodium bicarbonate based on the results.

H. Administer corticosteroids: prednisolone sodium succinate (Solu-Delta-Cortef) or methyl prednisolone sodium succinate (Solu-Medrol) 30 mg/kg and dexamethasone sodium phosphate 5 mg/kg intravenously.

 I. Administer deferoxamine (Desferal) 30 mg/kg intramuscularly to minimize ischemia or reperfusion-induced injury.

 J. Evaluate fluid balance. Diuresis may be necessary to eliminate excessive fluid load. Renal failure may develop as a result of ischemia.

VI. External cardiac massage

A. The dog should be turned onto its right side and a pad placed under its thorax. The resuscitator should face the spine of the animal during cardiac massage and use his or her body to immobilize the patient.

B. Alternatively, the resuscitator can stand on the sternal side of the patient, and the animal's spine can be stabilized by a second person or a solid object.

C. External lateral compression should be applied to the chest between the fourth and sixth ribs, one third of the distance up the chest, at a rate of 100 per minute. The palms of both hands should be used together, with the weight of the operators' shoulders included in the force of massage for a big dog. The compressions should be smooth and regular, with a 1:1 time ratio between compression and relaxation, and with complete release between compressions (no pressure on the chest) to allow flow of blood into the heart. The rhythm of massage should not be interrupted; inflation of the lungs should be interposed between compressions.

D. If one person only is available to ventilate and apply cardiac massage, it is usual to follow a sequence of 2 breaths, 20 compressions, 2 breaths, 20 compressions, and so on.

E. Interposed abdominal compression with thoracic pressure may increase cerebral blood flow. Care must be taken to avoid pressure around the liver that may cause liver damage during massage. Outcome studies reveal no differences in survival rate at 24 hours from CPR including abdominal compression over standard CPR.

F. Binding of the abdomen and hindlimbs is not recommended as it decreases blood flow through the heart by increasing intracranial pressure and right atrial pressure.

G. External cardiac massage can also be performed with the dog on its back and the resuscitator facing the dog's head. Massage is accomplished with one hand on either side of the chest, fingers interlocking across the sternum, and pressure applied with the heel of the hand. For the pressure to be applied at the correct site in large dogs, a 4–6 inch strip of rope or canvas, with a loop on either end for handholds, should be substituted for interlocking fingers.

H. Adequate cardiac massage can be accomplished in small dogs and cats using one hand, with the thumb placed on the left side and the fingers on the right side of the chest. The other hand is laid alongside the spine to support the body during massage.

VII. Internal cardiac massage

A. Time should not be wasted clipping hair and prepping the skin. A single sweep of the clippers may be satisfactory; hair of a long-haired dog may be parted and wetted.

B. The thorax should be entered on the left side at the fourth or fifth intercostal space. The pericardium should be incised longitudinally below the phrenic nerve and the ventricles massaged from the apex toward the base of the heart. The aorta may be cross-clamped or compressed with fingers during cardiac compression to improve coronary and cerebral blood flow. Pressure should be applied with the palmar surfaces of the fingers and palm(s), as pressure from the fingertips may lacerate the myocardium. The heart must be held in a relatively normal position to avoid kinking the vena cava and pulmonary veins.

C. After successful resuscitation, the pericardium may be left open, the thoracic cavity lavaged with warm saline, and the thoracotomy closed.

VIII. Cardioversion

A. With the animal on its back, one paddle (electrode) should be placed over the left sixth intercostal space near the sternum and the other more dorsally over the right fourth intercostal space. Saline or paste should be used for good contact, not alcohol. No one should touch any part of the animal, or the table, during application of current. Use 200–400 joules (watt/sec) for a large dog, 100–200 J (watt/sec) for a medium dog, and 50 J (watt/sec) for a small dog or a cat. The power should be less for cardioversion through a thoracotomy; 10 J (watt/sec) for a small dog, to 50 J (watt/sec) for a large dog.

B. When defibrillation is unsuccessful, ventilation and cardiac massage should be resumed, and epinephrine should be injected to coarsen the fibrillation. If sinus rhythm is restored but quickly relapses, inject lidocaine at 2 mg/kg before the next attempt. After several attempts, inject sodium bicarbonate at 1 mEq/kg to correct acidosis before the next attempt.

Dysrhythmias: General Considerations

Abnormalities of rate and rhythm existing before anesthesia induction should have been identified by the preanesthetic physical examination so that the most appropriate anesthetic management is chosen. Evaluation and treatment of dysrhythmias occurring during anesthesia should not be restricted to cardiac rhythm alone, but should include total assessment of the patient and anesthetic equipment. The following descriptions are intended to enable rapid identification of abnormal rhythm and selection of the most appropriate treatment.

Atrial Premature Depolarizations

I. Identification
  A. P wave occurs early, such that it may be obscured by previous QRST complex and may be inverted.
  B. These P waves are followed by normal QRST complexes.
  C. Beats may occur singly, in pairs, or in runs (paroxysmal atrial tachycardia).
II. Treatment
  A. Isolated atrial premature contractions do not require treatment if measurements of cardiovascular function are normal.
  B. Assess adequacy of ventilation and institute controlled ventilation if necessary.
  C. Improve cardiovascular status.
  D. The patient may be treated with propranolol if frequency of premature contractions is increasing despite conservative treatment.

Atrioventricular Heart Block

I. Definition: atrioventricular (AV) heart block is impaired conduction of electrical impulse through the AV node, bundle of His, or bundle branches.
II. Identification
  A. First-degree AV block is identified as prolongation of PR interval.
  B. Second-degree AV block consists of a P wave without a QRST complex (Fig. 8–7). This pattern may or may not be preceded by progressive prolongation of the PR interval.
  C. Advanced AV block consists of P waves only, no QRST waves.
  D. Third-degree AV block consists of QRS complexes unrelated to P waves; QRS complexes are abnormal, irregular, and less than 40 per minute.
III. Causes
  A. Degenerative disease: cardiac disease, myocardial contusions
  B. Infectious myocarditis
  C. Autonomic nervous system stimulation
    1. Painful procedures
    2. Dobutamine
  D. Hyperkalemia
  E. Hypoxemia
  F. Anesthetic drugs: xylazine
IV. Treatment
  A. Treat hypoxemia; stop infusion of dobutamine.

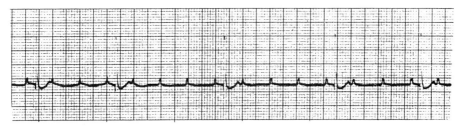

Figure 8–7. Second-degree atrioventricular heart block. P waves without QRS complexes are interspersed between normal beats.

B. Administer atropine 0.02 mg/kg intravenously. Repeat in 3–4 minutes if necessary.

C. Administer dopamine 7 μg/kg per minute (50 mg in 500 ml 0.9% saline, 100 μg/ml solution).

D. Institute transvenous pacing.

Ventricular Premature Depolarizations

I. Identification
  A. Premature wide and bizarre QRS complex (Fig. 8–8)
  B. No associated P wave
  C. May or may not be a pulse deficit

II. Causes
  A. Increased circulating catecholamines: excitement before induction of anesthesia, endotracheal intubation, pain, hypercarbia, hypoxemia, administration of epinephrine for hemostasis, administration of dopamine or dobutamine, pheochromocytoma, malignant hyperthermia
  B. Myocardial damage: traumatic myocarditis, gastric dilatation-volvulus, endotoxemia, cardiomyopathy
  C. Anesthetic drugs: thiopental
  D. Surgical manipulation of the heart: intrathoracic surgery

III. Treatment
  A. Check depth of anesthesia (too light or too deep), and deepen or lighten as necessary.
  B. Supply oxygen. Evaluate adequacy of ventilation. Hypercarbia is a common cause of premature ventricular depolarizations during inhalation anesthesia. Institute controlled ventilation.
  C. Measure or assess arterial pressure and peripheral perfusion. If they are decreased, improve cardiovascular function by any of the following:
    1. Decreasing anesthetic administration
    2. Providing adequate ventilation
    3. Increasing intravenous fluid administration
    4. Correcting metabolic acidosis
  D. Dobutamine is a better choice than dopamine for improving cardiovascular function in the presence of premature ventricular contractions associated with cardiac disease or damage.
  E. Administration of lidocaine is recommended if the premature ventricular depolarizations do any of the following:

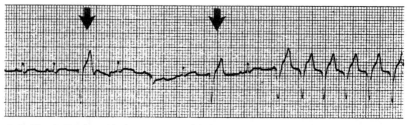

Figure 8–8. Two isolated ventricular premature depolarizations (arrows) followed by a run of premature beats (ventricular tachycardia).

1. Occur at a rate of 15 or more per minute or at a rate that causes a significant decrease in arterial blood pressure
2. Occur frequently and are multifocal (QRS complexes are of different configurations, indicating more than one ventricular origin)
3. Appear in pairs (two consecutive premature beats) or in runs (three or more consecutive beats)
4. Are superimposed on the previous T wave (R-on-T phenomenon)

F. Lidocaine at 1–2 mg/kg is used as an intravenous bolus. Usually less drug is needed in the cat, and a 1 ml graduated syringe with a 25-gauge needle should be used to provide accurate administration and avoid overdosage.
   1. Duration of antiarrhythmic action may be as short as 10 minutes, but a single dose may be sufficient if the inciting cause can be corrected.
   2. Additional lidocaine can be administered: up to 8 mg/kg in dogs and 6 mg/kg in cats over a period of 10 minutes. Blood lidocaine concentration may be maintained by infusion of lidocaine up to 0.08 mg/kg per minute in dogs and 0.04 mg/kg per minute in cats (25 ml 2% lidocaine or 12.5 ml 4% lidocaine in 500 ml 0.9% saline, 1 mg/ml solution).
   3. Lidocaine will reduce the requirement for other anesthetic drugs.

G. Change from halothane to isoflurane if it is available.

Ventricular Tachycardia

I. Identification
   A. Wide, abnormal QRS complex (Fig. 8–8)
   B. Ventricular rate greater than 100 per minute
   C. Rhythm may be regular
   D. Independent or retrograde P waves
II. Causes: same as for premature ventricular depolarizations
III. Treatment
   A. Discontinue anesthetic administration.
   B. Immediately institute treatment of this serious, potentially fatal dysrhythmia (see treatment of premature ventricular depolarizations).
   C. Identify cause of ventricular tachycardia, and treat.
   D. Consider other factors if usual treatment is unsuccessful.
      1. Mistaken diagnosis
      2. Hypoxia
      3. Hypovolemia
      4. Acidosis
      5. Hypokalemia

Hemorrhage

I. General considerations
   A. Oxygen delivery to tissues depends on (1) oxygen-carrying capacity of the blood, (2) cardiac output, and (3) peripheral perfusion. The oxygen-carrying capacity of the blood is determined by the concentration of hemoglobin and the arterial oxygen saturation. Thus, the blood of an animal with a low hematocrit may not be able to carry sufficient oxygen to the tissues, even though it has a normal heart and normal lungs. Acute decreases in hematocrit to 25% are compensated by increases in organ blood flow,

provided that blood volume is adequate (normovolemia). When the hematocrit decreases below 20%, oxygen extraction by the tissues increases, but oxygen supply becomes progressively restricted.

B. Anesthesia decreases cardiac output, and the normal physiologic response to blood loss is thus modified or lost. Therefore, a smaller volume of blood loss is significant when the animal is anesthetized than when it is conscious. Blood loss exceeding 20% of blood volume usually results in shock despite infusion of balanced electrolyte solution. Normal blood volume of the dog is 88 ml/kg and of the cat is 56 ml/kg. Furthermore, when blood loss occurs during anesthesia, the cardiac output decreases significantly before blood pressure decreases.

C. Transfusion reactions are uncommon during the first blood transfusion from a universal donor, but cross-matching is advisable unless immediate blood replacement is considered essential for survival of the patient.

D. Severe systemic effects may be produced by infusion of feline type A blood into a type B cat.[3]

E. Autotransfusion may be possible when hemorrhage into the thorax or abdomen is severe. Detailed accounts of canine and feline blood groups and autotransfusion are available.[4-6]

II. Clinical signs

A. Free blood in operative site, on swabs and drapes, in the suction bottle

B. Tachycardia: a normal response to blood loss in an awake animal but may not occur during anesthesia

C. Hypotension, weak pulse

D. White mucous membranes

E. Labored breathing (in response to decreased oxygen delivery to tissues)

III. Treatment

A. When severe hemorrhage occurs during inhalation anesthesia, administration of the anesthetic agent should be decreased or discontinued until hemorrhage is controlled and the circulation is stable.

B. Infuse lactated or acetated Ringer's solution at a rate of 2.5 times the volume of blood lost. Add to maintenance infusion rate of 10 ml/kg per hour.

C. Administer hypertonic saline solution or colloid solution (hetastarch, dextran 70, or blood) intravenously when blood loss exceeds 20% of blood volume or when hypotension is present despite decreased anesthetic administration and infusion of electrolyte solution. A colloid should be used when the patient is hypoproteinemic. Hematocrit should be monitored.

1. Infuse hypertonic 7.5% saline 4 ml/kg, intravenously over 10 minutes. Hypertonic saline expands blood volume by drawing fluid from interstitial tissues. Cardiac output and blood pressure should be improved for 1–2 hours, which is usually sufficient time to obtain blood for transfusion or to complete surgery and allow the patient to recover from anesthesia, thus removing the cardiovascular depressant effects of anesthetic agents. Dehydration must be prevented by additional infusion of lactated Ringer's solution. Note that when the source of the bleeding is not controlled, administration of hypertonic saline will increase blood loss. Repeating the dose after 2 hours is associated with a smaller improvement in cardiovascular function.

2. Infuse hydroxyethyl starch (hetastarch) up to 20 ml/kg intravenously over 30 minutes. Hetastarch increases intravascular volume by an amount equal to or greater than the volume infused and increases the colloid osmotic pressure.[7] Activated prothrombin time may be in-

creased, but with little clinical evidence of increased hemorrhage unless multiple doses of hetastarch are administered.

3. Infuse 6% dextran 70 up to 20 ml/kg intravenously over 30–60 minutes (maximum dose 20 ml/kg per 24 hours). Dextran 70 increases the plasma volume in normal dogs by a volume slightly greater than the volume infused. Minimal hemostatic abnormalities are produced in normal dogs, but bleeding may be increased in dogs with abnormal function.[8]

4. Blood transfusion during anesthesia is indicated when blood loss exceeds 20% of blood volume or when hematocrit (Hct) decreases to less than 20%.

   a. The volume of blood needed may be determined by estimating blood loss, or the following formula may be used:

   $$\text{Milliliters of Blood Needed} = \text{Patient's Body Weight (kg)} \times 70 \times \frac{\text{Hct Desired} - \text{Hct of Patient}}{\text{Hct of Donor in Anticoagulant}}$$

   b. Administer diphenhydramine (Benadryl) 2.2 mg/kg intravenously before infusion of plasma or blood. Start infusion extremely slowly for the first 2–3 minutes to minimize severity of the reaction should it occur. The infusion rate should not exceed 20 ml/kg per hour when the patient is normovolemic, but more rapid administration is indicated when severe blood loss has occurred. Rapid infusion of blood can cause a decrease in blood pressure. If decreased blood pressure is suspected to be due to transfusion and not to continuing blood loss, stop transfusion until blood pressure has stabilized, then restart at a slower infusion rate.

IV. Autotransfusion

Blood may be collected aseptically from the patient's thorax or abdomen into blood bottles or bags for reinfusion. The origin of blood should be observed during surgical operation to confirm that contamination with urine, intestinal fluid, bile, or penetrating wound has not occurred. A micropore filter with pore size of 40 μm should be used with the blood transfusion set to prevent infusion of microemboli.

Hypertension

I. Clinical signs
  A. Systolic pressure of greater than 180 mm Hg
  B. Diastolic pressure of greater than 110 mm Hg
  C. Heart rate decreased, normal, or increased
  D. Dysrhythmias

II. Causes
  A. Erroneous reading
    1. Blood pressure cuff loose
    2. Manometer or transducer for direct pressure measurement below the level of the heart; clotting of blood in the arterial catheter
  B. Sympathetic nervous system stimulation
    1. Hypercarbia
    2. Pain, including tourniquet pain; awareness
    3. Anesthetic drugs (xylazine, medetomidine, ketamine)

> 4. Intravenous injection or infusion of dopamine, dobutamine, epinephrine, or doxapram
> 5. Catecholamine release from pheochromocytoma
> 6. Malignant hyperthermia syndrome

C. Preexisting disease
1. Chronic renal disease
2. Hyperthyroidism
3. Hypoadrenocorticism
4. Cardiac disease
5. Increased intracranial pressure

III. Treatment
A. Check accuracy of measurement.
B. Assess depth of anesthesia: deepen if appropriate, or include intravenous opioid (oxymorphone 0.025–.05 mg/kg, butorphanol 0.05–0.1 mg/kg) or nitrous oxide to ensure analgesia.
C. Evaluate adequacy of ventilation, and consider controlled ventilation to decrease arterial carbon dioxide concentration.
D. Hypertension arising from induction of anesthesia with diazepam-ketamine will dissipate after approximately 30 minutes. Discontinuation of dopamine and dobutamine infusion should be followed by a decrease in blood pressure within 10 minutes.
E. Hypertension from pheochromocytoma can be treated with phentolamine (Regitine) 10 mg in 100 ml 5% dextrose in water infused in 1 ml increments to the desired effect. Tachycardia should respond to propranolol administration.
F. Specific treatment for malignant hyperthermia is recommended (see item IV, D, under "Other Complications During Anesthesia" for details).

Hypotension

I. General considerations
A. The mean arterial pressure in awake, healthy dogs and cats is 90–100 mm Hg (135–160 mm Hg systolic and 65–80 mm Hg diastolic). General anesthesia decreases cardiovascular function and arterial pressure. Deep anesthesia with an inhalation agent in dogs decreases mean arterial pressure to 60 mm Hg through decreased myocardial contractility and peripheral vasodilation. Autoregulatory mechanisms of blood flow in specific organ circulations may be impaired by anesthetic drugs, and are inactive when the arterial pressure is less than 70 mm Hg. Frequently, the start of surgery initiates vasoconstriction, and mean arterial pressure increases.
B. The normal physiologic response to decreased blood pressure resulting from decreased blood volume is an increase in sympathetic nervous system activity, which produces an increase in heart rate and myocardial contractility and causes vasoconstriction. Anesthetic agents decrease or abolish this response, and hypotension developing during anesthesia may not be marked by an increase in heart rate.
C. The consequences of a period of hypotension vary considerably. After 10 minutes of hypotension, one animal may be treated and suffer no lasting effect, whereas another may develop blindness or renal failure. At some point, tissue damage from hypoxia becomes irreversible. Inadequate splanchnic blood flow results in intestinal ischemia and loss of the mucosal barrier to intraluminal endotoxin. Other factors, such as stimulation of

the coagulation cascade and prostaglandin production, contribute to the development of shock.

II. Clinical signs
    A. Weak pulse in peripheral artery
    B. Prolonged capillary refill time
    C. Tachycardia present or not
    D. Diminished bleeding at the operative site
    E. Systolic arterial pressure of less than 75 mm Hg and mean arterial pressure of less than 60 mm Hg

III. Causes
    A. Anesthetic drugs
        1. Phenothiazine tranquilizers cause vasodilation and expand the vascular space, causing a relative hypovolemia. Only a minor decrease in blood pressure should occur in young, healthy animals with recommended preanesthetic dosages, but hypotension may develop in old, sick, or hypovolemic patients and in dogs with renal hypertension.
        2. Rapid intravenous injection of morphine or meperidine
        3. Deep halothane, isoflurane, or sevoflurane anesthesia
        4. General anesthesia in patients with abnormal fluid, electrolyte, or acid-base balance or in patients with cardiac disease
    B. Decreased venous return to the heart
        1. Hemorrhage without fluid replacement
        2. Progressive fluid loss from evaporation from viscera without fluid replacement
        3. Compression of the caudal vena cava by a tumor or enlarged organ when the animal is placed on its back
        4. Increased intra-abdominal pressure (introduction of carbon dioxide during laparoscopy, inflation of intestines during proctoscopy, colonoscopy, and gastroscopy)
        5. Increased intra-abdominal pressure from gastric dilatation or volvulus
        6. Controlled ventilation: when inspiratory time is greater than 2 seconds, cardiac output is decreased because the increase in intrathoracic pressure limits blood return to the heart.
        7. Hyperinflation of the lung occurring during apposition of a thoracotomy incision or as a result of failure to exhale (high pressure in anesthesia circuit)
        8. Tension pneumothorax
        9. Change in posture (e.g., from lateral to lateral, lateral to dorsal, or dorsal to prone position) during surgical-depth anesthesia
      10. Head-up or head-down tilt greater than 30° to the horizontal
      11. Ruptured diaphragm repair (during removal of abdominal organs from the thoracic cavity)
      12. Radiographic contrast media causing peripheral vasodilation
    C. Cardiac disease or drugs used in the treatment of cardiac disease
        1. Valvular insufficiency
        2. Arrhythmias
        3. Cardiomyopathy
        4. Congestive heart disease
        5. Pericardial effusion
        6. Enalapril (Enacard): hypotension occurs during anesthesia in dogs re-

ceiving treatment with enalapril for valvular insufficiency. Recommendations for anesthesia in human patients receiving the same drug include omission of treatment on the morning in which anesthesia is scheduled.

   D. Antibiotics

      1. Decreased cardiac contractility from intravenous injection of sodium or potassium penicillin

      2. Decreased cardiac output from rapid intravenous injection of cephalosporins or gentamicin

   E. Endotoxic shock/release of vasoactive substances

      1. Hypotension can develop at the onset of anesthesia in patients in septic or endotoxic shock (gastric dilatation or volvulus, intestinal obstruction, trauma).

      2. Sudden cardiovascular collapse may occur after manipulation of a pancreatic abscess, torsed stomach, intussusception, massive muscle damage adjacent to a fractured humerus or femur, bronchial carcinoma, or carcinoma of the gastrointestinal tract.

   F. Anaphylactic or anaphylactoid shock

      1. Barbiturates

      2. Blood or plasma transfusion reaction

      3. Antibiotics

IV. Treatment

   A. Eliminate mechanical cause of hypotension (check whether pop-off valve on anesthesia machine is open and rebreathing bag is not overdistended).

   B. Assess depth of anesthesia; it may assist in diagnosis of the cause.

   C. Correct the cause of the hypotension (Fig. 8–9).

   D. If the cause is not immediately obvious and correctable, administration of anesthetic should be reduced.

   E. Supply 100% oxygen and maintain normal arterial carbon dioxide concentrations by controlled ventilation (spontaneous ventilation progressively decreases in effectiveness during hypotension).

   F. Maintain or expand blood volume by intravenous infusion of lactated or acetated Ringer's solution or, in the case of severe hemorrhage, hypertonic saline or blood. Inject diphenhydramine (Benadryl) 2.2 mg/kg intravenously before blood transfusion.

   G. Myocardial contractility should be increased by infusion of dopamine or dobutamine at 3–7 μg/kg per minute; 50 mg dopamine added to 500 ml 0.9% saline produces a solution of 100 μg/ml. The infusion rate is more easily controlled when a pediatric infusion set (60 drops/ml) is used.

   H. Sodium bicarbonate can be given at 1 mEq/kg intravenously for every 10 minutes of hypotension.

   I. In patients at risk for reperfusion injury (gastric dilatation-volvulus, intestinal obstruction, splenic torsion), inject deferoxamine (Desferal) 30 mg/kg intramuscularly before or at the start of anesthesia.

Tachycardia

I. Identification

   A. Heart rate is rapid, exceeds 180 beats/min in dogs and 200 beats/min in cats.

   B. Sinus tachycardia is regular and continuous except for respiratory variation.

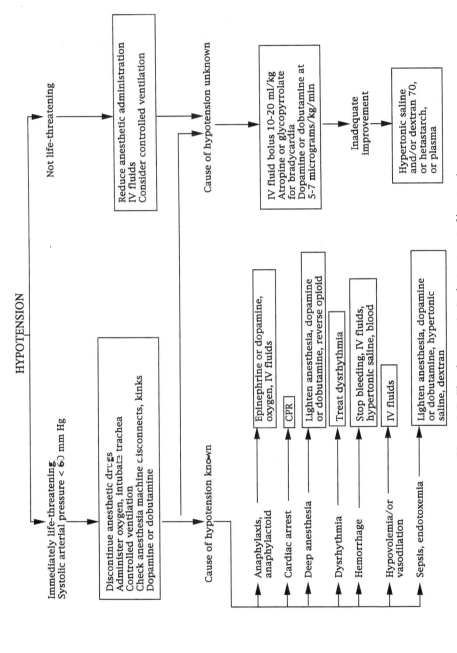

HYPOTENSION

Immediately life-threatening
Systolic arterial pressure < 60 mm Hg

Discontinue anesthetic drugs
Administer oxygen, intubate trachea
Controlled ventilation
Check anesthesia machine disconnects, kinks
Dopamine or dobutamine

Cause of hypotension known

Anaphylaxis, anaphylactoid	Epinephrine or dopamine, oxygen, IV fluids
Cardiac arrest	CPR
Deep anesthesia	Lighten anesthesia, dopamine or dobutamine, reverse opioid
Dysrhythmia	Treat dysrhythmia
Hemorrhage	Stop bleeding, IV fluids, hypertonic saline, blood
Hypovolemia/or vasodilation	IV fluids
Sepsis, endotoxemia	Lighten anesthesia, dopamine or dobutamine, hypertonic saline, dextran

Not life-threatening

Reduce anesthetic administration
IV fluids
Consider controlled ventilation

Cause of hypotension unknown

IV fluid bolus 10-20 ml/kg
Atropine or glycopyrrolate for bradycardia
Dopamine or dobutamine at 5-7 micrograms/kg/min

Inadequate improvement

Hypertonic saline and/or dextran 70, or hetastarch, or plasma

Figure 8–9. Flowchart to assist in the treatment of hypotension.

When rhythm originates outside the SA node (atrial tachycardia), P waves may be abnormal. Tachycardia may be continuous or paroxysmal.

   C. QRST complexes are normal.

II. Causes

   A. Physiologic: pain, awareness, excitement during induction of anesthesia

   B. Pathologic: hypoxemia, hypercarbia, hypotension, catecholamine release from endotracheal intubation, fever, hyperthyroidism, congestive heart failure

   C. Drugs: atropine, ketamine, epinephrine, isoproterenol, dopamine, dobutamine

III. Treatment

   A. No treatment may be necessary when tachycardia occurs immediately after induction of anesthesia, especially after injection of diazepam-ketamine, and blood pressure is adequate.

   B. Eliminate surgical stimulus, hypercarbia, and hypoxemia as causes of tachycardia by temporarily stopping surgery and starting artificial ventilation.

   C. Slow or stop infusion of an cardiostimulatory drug.

   D. Find and treat cause of tachycardia (Fig. 8–10).

   E. Propranolol may be used to treat tachyarrhythmias, but it decreases cardiac contractility and must be used cautiously in the anesthetized patient. Inject 0.04–.06 mg/kg intravenously and slowly.

   F. Evaluate for underlying cardiac disease.

OTHER COMPLICATIONS DURING ANESTHESIA

Hyperthermia

I. Clinical signs

   A. Panting

   B. Patient hot to touch

   C. Rectal temperature of more than 39°C (102.5°F).

II. Causes

   A. Excessive application of heat: patient with a heavy hair coat lying on a hot-water pad or in an excessively warm environment

   B. Inability to lose heat: closed system of administration of inhalation anesthetics (circle system or to-and-fro system with low oxygen inflow)

   C. Increased metabolic rate

      1. Bacteremia or endotoxemia

      2. Inherited defect of skeletal muscle that results in a massive increase in metabolism when triggered by emotional stress or anesthetic drugs.

         a. The syndrome of malignant hyperthermia is initiated and maintained by excess myoplasmic calcium and is characterized by increased carbon dioxide production, lactic acidosis, hyperkalemia, and increased circulating concentrations of catecholamines.

         b. Rectal temperature may increase to more than 44°C (>110°F). Initial cardiovascular stimulation progresses to cardiovascular failure.

         c. This syndrome is rare in dogs, most often reported in greyhounds, and extremely rare in cats.

      3. Increased circulating concentrations of thyroid hormones (thyrotoxicosis, hyperthyroidism) are due in most cases to thyroid carcinoma in dogs and functional thyroid adenoma in cats.

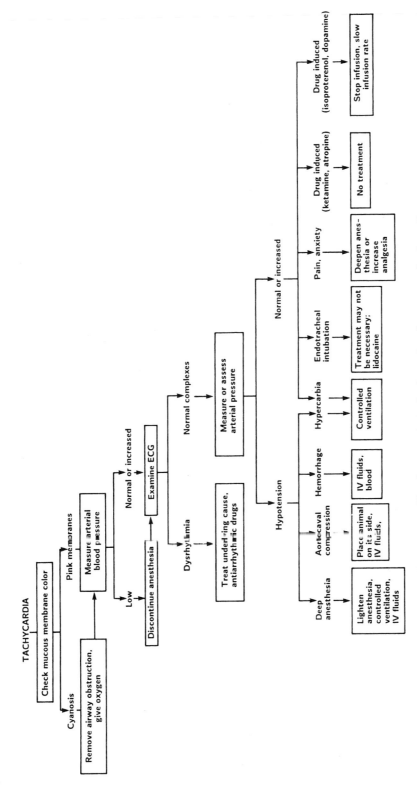

Figure E–10. Flowchart to assist in the diagnosis and treatment of tachycardia.

D. Failure of central thermoregulation: xylazine, ketamine, tiletamine-zola-zepam (Telazol), inhalant anesthetics, antibiotics

III. Differential diagnosis

A. Heat stroke

  1. The only abnormal clinical signs should be an elevated rectal temperature and panting if heat stroke developed during anesthesia.

B. Bacteremia/endotoxemia

  1. The patient may have a history of a septic process or ischemic tissue.

C. Malignant hyperthermia

  1. Onset of signs may be insidious or may be dramatic.

  2. Panting, tachycardia, hypertension, and arrhythmias occur. Rectal temperature may exceed 41°C (105.8°F). Increased carbon dioxide production results in a more rapid than usual change in soda lime color, and the canister feels hotter. The pH and blood gas analysis will reveal a severe metabolic acidosis. Muscle rigidity is not usual in dogs.[9]

  3. Cyanosis and cardiovascular collapse ensue. Rigor mortis develops rapidly.

D. Thyrotoxicosis/hyperthyroidism

  1. Clinical signs referable to hyperthyroidism are usually present before induction of anesthesia.

  2. A moderately elevated temperature is accompanied by tachycardia and arrhythmias that can be difficult to differentiate from malignant hyperthermia.

  3. Massive carbon dioxide production and lactic acidosis are not a feature of hyperthyroidism.

IV. Treatment

A. All heating devices should be removed.

B. If anesthesia is maintained by an inhalation agent via a circle circuit, the oxygen flow rate should be increased to flush the warm gases and water vapor from the system. The soda lime should be changed.

C. Active cooling of the patient may be necessary with ice packs and infusion of cold fluid intravenously.

D. Malignant hyperthermia (MH) should be treated as follows.

  1. Avoid inhalation anesthetics and succinylcholine and pretreat with dantrolene (Dantrium) if a familial incidence of malignant hyperthermia is known.

  2. If the syndrome developed during anesthesia, administration of the inhalation agent should be discontinued, the soda lime and circuit hoses changed, and the patient ventilated with 100% oxygen using a larger than normal tidal volume.

  3. The patient should be placed in an ice-water bath if possible. Alternatively, cooling should be attempted by placing ice packs in the groin and axillae, instilling cold-water enemas, and infusing cold saline intravenously.

  4. Metabolic acidosis should be corrected by injection of sodium bicarbonate 1.5 mEq/kg initially, with additional amounts preferably determined by laboratory analysis of pH and P_{CO_2}.

  5. Specific treatment of MH is intravenous injection of dantrolene, which acts within the muscle cell to cause relaxation. Dantrolene 3 mg/kg should be given by rapid intravenous injection.[9] Other researchers have recommended follow-up treatment with dantrolene 1 mg/kg every 6 hours.

6. Serum $[K^+]$ will be high early in the reaction but may drop to a low level as the syndrome progresses.

7. If the syndrome is aborted and rectal temperature begins to decrease, the patient should not be moved until danger of a reaction relapse has passed. Further treatment should be directed at supporting the cardiovascular system and maintaining renal function. Renal failure secondary to myoglobinuria may occur after an episode of MH.

Hypoglycemia

I. General considerations

    A. Hypoglycemia is almost impossible to diagnose during anesthesia without measurement of blood glucose. Only a short period of hypoglycemia can result in irreversible brain damage; therefore, it is important to identify patients at risk (diabetics, especially those undergoing cesarean section; newborns; patients with weight loss, liver disease, or insulinoma) beforehand and take steps to prevent hypoglycemia or be prepared to treat it.

II. Clinical signs

    A. None may be apparent.

    B. Tachycardia, hypertension, hypotension, and sweating may occur.

    C. Seizures will probably be masked by the anesthetic drugs.

    D. Blood glucose levels are less than 60 mg/dl.

III. Prevention and treatment

    A. Replace part of the intraoperative fluid requirements with 5% dextrose in water, 2–5 ml/kg per hour. An alternative solution is 0.45% saline or half-strength lactated Ringer's solution with 2.5% dextrose.

    B. Measure blood glucose before anesthesia and, if low, correct by administration of syrup orally or 5% dextrose in water intravenously. Measure blood glucose every 2 hours during anesthesia (more frequently in the uncontrolled diabetic) and adjust infusion of 5% dextrose in water to maintain blood glucose at 100–250 mg/dl. Measure blood glucose several hours after anesthesia and ensure that the patient either eats its evening meal or receives supplementary glucose.

Hypothermia

I. General considerations

    A. A retrospective study of body temperature change during anesthesia in cats revealed that (1) the greatest temperature drop occurred from induction of anesthesia to the start of surgery, while the cat was being clipped and prepped; (2) once the cat was placed on a hot-water circulating pad for surgery, the rapid decline in body temperature was stopped; and (3) there was no significant difference in temperature decrease among anesthetic drug combinations (drugs used included acepromazine, thiamylal, ketamine, halothane, and methoxyflurane).[10]

    B. Hypothermia during general anesthesia has several consequences.

        1. Anesthetic drug requirement is decreased; a decrease of 50% has been measured in dogs during a decrease in temperature from 38°C (100.4°F) to 28°C (82.4°).

        2. Ventilation is decreased, and ventilatory drive to hypercapnia and hypoxemia is decreased.

3. The oxygen-hemoglobin dissociation curve is shifted such that less oxygen is available to the tissues.

4. Metabolism is slowed, and elimination of anesthetic drugs may be delayed, prolonging recovery.

5. In addition, during recovery from anesthesia, increased oxygen demand caused by shivering may not be met by the depressed cardiovascular and respiratory systems. Hypoxia may result.

C. During convalescence, hypothermia during surgery is associated with increased incidence of postoperative infections, delayed wound healing, and weight loss.

D. Prevention of hypothermia is much easier to accomplish than rewarming during anesthesia and surgery.

II. Causes

A. Decreased rate of heat production

1. Decreased metabolic rate caused by anesthetic drugs

2. Lack of muscle tone and muscle movement

B. Increased heat loss

1. Absence of nasal warming of inspired gases during endotracheal intubation is most apparent when a non-rebreathing system is used, whereas inspired gas from a circle circuit is partially humidified and warm. Conservation of moisture and heat in a circle is greatest when the oxygen inflow rate is low.

2. Vasoconstriction, which would normally occur in an air-conditioned environment, is blocked by anesthetic drugs. Heat is lost from the skin to the environment and to a cold table surface.

3. Loss of heat may occur from the surgical site owing to clipping of hair, application of cold prepping solutions and alcohol, and exposure of visceral surfaces during surgery.

III. Prevention

A. Minimize anesthesia time by clipping the animal before induction of anesthesia.

B. Place the patient on a hot-water circulating pad immediately after induction of anesthesia. Use of a sheepskin or foam pads will slow heat loss but will not prevent it.

C. Use a hot-water circulating pad during surgery. Do not turn the thermostat above 40°C (104°F), or skin burn may result. It is possible during some procedures to place a second hot pad over part of the patient. Place heated gel packs or examining gloves filled with warm water around and over the head, neck, and limbs. Patient's limbs or body can be wrapped in plastic (Saran Wrap).

D. Insert disposable humidifier (Humid-Vent, Gibeck) between the endotracheal tube and adaptor of a non-rebreathing circuit to warm and moisten inhaled gases. Use of low flow in a circle circuit may help to retain warmth and moisture in breathed gases.

E. Maintain operating room temperature at 21–23.9°C (70°–75°F).

F. Use warm intravenous fluids. Use a warmer on the fluid-administration tubing.

G. Use warm saline for abdominal lavage.

H. Perform surgery as rapidly as is compatible with good surgical technique.

References

1. Tillson DM: Thoracostomy tubes. Part I. Indications and anesthesia. Comp Contin Ed 19:1258–1275, 1997.
2. Clutton E: Management of perioperative cardiac arrest in companion animals. Part 2. In Practice 16:3–10, 1994.
3. Norsworthy GD: Clinical aspects of feline blood transfusions. Comp Contin Ed 14:469–475, 1992.
4. Griot-Wenk ME, Giger U: Feline transfusion medicine: Blood types and their clinical importance. Vet Clin North Am Small Anim Pract 25:1305–1322, 1995.
5. Hale AS: Canine blood groups and their importance in veterinary transfusion medicine. Vet Clin North Am Small Anim Pract 25:1323–1332, 1995.
6. Purvis D: Autotransfusion in the emergency patient. Vet Clin North Am Small Anim Pract 25:1291–1304, 1995.
7. Rudloff E, Kirby R: The critical need for colloids: Selecting the right colloid. Comp Contin Ed 19:811–826, 1997.
8. Concannon KT, Haskins SC, Feldman BF: Hemostatic defects associated with two infusion rates of dextran 70 in dogs. Am J Vet Res 53:1369–1375, 1992.
9. Nelson TE: Malignant hyperthermia in dogs. J Am Vet Med Assoc 198:989–994, 1991.
10. Haskins SC: Hypothermia and its prevention during general anesthesia in cats. Am J Vet Res 42:856–861, 1981.

Postanesthetic Care and Complications

Cynthia M. Trim

ROUTINE CARE

Routine care at the end of anesthesia is straightforward for some patients (Table 9–1). Other patients may require special treatment. This chapter first deals with the routine care of dogs and cats after anesthesia and then details the clinical signs, causes, diagnosis, and treatment of complications that may develop at that time.

Analgesia

I. General considerations
  A. *Pain* is defined as an unpleasant sensory and emotional experience associated with actual or potential tissue damage.
  B. Evaluation of pain scores and measurement of catecholamines and cortisol concentrations have determined the value of "preemptive pain control" by administration of analgesia, such as an opioid, nerve block, or carprofen, before surgery. Such preoperative analgesia will block sensitization of the central nervous system (CNS) to noxious stimuli and allow the use of smaller doses of analgesics during recovery from anesthesia.
  C. We have an ethical responsibility to minimize pain and anxiety.
II. Consequences of uncontrolled pain
  A. Pain causes sympathetic nervous system stimulation and catecholamine release. Tachycardia and peripheral vasoconstriction result in increased cardiac work. Increased myocardial contractility may not be matched by myocardial oxygen supply and hence will result in ischemia, especially in patients with preexisting cardiac disease.
  B. Hypoventilation may occur when breathing is painful, particularly after thoracic or upper abdominal surgery. The decrease in ventilation may be compounded by decreased cardiovascular function from residual effects of anesthetic drugs. Hypoventilation may cause respiratory acidosis and hypoxemia, and lung collapse predisposes the patient to pneumonia.
  C. Pain results in decreased gastrointestinal motility. The patient in pain before anesthesia may have had delayed gastric emptying and be at risk for vomiting or regurgitation with pulmonary aspiration, either during induction of or recovery from anesthesia. Pain may also cause ileus postoperatively.
  D. Pain stimulates release of antidiuretic hormone and contributes to the changes in body fluid balance associated with surgery.
  E. Pain may result in prolonged recumbency, which predisposes the patient to lung collapse and pneumonia.
  F. The immediate effects of pain after surgical operation may include excitement, violence, and self-mutilation and may cause irreparable harm to the patient or to the surgical site (sutures torn out predisposing to infection, wound dehiscence, and breakage of surgical implants).

Table 9–1. Routine Patient Care at Termination of Inhalation Anesthesia

- Administer drugs to control pain postoperatively, if not done already.
- Supply oxygen for 5 minutes after discontinuing nitrous oxide.
- Administer oxygen after turning vaporizer off and until depth of breathing increases.
- Empty urinary bladder by palpation or catheterization; note volume of urine.
- Flush catheter with heparinized saline after fluids are discontinued.
- Wait for swallowing reflex before extubating trachea.
- Check temperature and apply warmth if ≤36°C (≤97°F).
- Keep under observation.

III. Signs of pain
   A. The degree of pain appears to be related to the origin of pain, with superimposed individual variation in tolerance. Some generalizations of surgery-induced pain include the following:
      1. Pain is most severe after thoracic or upper abdominal surgery, ophthalmologic procedures, and operations on the nasal cavity and perineum.
      2. Surgery on the lower abdominal region or major joints is less painful.
      3. Least painful are superficial surgery and surgery on extremities.
   B. Pain may be potentially assessed by observed changes in behavior. These changes may depend on the origin of the pain, the species and breed of animal, and the personality of the patient. Behavior associated with pain includes shivering, reluctance to move, guarding or avoidance of human touch, excitement, aggression, vocalization, mutilation of a painful area, and excessive salivation.
   C. Other parameters used in the assessment of pain are physiologic: dilated pupils, tachycardia, and hypertension. Respiratory rate may also be increased.
   D. Other measurements that have been used to document the existence of pain involve plasma beta endorphin, catecholamine, and cortisol concentrations and recordings of the electroencephalogram or evoked potentials.
IV. Options for pain control
   A. Distraction of the animal's attention by holding or talking to it. This may be particularly applicable in the immediate recovery period when the patient appears to be disoriented.
   B. Administration of a nonsteroidal anti-inflammatory drug such as carprofen before surgery
   C. Systemic administration of an opioid
   D. Epidural injection of an opioid, alpha-2 agonist, or local anesthetic
   E. Use of adjunct drugs to provide tranquilization or sedation
   F. Regional analgesia by nerve blocks such as epidural or brachial plexus block.
   G. Application of hot or cold compresses
   H. Mechanical assistance, for example, immobilization of a fractured limb
   I. Transcutaneous electrical nerve stimulation
V. Treatment of pain with systemic drugs
   A. A smaller drug dose can be used when the analgesic drug is administered before the patient regains consciousness and feels pain. Once the animal is awake, catecholamine release results in increased dose requirement.
   B. The timing of administration depends on the rate at which the animal is expected to recover from anesthesia, the route of administration, the time

of onset of action of the drug used, and time elapsed from administration of opioid for premedication or intraoperative analgesia. Administration should be timed so that drugs for postoperative analgesia have taken effect before the patient regains consciousness. Dose rates for postoperative analgesia may be less than for premedication (Table 9–2).

C. In some patients the provision of analgesia alone is insufficient to prevent excessive movement or vocalization; sedation may also be required. A small dose of acepromazine (0.03 mg/kg) given intravenously or a small dose of diazepam may facilitate analgesia.

D. A fentanyl patch applied 12 hours before anesthesia will provide some analgesia, but additional opioid administration is usually necessary for the first few hours after surgery. Morphine, meperidine, and oxymorphone are compatible with fentanyl.

VI. Precautions

A. Meperidine and morphine will cause hypotension if injected intravenously as a bolus. This effect can be avoided if the drug is injected intramuscularly or is injected over several minutes when given intravenously.

B. Opioids cause respiratory depression, especially when combined with the residual effects of general anesthesia. The rate and depth of breathing must be critically evaluated as the drugs attain their full effect.

C. Some opioids may cause excitement when used alone in cats. Buprenorphine, butorphanol, meperidine, and oxymorphone can be administered for postoperative pain control in cats.

VII. Opioids in the epidural space

A. Morphine 0.1 mg/kg or oxymorphone 0.05 mg/kg can be injected epidurally at the lumbosacral junction to provide pain relief for pelvic and hindlimb surgery for 12–24 hours and 10 hours, respectively. Pain relief after thoracotomy has also been documented with epidural opioid administration.

Table 9–2. Opioids for Postoperative Analgesia

Drug	Dosage	Comment
Buprenorphine (Buprenex) 0.3 mg/ml	0.006 mg/kg IM; 40 minutes before end of anesthesia	Dosing interval 4–6 hours; dose increased to 0.01 mg/kg after recovery from anesthesia
Butorphanol (Torbugesic) 10 mg/ml	0.1–.2 mg/kg IM; 10 minutes before end of anesthesia	Duration 1–1.5 hours
Fentanyl (Duragesic transdermal system)	Cats 25 µg/hour patch; dogs 10–20 kg 50 µg/hour; 20–30 kg 50–75 µg/hour; >30 kg 75–100 µg/hour; onset time 12 hours; apply 12 hours before anesthesia	Not sufficient for immediate postoperative analgesia; duration 72 hours; somnolent = overdose
Meperidine 50 mg/ml	2.0 mg/kg IM; 20 minutes before end of anesthesia	Do not inject IV; duration 1–1.5 hours
Morphine 15 mg/ml	0.2–.5 mg/kg IM; 30 minutes before the end of anesthesia	Do not inject IV Duration 4 hours
Morphine (Duramorph for epidural) 1 mg/ml	0.1 mg/kg epidural; 45 minutes before surgery	Duration up to 24 hours
Oxymorphone (Numorphan) 1.5 mg/ml	0.05 mg/kg IM, IV; IM 15 minutes before end of anesthesia	Duration 2–4 hours
Oxymorphone (Numorphan) 1.5 mg/ml	0.05 mg/kg epidural; 45 minutes before surgery	Duration 10 hours

B. A long-acting (5–6 hours) local anesthetic drug such as bupivacaine can be added to the opioid.

VIII. Treatment of pain with nerve blocks

A. Intercostal nerve blocks can be performed to control pain from a thoracotomy. Bupivacaine 0.5% solution (0.5 ml/nerve for a large dog; maximum total dose 2 mg/kg) may be injected before the incision is closed by direct viewing of the intercostal nerves beneath the pleura on the caudal border of the rib. Two nerves cranial to the incision and two nerves caudal should be blocked.

B. Intrapleural bupivacaine may also block pain from a thoracotomy and chest tube friction. Bupivacaine 1.5 mg/kg is infused down the chest tube. The block is most predictable when the dog is restrained with the infused side down or is in the dorsal-lateral position for approximately 15 minutes.

Breathing After Controlled Ventilation

I. General considerations

A. The patient should not be removed from ventilatory support until the surgery is almost completed if hypoventilation was the initial reason for instituting controlled ventilation.

B. Lighten the depth of anesthesia first.

C. Residual neuromuscular blockade from a nondepolarizing neuromuscular blocking agent should be antagonized by the administration of edrophonium, neostigmine, or pyridostigmine along with an anticholinergic drug.

D. Decrease respiratory rate to 4–6 breaths per minute (either using the ventilator control or by manual squeezing of the rebreathing bag) to allow the arterial carbon dioxide (CO_2) concentration to increase to a level that will stimulate breathing. Leave the tidal volume the same to minimize alveolar collapse.

E. When an assist mode is present on a ventilator, the sensitivity of the ventilator can be increased. Return of spontaneous breathing can then be recognized by an increase in respiratory rate.

F. Check that the animal's position will not impair breathing. For example, a patient in a prone, head-down position for perineal surgery should be placed on its side before being allowed to breathe spontaneously.

G. It should be remembered that pain, especially after thoracic or upper abdominal surgery, and hypothermia cause hypoventilation.

H. An opioid administered for maintenance of anesthesia or for postoperative pain usually decreases ventilation.

1. The patient should be observed for adequacy of breathing, including both rate and depth of breathing.

2. When the patient is hypoventilating and depth of anesthesia has lightened such that the animal must be removed from the anesthesia machine and extubated, oxygen should be supplied. The oxygen can be administered by face mask or insufflated through a nasal tube, or the animal can placed in an oxygen cage or incubator.

3. If necessary, the respiratory depression can be partially reversed by naloxone given in small increments intravenously.

I. Injection of a mixed opioid agonist such as butorphanol will reverse the respiratory depression caused by morphine or oxymorphone and provide some analgesia.

II. How long should you wait?

A. The time lapse between discontinuation of controlled ventilation and restoration of spontaneous breathing that can be safely tolerated by the patient varies according to the percent of inspired oxygen used and the ventilatory status of the patient.

B. Arterial CO_2 tension may not increase sufficiently to stimulate spontaneous breathing for as long as 5 minutes after cessation of controlled ventilation. Hypoxemia may or may not develop during apnea. Artificial ventilation should be resumed if cyanosis occurs or if hemoglobin oxygen saturation decreases to 90%.

C. When a patient has been ventilated for several minutes using a slow (4–6 breaths per minute) respiratory rate and spontaneous breathing has not resumed, causes of apnea other than hypocarbia should be investigated. Severe accumulation of CO_2 should be avoided.

III. Causes of apnea or hypoventilation after controlled ventilation

A. Arterial CO_2 concentration too low to stimulate breathing (hypocarbia)

B. Depression of respiratory centers by anesthetic drugs

C. Inadequate reversal of neuromuscular blockade

D. CNS injury: hypoxia, cerebellar herniation, high cervical transection

E. Pain after thoracic or upper abdominal surgery

F. Hypothermia

IV. Diagnostic approach to failure to resume breathing or hypoventilation

A. Anesthesia history

1. Apnea or hypoventilation may be the result of high dosage of anesthetic drugs used for maintenance, especially opioids.

2. Whenever neuromuscular blocking agents have been used, they must be suspected as a cause of hypoventilation postoperatively.

3. Cardiac arrest or an episode of hypotension may have resulted in cerebral hypoxia.

4. Patients with head trauma present before anesthesia or patients undergoing cervical disk surgery, stabilization of cervical vertebrae, or ventriculography may suffer cerebral or spinal cord damage during anesthesia by direct trauma, increased intracranial pressure, or cerebellar herniation.

B. Physical examination

1. The patient should be observed for depth of anesthesia.

a. Presence of palpebral reflex, limb withdrawal to toe pinch, and spontaneous movement all indicate a light plane of anesthesia.

b. The eyeball positioned central in the orbit and a strong palpebral reflex indicate a light plane of anesthesia. The eyeball rolled down, showing part of the sclera, indicates moderate plane of anesthesia. At either of these levels, adequate breathing should be possible.

2. Pupillary dilation may be caused by anxiety, pain, deep anesthesia, cerebral damage, or ketamine administration.

3. Persistent neuromuscular blockade may be difficult to confirm without the use of a peripheral nerve stimulator. Any one of the following situations may develop after administration of edrophonium or neostigmine to antagonize the action of a neuromuscular blocking drug:

a. Adequate rate and depth of spontaneous breathing may return.

b. Apnea may persist because of hypocapnia or because of opioid or anesthetic drug depression of the respiratory centers.

      c. Respiratory rate may be normal but the depth of breathing shallow, resulting in respiratory acidosis.

      d. Normal spontaneous breathing may not resume. Instead, accumulated CO_2 or hypoxia results in "tracheal tug" (jerky inspiratory movements accompanied by flexion of the head and ventral movement of the mandible). In this case, inadequate reversal of neuromuscular blockade exists.

      e. Spontaneous breathing may be adequate, and the patient may be able to swallow, but it may not be able to lift its head or blink. This could be an indication that insufficient antagonist was administered. Not all muscles regain full function at the same rate after administration of the antagonist. The muscles of respiration are the first to be restored and the muscles of the face and jaw the last.

      f. "Dual block" may sometimes develop after multiple doses of succinylcholine, resulting in persistent paralysis. In this situation, neuromuscular blockade is characterized by both depolarization and nondepolarizing features.

        (1) Succinylcholine may be antagonized by neostigmine when dual block has been confirmed by use of a peripheral nerve stimulator.

        (2) When this equipment is not available, controlled ventilation should be continued until neuromuscular blockade wears off.

V. Treatment of inadequate ventilation

  A. Resume controlled ventilation.

  B. Continue administration of inhalation anesthetic agents at a low level while neuromuscular blockade is present. Antagonize neuromuscular blockade if appropriate.

  C. Assess depth of anesthesia; lighten it if it is deep.

  D. Decrease respiratory rate and again attempt weaning to spontaneous breathing.

  E. If respiratory movements start but ventilation is inadequate, follow steps described in section on abnormal respiratory movements under "Complications."

Extubation

I. Procedure

  A. Extubation should be performed after the swallowing reflex has returned.

  B. The pharynx should be cleaned of blood, water, and debris before extubation.

  C. The patient should remain attached to the anesthesia machine for 10 minutes or as long as possible after termination of inhalation anesthesia. This allows continued scavenging of exhaled anesthetic gas and provides the patient with oxygen to breathe while the respiratory system is depressed.

  D. In most patients, the endotracheal tube cuff should be deflated before the tube is removed.

  E. The tube should be removed with the cuff still inflated when fluid may have entered the trachea and become sequestered proximal to the cuff. The cuff should be slightly deflated to avoid tearing the tracheal mucosa. The patient should be extubated with its head hanging over the edge of a table.

II. Precautions

    A. The coughing reflex may be present for some time before the swallowing reflex returns. The patient should be allowed to lie quietly so that the tube will not move in the trachea and stimulate coughing.

    B. Aspiration can still occur in the patient that can swallow. The patient may asphyxiate or aspirate fluid or solid material into the lungs if it is too depressed to lift its head when regurgitating or vomiting. A dog that has refluxed during anesthesia may have gastric fluid in the nasal passages. Inhalation of this fluid may occur when the animal takes its first breath after extubation. Complete protection against aspiration may not return for several hours after the patient has regained consciousness.

    C. The depth of anesthesia should not be lightened prematurely so that the patient regains consciousness while restrained on its back. It will be difficult to manage complications if extubation is performed with the patient in this position.

    D. Failure to monitor the patient adequately during recovery may result in the patient chewing and severing the endotracheal tube. The free pieces may be inhaled or swallowed.

    E. A pharyngostomy tube should be properly placed and not in a position to obstruct the entrance to the larynx.

    F. Arrangements should be made to treat or prevent airway obstruction after extubation in those patients who are at increased risk because of their anatomy or surgical problem.

Monitoring

I. Central nervous system

    A. Return of reflexes (palpebral, pedal), muscle movement, awareness and behavior should be observed.

    B. Stimulation during early recovery by patting or rubbing the patient or by use of verbal commands may enhance recovery from inhalation agents by increasing respiration and therefore elimination.

    C. Avoid turning a dog from side to side while it is still anesthetized, because the change in body position when the cardiovascular system is depressed may result in hypotension or even cardiac arrest.

II. Respiratory system

    A. Respiratory rate, depth, and character as well as mucous membrane and skin color should be noted.

    B. Cyanosis may not be obvious when a dog is hypoxic. Pulse oximeter with tongue or rectal probe is useful to monitor arterial oxygenation.

III. Cardiovascular system

    A. Pulse rate and rhythm, mucous membrane color, and capillary refill time should be noted.

    B. Arterial blood pressure and the electrocardiogram (EKG) should be monitored in those patients at risk for cardiovascular complications.

    C. Continuation of intravenous fluid administration into recovery will depend on the condition of the patient.

IV. Temperature

    A. Body temperature should be monitored for up to several hours after surgery.

    B. Hypothermia will prolong recovery. Patients with temperature of less than

36°C (97°F) should be warmed by use of hot-water-circulating pads or heated cages or by warming the surrounding air with a heat lamp or hot air from a dryer attached to the cage door.

V. Urine production

A. Expressing the bladder at the end of anesthesia, either by abdominal compression or catheterization of the bladder, provides an estimate of urine production during anesthesia. This information aids the decision on whether fluid therapy is needed during recovery.

Oxygen Therapy

I. General considerations

A. This section deals with methods of increasing the inspired concentration of oxygen above that of room air for conscious or sedated patients. This treatment is for poor oxygenation and not for hypoventilation (hypercarbia).

II. Indications

A. Cyanosis of mucous membranes or a pulse oximeter reading of less than 90% saturation in a spontaneously breathing patient

B. Patients in the following categories:
   1. Geriatric patients
   2. Obese patients
   3. Brachycephalic breeds
   4. Patients with CNS depression before anesthesia
   5. Patients with pulmonary contusions or thoracic trauma
   6. Patients with pneumonia
   7. Patients with cardiac disease

C. Patients who have undergone surgical procedures that may contribute to impaired oxygenation such as the following:
   1. Thoracotomy
   2. Ruptured diaphragm repair
   3. Upper abdominal surgery

III. Procedures

A. Face mask
   1. Supply oxygen from an anesthesia machine via a face mask and either a non-rebreathing or a circle circuit.

B. Oxygen cage
   1. Several types of oxygen cages and pediatric incubators are available commercially. They will provide a controlled environment of temperature (75°F) and humidity (50%).
   2. The oxygen flow rate should be adjusted to provide the patient with an oxygen concentration of 40–60%.

C. Nasal catheter
   1. Oxygen is insufflated through a catheter placed in the ventral nasal meatus. Ideally, the catheter is placed before the animal is allowed to recover from anesthesia. Alternatively, a small amount of 2% lidocaine (1 mg/kg) can be instilled into the nostril and 2 minutes allowed for analgesia to develop.
   2. A rubber (urethral) catheter or a polyurethane catheter (pediatric nasogastric tube) with a nylon stylet should be lubricated and inserted

gently into the ventral nasal meatus to the level of the carnassial tooth. Direct the tube dorsally for the first centimeter, then ventrally.

3. The catheter should be sutured to the skin immediately after it exits from the nostril and again further back on the forehead.

4. An Elizabethan collar may be used to prevent the animal from scratching, resulting in extubation.

5. Oxygen should be bubbled through a half-full bottle of sterile water or saline for humidification. An intravenous administration set and extension tubing make a convenient connection between the saline bottle and the nasal catheter.

6. Oxygen flow rates of 50–100 ml/kg per minute should increase the tracheal oxygen concentration to 40%.

D. Transtracheal

1. Oxygen may also be administered through a catheter inserted between tracheal rings into the lumen of the trachea.

2. Potential complications are bleeding from the insertion site, subcutaneous emphysema, local cellulitis, mucosal damage from "whipping" of the catheter, or bronchospasm if the catheter is inserted into the bronchial tree.

3. A 30-cm catheter usually used in the jugular vein for fluid infusion may be used for transtracheal oxygen administration. After surgical preparation of the skin, a few inches of catheter may be inserted aseptically midline into the trachea. The catheter should be secured to the skin so that it cannot be accidently pulled out.

4. Humidified oxygen may be supplied as previously described at a rate of 50 ml/kg per minute.

E. Tracheostomy

1. Oxygen may be administered via a tracheostomy tube (a) through a catheter inserted into the tube, (b) by connecting an anesthesia machine circuit to the tracheostomy tube, (c) as assisted or controlled ventilation delivered from a Bird ventilator, or (d) using a high-frequency jet ventilator.

2. Hypoventilation can also be treated with a Bird ventilator or a high-frequency jet ventilator. (See Chapter 8 for technique of insertion of tracheostomy tube.)

F. Endotracheal intubation

1. Endotracheal intubation may be necessary in some patients to provide 100% oxygen and controlled ventilation.

2. For most of these patients, propofol is the drug of choice, along with an opioid such as morphine or oxymorphone for analgesia. A light plane of anesthesia can be maintained with propofol using small bolus doses or a continuous infusion of up to 0.3 mg/kg per minute.

IV. Precautions

A. Oxygen toxicity

1. Efforts should be made to restrict the patient to breathing 40–60% oxygen when oxygen therapy is to continue for more than a few hours. Adverse changes in the lungs will develop in the patient breathing 100% oxygen, and these changes occur despite continuing cyanosis of mucous membranes.

a. Mucociliary clearance is diminished after 3 hours.

b. Pulmonary capillary endothelial cell damage and alveolar fibrin deposits are present in dogs after breathing 100% oxygen for 24 hours.

    c. Other early signs may be refusal of food, nausea, and vomiting.

    d. Blindness (retrolental fibroplasia) will develop when newborn animals up to 2 weeks of age are allowed to breathe 100% oxygen for many hours.

B. Hypercarbia

    1. It should be remembered that during oxygen therapy the mucous membranes may be pink and yet the patient may be hypercarbic. Adequacy of ventilation (rate and depth) must be assessed frequently.

C. Accumulation of bronchial secretions

    1. Pulmonary secretions cannot be eliminated when a tracheostomy tube is present. Suctioning the tube may be necessary every 2–4 hours.

    2. The diameter of the suction catheter should not exceed one half that of the tracheostomy tube diameter, and suction should not be applied for more than 5 seconds. Otherwise hypoxia or lung collapse may occur.

    3. Ideally, oxygen should be supplied by face mask before and after the suctioning process.

    4. A sterile suction catheter (Superior, Healthcare Group Inc.; Argyle, Mallinckrodt Critical Care) should be introduced, using strict asepsis, until its tip is at the carina. Suction should then be applied by placing a thumb over the vacuum-control side port and the catheter withdrawn under continuous rotation to remove secretions from the trachea or tube surfaces.

D. Humidification

    1. The oxygen should be humidified to prevent drying of mucosa or secretions.

E. Gastric inflation

    1. Oxygen supplied at a high flow rate through a nasal catheter may cause the stomach to inflate.

F. Hyperthermia

    1. Large dogs in a closed oxygen chamber may overheat.

COMPLICATIONS

Surveys of postoperative complications in human hospitals indicate that the incidence of complications is related to the following factors:

I. The preoperative physical status of the patient, with more complications occurring in higher-risk categories.

II. The duration of anesthesia, with an increase in complications occurring with increased length of time of anesthesia.

III. The experience of the anesthetist; the greater the experience of the anesthetist, the less the risk is of postoperative problems.

Abnormal Respiratory Movements or Labored, Difficult Breathing

I. General considerations

A. Hypercarbia or hypoxemia may initiate signs of abnormal breathing or be the result of inadequate breathing. It should be remembered, however, that hypercarbia or hypoxemia can be present without signs of difficult breathing when the patient is depressed by anesthetic drugs. Furthermore, circulatory failure can result in hypoxia, and hypoxia from inadequate ventilation can initiate circulatory failure.

II. Clinical signs
  A. Absence of air movement in or out of lungs
  B. Cyanosis of mucous membranes or muzzle
  C. Grimace of facial muscles, lips drawn back, and mouth-breathing (signs of hypoxia)
  D. Flexion of head and neck during inspiration, with a ventral jerk of the lower jaw
  E. Crowing, or harsh inspiratory noise produced by partial airway obstruction (stridor)
  F. Prolonged inspiratory time
  G. Exaggerated thoracic movement
  H. Inward movement of intercostal muscles and outward movement of abdomen during inspiration (paradoxic breathing)
  I. Excitement or restlessness accompanying a low arterial P_{O_2}
  J. Gasping
  K. Apneustic breathing pattern
  L. Slow, shallow breathing

III. Causes
  A. Airway obstruction
    1. Anatomic predisposition to obstruction in brachycephalic breeds (elongated soft palate, eversion of the ventricles, anatomic distortion of the larynx in bulldogs)
    2. Displacement of the soft palate (common in dogs)
    3. Laryngospasm (occurs sometimes in cats, rare in dogs)
    4. Malplacement of a pharyngostomy tube (the pharyngostomy tube should not pass over the epiglottis or the entrance to the larynx)
    5. Tongue rolled back into the pharynx (occasionally a dog will lick its lips excessively and curl its tongue during recovery from anesthesia; the tongue may become rolled up, and swallowing action then causes it to be wedged in the back of the pharynx)
    6. Pharyngeal swelling (trauma during surgical repair of jaw fracture, swelling after cryotherapy)
    7. Laryngeal hemiplegia (trauma to laryngeal nerve during neck surgery)
    8. Laryngeal or tracheal mucosal swelling (trauma during intubation, prolonged inflation of the endotracheal tube cuff, chemical irritation from residue in an ethylene-oxide-sterilized endotracheal tube, trauma from retraction or manipulation during neck surgery)
    9. Tracheal collapse
    10. Aspiration of a solid object (gauze packing, blood clot, loose tooth, chewed-up endotracheal tube, esophageal stethoscope, or temperature probe)
    11. Bandage around head, neck, or thorax too tight
  B. Central depression of respiratory control
    1. Residual effects of drugs used for anesthesia
    2. Opioids
    3. Hypothermia

C. Inadequate arterial oxygenation or increased CO_2
  1. Failure to supply oxygen after nitrous oxide has been discontinued
  2. Circulatory failure
  3. Pulmonary pathologic condition
  4. Pneumothorax
  5. External compression of thorax
  6. Inadequate reversal of neuromuscular blockade
D. Stimulation of respiratory centers
  1. Hyperthermia
  2. Metabolic acidosis
  3. Some opioids
  4. Pain
E. Failure of neural control
  1. Inadequate reversal of neuromuscular blockade
  2. Cerebellar herniation
IV. Differential diagnosis and treatment
  A. Time of onset of abnormal breathing may rule in or rule out some causes (Table 9–3).
  B. Apnea, no chest movement
    1. Check for absence of peripheral pulse indicating cardiac arrest. Institute cardiopulmonary resuscitation (see Chapter 8).
    2. A dog that receives a nondepolarizing neuromuscular blocking drug during anesthesia and an aminoglycoside antibiotic in recovery may become reparalyzed. Artificial ventilation should be started and neostigmine administered.
    3. Cerebellar herniation may follow an increase in intracranial pressure in a neurologic patient.
    4. Depression of respiratory centers can be caused by anesthetic agents.
  C. Endotracheal tube present, no air movement, chest movement present
    1. Examine endotracheal tube for kinks or compression by clenched jaws.
    2. Patency of the tube within the trachea should be checked by artificially inflating the lungs using a resuscitator (Ambu bag) or an anesthesia machine and circuit.
    3. Remove the cause of obstruction.
  D. After extubation, no air movement, chest movement present
    1. After the endotracheal tube has been removed, absence of air movement at the nose or mouth should be identified by listening or feeling.
    2. The head and neck should be extended, the patient's mouth opened, and the tongue pulled rostrally. This action helps in treatment of brachycephalic breeds and animals with soft-palate displacement or laryngospasm.
    3. The animal should be placed sternal. This positioning helps treat soft-palate displacement.
    4. A bandage encircling the neck should be cut, unless it is obviously very loose.
    5. The laryngeal entrance should be examined for laryngospasm. The position of a pharyngostomy tube should be observed.
    6. If obstruction is still present, the trachea should be reintubated. Administration of a small amount of oxymorphone-diazepam, diazepam/ketamine, propofol, or barbiturate may be necessary. Use of a

Table 9–3. Causes of Abnormal Respiratory Movements or Labored, Difficult Breathing During Recovery from Anesthesia

---

A. Endotracheal tube present; recent disconnection from anesthesia machine

No air moving in/out of trachea

1. Cardiac arrest
2. Airway obstruction
   a. Kinked endotracheal tube
   b. Teeth clenched, compressing tube
   c. Mucus in lumen of tube

Air movement present; cyanosis may or may not be present

1. Hypoventilation
   a. Anesthetic drug depression
   b. Inadequate reversal of neuromuscular blockade
   c. Compromise by positioning
   d. Tight chest or abdominal bandage
   e. Pneumothorax
2. Diffusion hypoxia from N_2O elimination
3. Circulatory failure
   a. Persistent hemorrhage
   b. Congestive heart failure
4. Pulmonary edema

B. Immediately after removal of endotracheal tube

1. Complete or partial airway obstruction
   a. Anatomic predisposition (brachycephalic)
   b. Soft-palate displacement
   c. Laryngospasm
   d. Pharyngostomy tube malpositioned
   e. Tracheal collapse
   f. Compression by tight bandage
   g. Aspiration of blood clot, gauze, esophageal stethoscope, or broken endotracheal tube
   h. Laryngeal hemiplegia

C. Delayed onset; minutes or hours after extubation

1. Airway obstruction
   a. Laryngeal edema
   b. Pharyngeal edema
   c. Tracheal edema
   d. Pharyngostomy tube
2. Pain, fear
3. Circulatory failure
4. Pulmonary edema
5. Pneumothorax
6. Shock lung
7. Hyperthermia
8. Return of neuromuscular blockade
   a. Aminoglycoside antibiotic
   b. Delayed elimination

---

nondepolarizing neuromuscular blocking drug such as atracurium is not recommended. Such a drug should be used only if the veterinarian is sure that endotracheal intubation can be accomplished and that facilities for artificial ventilation are immediately available.

E. Cyanosis or oxygen saturation of less than 90%

1. Look for and correct airway obstruction.

2. Check peripheral pulse; if it is absent, institute cardiopulmonary resuscitation.

3. When a pulse is present, supply oxygen by face mask if the patient is breathing spontaneously. Intubate the trachea and artificially ventilate if the patient is apneic.

4. When cyanosis is not corrected by administration of oxygen, evaluate the circulation using pulse rate and palpable pressure, capillary refill time, and measurement of blood pressure. Supportive treatment should be started if poor cardiovascular function is present.

5. The adequacy of spontaneous breathing should be assessed. When either rate of breathing or depth of breathing are severely inadequate, immediate treatment is indicated. Options follow:

   a. The trachea can be intubated and controlled ventilation instituted.

   b. When a thoracotomy or ruptured diaphragm repair has been performed, the chest tube should be aspirated or thoracentesis performed to measure and remove air from the thoracic cavity. Spontaneous pneumothorax may develop during or after other types of surgery owing to rupture of a pulmonary bleb or bulla that accompanies pulmonary contusions caused by traumatic accident. Thoracic radiography may be indicated.

   c. Respiratory depression caused by administration of an opioid can be antagonized by naloxone. An intravenous bolus dose may restore breathing in 1–2 minutes. The dose may, however, result in an abrupt return to consciousness accompanied by struggling, vocalization, and increased circulating catecholamine concentrations.

   d. When cyanosis has been corrected by administration of oxygen, partial opioid reversal can be attempted by intravenous injections of small doses of naloxone at 2-minute intervals.

F. Jerky or abnormal respiratory movements

   1. Mucous membrane color should be checked. Oxygen should be supplied by face mask if cyanosis is present and oxygen administration continued during examination of the patient and until the cause of the abnormal breathing is identified.

   2. Consider the possibility of partial airway obstruction.

      a. The clinical signs may vary according to the degree of CNS depression from anesthetic drugs.

      b. A harsh inspiratory noise may or may not be present, inspiratory time may be prolonged, the head and neck may be flexed, and the mandible may be moving ventrally during inspiration.

      c. The patient should not be stimulated or excited; partial airway obstruction may not be critical if the patient's breathing remains quiet.

      d. The patient's mouth should be opened and the tongue pulled rostrally. The head and neck should be extended. This action helps in treatment of brachycephalic breeds and animals with soft-palate displacement or partial laryngospasm.

      e. Using good lighting or a laryngoscope, examine the pharynx and larynx for the possibility of a displaced pharyngostomy tube or laryngeal paralysis.

      f. The neck bandage should be loosened.

      g. If the cause of partial airway obstruction has not been identified, bronchoscopy, radiography, or fluoroscopy may provide additional information, such as evidence of tracheal collapse or a foreign body.

   3. Consider the possibility of pain.

      a. Pain may be suspected from the degree of surgical trauma and knowledge of the type and amount of anesthetic drugs administered.

      b. Signs associated with pain may include pupillary dilation, excessive salivation, tachycardia, excitement or immobility, vocalization, deep breathing, or rapid, shallow breathing.

   4. Consider the possibility of circulatory failure.

    a. Check for air movement in and out of the lungs and absence of inspiratory noise.

    b. The peripheral pulse should be palpated for abnormal rate, rhythm, or strength (to identify bradycardia, dysrhythmias, or hypotension).

    c. Capillary refill time should be assessed (to identify poor peripheral perfusion or hypotension).

    d. Arterial blood pressure should be measured (to confirm hypotension) unless the patient is in critical condition and valuable time cannot be wasted.

    e. An EKG should be taken (to reveal dysrhythmias).

    f. The patient should be observed for signs of bleeding. Abdominocentesis, thoracocentesis, or aspiration of the chest drain should be considered where appropriate (to rule out hemorrhage).

    g. See section on circulatory shock.

5. Consider the presence of a pulmonary pathologic condition.

    a. This condition may be indicated by froth and fluid in the endotracheal tube (indicating pulmonary edema or congestive heart failure).

    b. Fluid sounds may be auscultated over lung field (indicating pulmonary edema or hemorrhage).

    c. Absence of air sound by auscultation over lung field may be noted (indicating pneumothorax or hemorrhage).

    d. Radiography should be used to confirm pneumothorax, pulmonary edema, or shock lung. It is advisable to supply oxygen by face mask during the radiographic procedure and to monitor the patient closely when it is positioned on its side. Positioning the patient on its back may result in cardiac arrest.

    e. Thoracentesis may be carried out (to confirm pneumothorax or pleural effusion).

    f. Treat the abnormality.

6. Consider the possibility of persistent neuromuscular blockade if the patient received a neuromuscular blocking drug during anesthesia.

    a. Supply oxygen by face mask or endotracheal tube to ensure arterial oxygenation.

    b. Assess the degree of neuromuscular blockade (confirm by use of a peripheral nerve stimulator; suspect on the basis of absent palpebral reflex or on the inability to lift the head; suspect on the basis of a history of decreased hepatic or renal function).

    c. Administer additional antagonist.

    d. Patients with decreased ability to detoxify a neuromuscular blocking drug may have to be artificially ventilated for up to 12 hours after anesthesia. Sedation with oxymorphone or butorphanol may be necessary. Intubate trachea and institute controlled ventilation if ventilation is moderately or severely decreased.

    e. Meticulous care must be taken to avoid aspiration pneumonia.

7. Hyperthermia may be confirmed or discounted after measurement of temperature.

8. Metabolic acidosis should be considered.

    a. It is often accompanied by deep breathing.

    b. It may be only suspected, or it may be confirmed by calculating the base deficit after measuring arterial pH and P_{CO_2}.

V. Prevention of airway obstruction
  A. Laryngeal and tracheal trauma should be avoided. Tracheal intubation should be facilitated by good lighting and correct positioning of the patient. Endotracheal tubes with high-volume, low-pressure cuffs should be used. Excessive inflation of the cuff should be avoided. Instruments to test cuff pressure are available.
  B. Repositioning the cuff within the trachea after 3 hours of anesthesia, unless gastric reflux has occurred, may limit local mucosal damage.
  C. Anesthetic drugs administered to brachycephalic patients should be chosen to allow a rapid return of muscle tone when anesthesia is discontinued. Sedation after anesthesia with an opioid will often result in a dog tolerating the presence of an endotracheal tube for longer than usual. During this time, halothane or isoflurane is being expelled so that airway obstruction is less likely to occur when the endotracheal tube is finally removed.
  D. The mouth and pharynx should be thoroughly cleaned after oral surgery and before extubation.
  E. The patient should not be allowed to regain consciousness while restrained on its back. The depth of anesthesia must be closely assessed to prevent the patient chewing on the tube.
  F. The head and neck should not be bandaged too tightly. The bandage should be applied with the patient sternal and its head and neck held in a normal position.

Behavior Change

I. General considerations
  A. Ketamine and alphaxalone-alphadolone often result in a behavior change for a few hours after anesthesia.
  B. Behavior change lasting more than 24 hours has been reported with oxymorphone-acepromazine, fentanyl-droperidol (Innovar-Vet), etorphine-methotrimeprazine (Immobilon), and ketamine. The incidence of prolonged, severe change is rare.
II. Types of behavior change
  A. Excitement during recovery from anesthesia
    1. Excitement occurring before return of consciousness may include paddling of limbs, running in place, whining, yelping, howling, spasmodic total body contractions. These actions are more likely to occur when preanesthetic sedation is omitted, and they are more prevalent in young, vigorous patients. They also may occur when ketamine or tiletamine-zolazepam has been used for induction of anesthesia.
    2. Excitement occurring when consciousness returns rapidly may be triggered by sudden awareness of pain.
    3. Excitement in recovery is more likely in a patient that had a stormy induction of anesthesia.
  B. Hyperreflexia (exaggerated motor reflexes)
    1. This frequently occurs in cats during recovery from anesthesia with ketamine or alphaxalone-alphadalone.
  C. Disoriented behavior
    1. Abnormal behavior patterns commonly occur in cats recovering from ketamine anesthesia. These include clawing at the mouth with the forepaws; wide-mouth, tongue-rolling activity; and whole-body tremors.

    2. Confusion may also be caused by hypoxia, cerebral damage, electrolyte imbalance, hyperosmolality, fear, or pain.

    3. Behavior such as sudden starts or jerks and forward motions observed for several days after surgery, followed by attention to the operative site, is presumably initiated by sudden awareness of incisional discomfort.

D. Coughing (may be present early in recovery or may develop any time up to several days after anesthesia)

    1. Aspiration of foreign material

    2. Trauma of the larynx or trachea during intubation

    3. Sloughing of tracheal mucosa at the level of endotracheal tube cuff inflation

    4. Bacterial or viral tracheitis

E. Depression

    1. Decreased responsiveness from delayed elimination of anesthetic drugs

    2. Hypoglycemia (may not develop until 12 hours after anesthesia and is more likely to occur in young, small patients or diabetics)

    3. Sepsis

    4. Continued blood loss

    5. Cardiovascular disease

    6. Renal failure

F. Restlessness (developing within a few hours of anesthesia)

    1. Anxiety (from distended urinary bladder, unfamiliar surroundings, or awareness of other animals in close proximity)

    2. Pain (from the surgical site)

    3. Hyperthermia (from bacteremia, effects of myelography, or seizures)

    4. Hypoxia (from hypoventilation, progressive pneumothorax or hemothorax, pulmonary edema, or shock lung)

    5. Stimulation in some dogs from fentanyl absorbed from fentanyl patches (signs may also include decreased appetite)

G. Aggressive behavior

    1. Pain or fear

    2. Anesthetic agent

       a. Mutilation of newborn by bitches after cesarean section has been reported and attributed to the administration of fentanyl-droperidol (Innovar-Vet).

       b. Aggressive behavior in dogs and cats that were previously friendly has been reported after administration of oxymorphone-acepromazine, fentanyl-droperidol (Innovar-Vet), etorphine-methotrimeprazine (Immobilon), and ketamine.

H. Listlessness, lethargy, decreased appetite

    1. These symptoms have been observed in some hospitalized patients that are otherwise doing well or in which there is no organic reason for failure to recover more rapidly. The cause may be emotional withdrawal as a result of the stress of anesthesia and surgery, as some patients respond dramatically to increased sensory care and attention.

    2. At home, emotional disturbance may be reflected in the following:

       a. Distrust of the owner or increased dependence on the owner

       b. Altered sleeping, eating, or elimination habits

III. Treatment
  A. Ensure that the patient is free of moderate or severe pain by administering appropriate drugs.
  B. Avoid excessive adverse or painful manipulation of the patient during its return to consciousness.
    1. Maintain anesthesia until patient is untied from its position on the table.
    2. Apply bandages to a potentially painful site before consciousness returns.
    3. Take postoperative radiographs while the patient is still anesthetized, or wait until the patient is fully conscious, but do not take radiographs when the patient is only partially conscious.
    4. Express bladder while the patient is anesthetized.
  C. Prevent cats who are recovering after ketamine or tiletamine-zolazepam anesthesia from inflicting tongue or ear lacerations or corneal scratches on themselves by providing them with additional sedation, bandaging their forepaws, or attaching an Elizabethan collar. Confining the cat in a quiet, dark cage may improve the quality of recovery. Administration of butorphanol 0.2 mg/kg intramuscularly may be indicated.
  D. Dogs given tiletamine-zolazepam for induction of anesthesia may exhibit excessive uncontrolled muscle movement during recovery from anesthesia. This effect may be attributed to residual effects of tiletamine. Diazepam 0.2 mg/kg intramuscularly is usually effective treatment.
  E. Perform a thorough physical examination to identify other abnormalities such as hypoxia or hyperthermia, identify their cause, and institute appropriate treatment. Laboratory tests will be necessary to identify electrolyte imbalance, metabolic acidosis, and hypoglycemia.
  F. Institute accepted medical treatment of respiratory disease.
  G. Consider removal of fentanyl patch if signs so indicate.
  H. An aggressive animal may have to be tranquilized. Drug and dosage can be chosen according to individual judgment.

Blindness

I. Causes
  A. Cerebral hypoxia can be present owing to cardiac arrest, hypotension, or hypoxemia that occurred during anesthesia.
II. Treatment
  A. No treatment is indicated other than supportive therapy to restore cardiovascular function and respiration to normal as quickly as possible.
III. Prognosis
  A. If blindness is the only abnormality, sight should return within a few days. In at least one case, however, a dog was blind for 6 weeks after cardiac arrest.

Circulatory Shock

I. Clinical signs
  A. Cold extremities, decreased toe-web temperature
  B. Pallor of mucous membranes
  C. Prolonged capillary refill time

    D. Weak palpable pulse

    E. Tachycardia or bradycardia

    F. Decreased cerebral responsiveness

    G. Hypotension (systolic pressure of less than 75 mm Hg and mean pressure of less than 60 mm Hg)

    H. Pulse deficits or irregular pulse

    I. EKG changes or ST segment elevation or depression

    J. Oliguria

II. Causes

    A. Cardiogenic shock

       1. Congestive heart failure

       2. Cardiomyopathy

       3. Dysrhythmia

       4. Pulmonary embolus

       5. Hypoxia

       6. Hypercarbia

    B. Hypovolemic shock

       1. Hemorrhage

       2. Inadequate intraoperative fluid administration

       3. Excessive vasodilation from hypercarbia, antibiotic administration, or pancreatic enzyme release, and from drugs such as phenothiazines and inhalants

    C. Endotoxic or septic shock

       1. Intussusception, intestinal volvulus, gastric volvulus

       2. Portocaval shunt

       3. Septic focus

    D. Anaphylactic or anaphylactoid shock

       1. Antibiotics: penicillin, cephalosporins, gentamicin

       2. Vaccination

III. Diagnosis

    A. Clinical signs

       1. Signs indicating decreased tissue perfusion, including mental depression, prolonged capillary refill time (CRT) of more than 2 seconds, weak peripheral pulse, tachycardia or bradycardia, and hypotension

    B. Obvious cause

       1. Collapse within minutes after administration of an opioid, antibiotic, or other agent

       2. External hemorrhage

       3. Hypoxia resulting from respiratory arrest

    C. Suspected cause

       1. Anesthesia-induced

          a. Cardiovascular depression resulting from analgesic agent administered to control postoperative pain

          b. Inadequate ventilation (note that hypoxemia may not develop for 10–20 minutes after patient is disconnected from oxygen)

       2. Surgical procedure associated with complications

          a. Paracentesis of thorax or abdomen to confirm blood loss or pneumothorax

      b. EKG to confirm dysrhythmias from myocardial contusions, gastric dilatation or volvulus, splenectomy, cervical decompression or fenestration

   3. Exacerbation of patient's preexisting problem; Class 3, 4, or 5 patients

      a. Cardiac failure: dysrhythmias, decreased contractility, mitral insufficiency

IV. Treatment (Fig. 9–1)

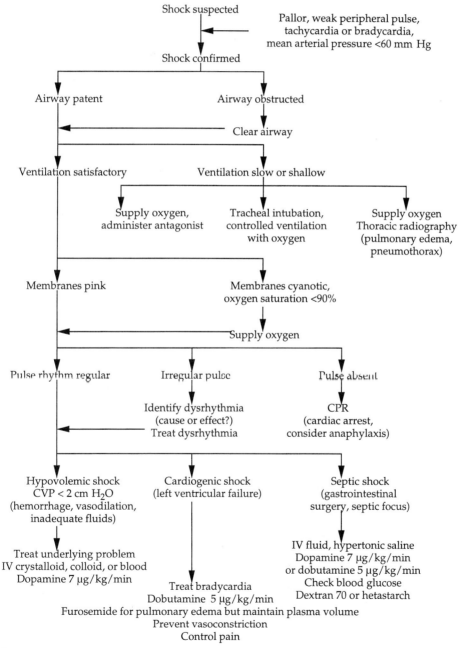

Figure 9–1. Management of circulatory shock during recovery from anesthesia (CVP = central venous pressure).

A. Xylazine or medetomidine should be antagonized. Naloxone should be injected to reverse collapse caused by administration of an opioid.

B. Check patency of airway. Oxygen should be supplied. The trachea should be intubated and artificial ventilation applied if respiration is severely depressed.

C. The underlying cause should be identified and treated.

D. The first priority of treatment is to increase mean arterial blood pressure to above 60 mm Hg so that perfusion of the brain and heart may be maintained. Ideally, fluid and drugs should be given intravenously. Intraosseous administration is as effective as intravenous.

  1. Bradycardia decreases cardiac output. Inject atropine 0.02 mg/kg or glycopyrrolate 0.005 mg/kg intravenously.

  2. Expand blood volume by intravenous infusion of balanced electrolyte solution and hypertonic saline, with dextran, hetastarch, or plasma (see recommendations for treatment of hypotension in previous chapter). Whole blood will be required in the treatment of major blood loss. Fluid overload may occur as a consequence of overenthusiastic treatment of hypovolemic shock and must be avoided in patients with cardiac failure or acute respiratory failure.

  3. Dopamine 7 μg/kg per minute may increase blood pressure and cardiac output in patients with hypovolemia or septic shock. Dobutamine 5–7 μg/kg per minute causes less peripheral vasoconstriction and may be a better choice for patients with cardiac disease.

  4. Acute adrenal crisis should be treated with prednisolone sodium succinate (Solu-Delta-Cortef) 10–30 mg/kg or dexamethasone sodium phosphate 0.5–2 mg/kg intravenously.

  5. Sodium bicarbonate 1 mEq/kg may be administered intravenously for every 10 minutes of hypotension (systolic pressure of less than 60 mm Hg) up to a total dosage of 3 mEq/kg unless laboratory measurement of metabolic acidosis is available.

E. Urine output should be monitored as a measure of effectiveness of treatment.

Hyperthermia

I. Clinical signs

  A. Panting

  B. Patient hot to touch

  C. Rectal temperature of more than 39.5°C (103°F)

II. Causes

  A. Excessive application of heat or failure to discontinue application of heat before desired temperature was reached during treatment of hypothermia, resulting in overshoot

  B. Increased metabolic rate

    1. Muscle activity during recovery from anesthesia, especially in cats after ketamine or tiletamine-zolazepam anesthesia

    2. Muscle activity during seizures

    3. Bacteremia or toxemia

    4. Malignant hyperthermia syndrome

  C. Failure of central thermoregulation: xylazine, ketamine, inhalant anesthetics, antibiotics

III. Treatment
   A. Treatment will vary according to the cause of increased temperature and the degree of hyperthermia. Hepatic, renal, and other bodily functions should be monitored for several days after hyperthermia has occurred.
   B. Treatment of specific causes of hyperthermia
      1. Cats with increased muscle activity during recovery from anesthesia can be sedated with butorphanol 0.2 mg/kg intramuscularly, with or without acepromazine 0.03–.1 mg/kg intramuscularly.
      2. Seizure activity following myelography should be controlled with diazepam or phenobarbital.
      3. Malignant hyperthermia is treated by dantrolene (Dantrium) 3 mg/kg intravenously (see previous chapter for more details). If the syndrome is advanced, the animal should be given oxygen to breathe and sodium bicarbonate 1–2 mEq/kg intravenously.
   C. Cooling
      1. Direct air from a fan into the cage.
      2. Place cold packs around the patient.
      3. Soak the skin with water. Soaking the skin with alcohol may improve cooling, but the patient may become intoxicated if it licks itself.
      4. The patient may be immersed in a cold-water or ice-water bath. Aggressive treatment should be stopped before the patient's temperature reaches 39.4°C (103°F); otherwise hypothermia may develop.
      5. Infuse with cool electrolyte solution intravenously.
      6. An antipyretic such as dipyrone may lower body temperature through an effect on the hypothalamus.

Hypoglycemia

I. Clinical signs
   A. Depression, coma, prolonged recovery from anesthesia
   B. Muscle weakness, muscle tremor, abnormal behavior
   C. Hypertension, hypotension
   D. Seizures
   E. Blood glucose of less than 60 mg/dl
II. Clinical causes
   A. Newborn or pediatric status
   B. Weight loss
   C. Pancreatic islet-cell tumor
   D. Diabetes mellitus
   E. Liver disease
   F. Extrapancreatic malignancies (large abdominal tumors, hepatic tumors)
III. Treatment
   A. Application of Karo syrup to tongue and gums
   B. Initial intravenous administration of 50% dextrose at 1–5 ml over 10 minutes.
   C. Continued intravenous infusion of 5% dextrose in water
   D. Serial measurements of blood glucose
   E. Administration of diazepam or dexamethasone, or both, if glucose administration does not control the CNS signs

Oliguria

I. Clinical signs
  A. Oliguria is indicated by a urine output of less than 0.5 ml/kg per hour. For some individuals an output of less than 1 ml/kg per hour is too low.
  B. An uncatheterized patient that has not voided urine for several hours after anesthesia should be examined for urine retention or failure to produce urine.
  C. A decrease in urine output should be monitored in a catheterized patient. An apparent decrease in urine volume may be produced by obstruction of the urinary catheter with mucus or a blood clot. A dog lying on a rack that sags in the middle may have an apparent decrease in urine output because the urine is pooling in the cranial end of the bladder and cannot drain.
  D. Signs of renal failure such as vomition or depression may not be manifested for 1–3 days.
II. Causes
  A. Prerenal factors causing an abrupt decrease in effective glomerular filtration rate (GFR)
    1. Preexisting abnormal body fluid balance resulting from dehydration, depression, vomiting, diarrhea
    2. Prolonged anesthesia or postanesthetic depression without (adequate) fluid administration
    3. Inadequate oral intake of water after anesthesia
  B. Postrenal obstruction causing back pressure and decreased GFR
    1. Obstruction of the urethra or urethral catheter by blood clots or calculi
    2. Unidentified urethral rupture (pelvic trauma)
    3. Inadvertent ligation of ureter(s) during laparotomy
  C. Hypoperfusion causing acute intrinsic renal failure
    1. Circulatory shock occurring after trauma (such as being hit by a car) but not identified before induction of anesthesia
    2. Severe decrease in cardiac output or arterial blood pressure during anesthesia
    3. Administration of epinephrine for hemostasis that causes intrarenal vasoconstriction
    4. Decreased cardiovascular function after anesthesia
  D. Nephrotoxicity
    1. Methoxyflurane anesthesia can result in decreased concentrating ability for 2–3 days. Increased urine production must be matched by increased fluid intake; otherwise hypovolemia and oliguria result.
    2. Aminoglycoside antibiotics, particularly gentamicin, create an increased potential for toxicity. Higher plasma gentamicin concentrations have been measured in patients for several hours after anesthesia compared with patients not receiving anesthesia.
  E. Chronic renal disease resulting in failure precipitated by the following:
    1. Alterations in fluid balance
    2. Changes in hormonal regulation and sympathetic nervous system tone caused by general anesthesia and surgery
III. Diagnostic approach
  A. History

1. Recent trauma to abdomen or pelvis
2. Several days of administration of antibiotics with potential nephrotoxicity
3. Documented preoperative renal disease
4. No fluid administration during anesthesia or during a prolonged recovery from anesthesia
5. Episode of hypotension during anesthesia
6. Intraoperative administration of epinephrine

B. Physical examination
1. Clinical signs of hypovolemia and dehydration may be nonspecific.
2. If a catheter cannot be passed into the urinary bladder, urethral obstruction may be present.

C. Radiography: excretory urography, contrast cystography, urethrography

IV. Treatment
A. Ensure that urethra is patent.
B. Placement of a urinary catheter may be advisable so that urine production can be monitored accurately. The patient should produce at least 1–2 ml/kg per hour of urine.
C. Treat hypovolemia and restore blood volume by intravenous administration of balanced electrolyte solution (lactated Ringer's solution, Normosol).
1. Measurements of packed cell volume (PCV) and plasma proteins (PP) or central venous pressure can be used as guides to avoid excessive hemodilution or fluid overload.
2. When the PCV is low initially, 10–20 ml/kg of fluid should be infused quickly and the patient's cardiovascular response evaluated before additional fluid is given. The additional fluid should be administered at a rate of 5–15 ml/kg per hour of 2.5% dextrose in 0.45% normal saline to promote diuresis.
D. Inject furosemide (Lasix) 2–5 mg/kg intravenously. Increased urine production should occur within 10 minutes.
E. Infuse dopamine intravenously at 2.5 μg/kg per minute. Dopamine 50 mg in 500 ml saline or 5% dextrose in water produces a concentration of 100 μg/ml. A 10 kg dog would need (10 × 2.5)/100 = 0.25 ml dopamine solution per minute. If an infusion set delivering 60 drops/ml is used, this dog would need 15 drops per minute.
F. Infuse mannitol 0.5–1.0 g/kg intravenously over 20 minutes.
G. Further laboratory tests are indicated.

Prolonged Return to Consciousness

I. General considerations
A. At worst, a prolonged return to consciousness may be an indication of a serious condition that will progress to death. More commonly, delayed recovery is due to excessive depth of anesthesia or slow elimination of anesthetic agents. Prolonged recovery results in continued organ depression necessitating continued monitoring and support. Thus prolonged recovery is not time-effective. Furthermore, depression of ventilation slows excretion of inhalation anesthetics, and hypothermia slows metabolism of injectable agents. It is neither necessary nor desirable for a patient

to be awake as soon as surgery is completed, but the patient should regain consciousness within 10–15 minutes.

II. Causes (see Table 9–4)

    A. CNS depression from drugs

        1. Relative drug overdose: drug calculations for an overweight dog made on the basis of its actual weight; administration of protein-bound drugs such as thiopental or ketamine to patients with low plasma protein

        2. Accumulated drug: deep plane of anesthesia maintained throughout surgery; anesthesia maintained by supplemental injections of thiopental or ketamine

        3. Increased CNS sensitivity: old age; hypothyroidism; hypothermia; individual variation that is reflected in an extremely decreased requirement for anesthetic agents in some individual dogs or litters

        4. Prolonged detoxification of drug

           a. Animals with low cardiac output may have a prolonged recovery because of poor delivery of drug to site of detoxification.

           b. Hypoventilation slows elimination of inhalation agents. Hepatic disease is associated with increased duration of effect of thiopental, opioids, succinylcholine, and pancuronium.

           c. Azotemia is associated with prolonged effect of thiopental, ketamine, opioids, and nondepolarizing neuromuscular blocking drugs (except atracurium).

Table 9–4. Causes of Delayed Return to Consciousness after General Anesthesia

Pathophysiology	Clinical Problems
Potentiation of anesthetic drug–induced CNS depression	Azotemia Hypoglycemia Hypothermia Hypothyroidism Individual sensitivity Old age Preexisting CNS depression
Prolonged elimination of anesthetic drugs	Acidosis Chloramphenicol Decreased cardiac output Decreased urine production Excessive administration Hepatic disease Hypothermia Hypoventilation (inhalants)
Brain damage occurring during anesthesia	Cardiac arrest Embolism Increased intracranial pressure Hypoglycemia Hypotension Hypoxemia
Muscle weakness	Neuromuscular blocking agents Neurologic disease
Circulatory shock	Endotoxemia/septicemia Hemorrhage Hypovolemia Severe pain Tension pneumothorax

      d. Concurrent administration of chloramphenicol prolongs the effect of thiopental or ketamine by competing at sites of metabolism in the liver.

B. Metabolic depression of the CNS
1. Hepatic failure is associated with increased sensitivity to opioids.
2. Hypothyroidism may be present.
3. Severe hypoglycemia may be present.
4. Hyperosmolar, hyperglycemic, nonketotic diabetes is a rare cause of prolonged recovery. The severe increase in blood glucose and sodium results in intracellular dehydration. The blood glucose exceeds 600 mg/dl, and the osmolality 375 mOsm/kg.

C. CNS damage
1. Cerebral ischemia as a result of hypotension or cardiac arrest
2. Increased intracranial pressure from hemorrhage or edema; cerebellar herniation
3. Hypoglycemia
4. Embolism

D. Muscle weakness
1. Continued paralysis from neuromuscular blocking drugs
2. Administration of an aminoglycoside antibiotic soon after the administration of neostigmine to reverse a nondepolarizing muscle relaxant
3. Neurologic disease (myasthenia)

E. Circulatory shock
1. Continued bleeding into thoracic or abdominal cavities
2. Inadequate fluid therapy during anesthesia
3. Tension pneumothorax
4. Endotoxemia or septicemia
5. Severe pain

III. Diagnosis and treatment
A. Oxygen should be administered to the patient when mucous membranes are cyanotic, oxygen saturation is less than 90%, or ventilation is obviously inadequate. The trachea should be intubated and controlled ventilation instituted when the depth of breathing is shallow or the respiratory rate is less than 5 breaths per minute if the jaws are relaxed sufficiently to allow intubation.

B. The following potential causes for prolonged recovery should be ruled out or treated.
1. Persistent effect of anesthetic agents
    a. Long duration of inhalation anesthesia at a deep plane of anesthesia. While the patient is connected to the anesthesia machine, increase oxygen flow to 3 L/min and assist ventilation to speed elimination of agent.
    b. Opioid depression should be suspected if an opioid was administered intraoperatively or at the end of surgery, more than 20 minutes have passed since the inhalant was discontinued, the palpebral reflex is brisk, and the swallowing reflex is minimal.
       (1) No treatment is necessary if cardiovascular function is good.
       (2) Partial reversal with naloxone can be attempted, but it is difficult to achieve a dose that will not result in complete arousal.
    c. Multiple dosing with thiopental or ketamine may be associated

with slow recovery. Propofol is unlikely to be the cause of prolonged recovery (cats are slower to recover from continuous infusion than dogs).

    d. Suspect prolonged elimination of anesthetic drugs as the cause of prolonged recovery when preoperative laboratory values of organ function (blood urea nitrogen, creatinine, hepatic enzymes) were abnormal. Supportive care should be instituted in all such patients.

2. Persistent neuromuscular blockade from neuromuscular blocking agent

    a. Absence of four equal twitches in response to train-of-four stimulation of ulnar, superficial peroneal, or tibial nerve by peripheral nerve stimulator

    b. Absence of palpebral reflex or swallowing reflex (even though spontaneous breathing may be present)

3. Inadequate cardiovascular function

    a. Check for hypotension (heart rate, arterial blood pressure, CRT).

    b. Seek cause of decreased function and treat appropriately.

4. Hypothermia

    a. Rectal temperature of less than 35°C (95°F)

5. Hypoglycemia

6. Determine electrolyte and acid-base status if laboratory facilities are available.

C. Suspect brain damage if the following conditions are present for an extended time after anesthesia has been discontinued.

1. Spontaneous breathing has not resumed despite slowing of artificial ventilation and CO_2 accumulation.

2. Pupils are fixed and dilated. Note that pupils can be normal size when brain damage is present. A dog with each pupil a different size may have brain damage, such as cerebellar herniation, or may make an uneventful recovery from anesthesia, with the pupils returning to the same size in 24 hours.

3. Voluntary movement is absent.

4. No involuntary movements (except spinal reflexes) are noted.

5. Involuntary movement is present, but the patient is still unresponsive after 4 hours of supportive therapy, and no other cause has been found.

D. Supportive therapy

1. Administer oxygen and artificial ventilation when needed.

2. Administer intravenous infusion of lactated Ringer's solution or 2.5% dextrose in 0.45% normal saline at 5 ml/kg per hour to maintain blood volume and to promote hepatic and renal perfusion. When the patient has not yet received intravenous fluid, 10 ml/kg of electrolyte solution should be infused in 10 minutes unless contraindicated (by moderate to severe cardiac disease or pulmonary contusions, for example). Additional fluid should be infused after evaluation of the cardiovascular system (see also Chapter 10).

3. Check blood glucose.

4. Maintain normal body temperature.

5. Turn patient hourly to decrease hypostatic congestion.

6. Apply ophthalmic lubricant to prevent corneal drying.

7. Monitor urine production. Catheterize or express urinary bladder.

8. Administer methylprednisolone sodium succinate (Solu-Delta-Cortef), 30 mg/kg intravenously when cerebral damage suspected. Mannitol 2 g/kg should be given intravenously over 30 minutes.
9. Doxapram (Dopram) will also cause some arousal in addition to its respiratory stimulant action.
   a. Doxapram causes release of norepinephrine and can cause tachycardia and dysrhythmias, particularly in patients that have been on inhalation anesthesia.
   b. Dosage should be 1 mg/kg intravenously after inhalation anesthesia and up to 5 mg/kg during anesthesia with injectable drugs.
   c. Doxapram should not be used as a substitute for good anesthetic management.
   d. Aggressive behavior has been observed in dogs sedated with xylazine and receiving doxapram.
10. Consider administration of antagonists.
   a. Naloxone for opioids
   b. Yohimbine or atipamezole for alpha-2 agonist sedatives
   c. Flumazenil for benzodiazepines

Pulmonary Edema

I. Clinical signs
  A. Anxiety, restlessness
  B. Dyspnea, coughing
  C. Cyanosis
  D. Pulmonary rales
  E. Froth in the endotracheal tube or at the nostrils
II. Causes
  A. Increased pulmonary capillary pressure
    1. Excessive intravenous infusion of fluid
    2. Cardiac failure
    3. Xylazine-ketamine anesthesia, xylazine-thiobarbiturate anesthesia
    4. Ligation of a patent ductus arteriosus with a fluid infusion rate that would not be excessive in a healthy patient
    5. Use of mannitol after treatment with epinephrine (renal shut-down)
  B. Increased capillary-alveolar permeability (acute respiratory failure)
    1. Pulmonary contusions
    2. Sepsis or endotoxemia
    3. Disseminated intravascular coagulation
    4. Aspiration of gastric fluid
    5. Fat embolism
    6. "Shock lung"
    7. Oxygen toxicity (inspired oxygen concentration of more than 60% for 24 hours)
  C. Decreased plasma oncotic pressure (hypoproteinemia)
    1. Hepatic disease
    2. Renal disease
    3. Protein-losing enteropathy
  D. Other causes

       1. Seizures

       2. Rapid expansion of collapsed lung "re-expansion pulmonary edema" (during repair of ruptured diaphragm)

III. Diagnosis

   A. History (facts to be considered)

       1. Recent aspiration of gastric fluid

       2. Administration of 60 ml/kg electrolyte fluid intravenously within 1 hour

       3. Cat anesthetized with or recovering from anesthesia with ketamine

       4. Surgical procedure that included repair of ruptured diaphragm or ligation of patent ductus arteriosus

       5. Hypoproteinemia

   B. Clinical signs

       1. Froth and fluid in the trachea or appearing at the nostrils

       2. Fluid sounds on auscultation of lungs

       3. Labored breathing

       4. Cyanosis

   C. Further examination

       1. Radiography may confirm the diagnosis of pulmonary edema, and the location of greatest density may identify the cause

       2. Oxygen should be supplied by face mask during the radiographic procedure or when dyspnea is present.

       3. Blood gas analysis showing low arterial Pa_{O_2} may confirm the diagnosis. Pa_{CO_2} may be normal to low when the patient hyperventilates in attempt to maintain oxygenation. Hypercarbia will develop when the edema becomes severe.

IV. Treatment

   A. The inspired oxygen concentration should be increased by placing the patient in an oxygen cage or insufflating the patient with oxygen via a nasal tube, transtracheal catheter, or tracheostomy tube. An endotracheal tube may have to be inserted when edema is severe. See section on oxygen therapy.

   B. In dogs, an opioid such as morphine 0.2–.5 mg/kg or oxymorphone 0.05–.2 mg/kg may be used to produce some sedation during treatment if necessary. The lowest effective dose should be used. Butorphanol or oxymorphone may be effective in cats. General anesthesia with propofol, tracheal intubation, and controlled ventilation may be necessary if edema is severe.

   C. Administer furosemide (Lasix) 4.4 mg/kg intravenously when pulmonary edema is life-threatening. Use lower doses when edema is less severe. Repeat dose in 1–2 hours if condition has not improved.

   D. Cardiac dysrhythmias should be controlled.

   E. Cardiac pulmonary edema may be improved by the administration of aminophylline 6–10 mg/kg intravenously or subcutaneously every 6 hours. (This drug has positive inotropic effect and produces bronchodilation; it also is arrhythmogenic.)

   F. The underlying process of noncardiac pulmonary edema must be identified and treated. Meanwhile, intensive care is necessary to support life. Breathing 100% oxygen with controlled ventilation may not provide adequate arterial oxygenation in some patients, in which case positive end-expiratory pressure (PEEP) will be necessary. Maintenance of a low level of positive pressure helps to keep small airways open that would otherwise collapse before the alveolae were emptied. PEEP can be created in the following ways:

1. By incorporating into the anesthetic system a specially designed, commercially available valve
2. By submerging the expiratory limb of the circuit 5–10 cm below the surface of water in a container
3. By partially closing the pop-off valve until the pressure gauge in the circuit reads between 5–10 cm H_2O pressure

Seizures

I. Causes
   A. Ketamine
   B. Radiographic contrast media
      1. Ventriculography
      2. Myelography
   C. Hypoglycemia
      1. Diabetes
      2. Insulinoma
      3. Newborn status or small size, together with a too-long withholding of food
   D. Epilepsy
   E. Increased intracranial pressure
II. Treatment
   A. Mucous membrane color should be observed during a seizure and 100% oxygen administered if membranes do not remain pink. The head and neck should be held in an extended position to preserve a patent airway. When an endotracheal tube is present, it should be checked to make sure that increased jaw tone has not compressed and occluded the tube.
   B. Check blood glucose. Treat hypoglycemia with 50% dextrose 1–5 ml over 10 minutes and 5% dextrose in water at 5 ml/kg per hour. If seizures are intermittent, corn syrup may be given orally. Recheck blood glucose.
   C. A cat having seizures after ketamine administration should be treated by intravenous infusion of fluid (lactated Ringer's solution 10 ml/kg over 10–20 minutes) to speed elimination of the ketamine. The seizures may be treated with diazepam 0.2 mg/kg intravenously or, alternatively, the cat can be lightly anesthetized with isoflurane or halothane for 15–20 minutes while fluid is infused.
   D. Inject diazepam 0.2–.5 mg/kg intravenously to control seizures caused by radiographic contrast medium. This dose can be repeated after several minutes. Intravenous fluid administration to cause diuresis and elimination of the drug is most important.
      1. Administration of phenobarbital 2–4 mg/kg intramuscularly may be necessary if seizures persist despite treatment with diazepam. The phenobarbital will usually result in partial anesthesia, and the animal must have the appropriate intensive care.
         a. Hydration must be maintained, ophthalmic ointment applied to prevent corneal drying, and the patient turned hourly to minimize hypostatic congestion of the lungs.
         b. Check rectal temperature frequently for hyperthermia.

           c. Atropine or glycopyrrolate may be necessary to control excessive salivation.

   E. If cerebral edema suspected, inject methylprednisolone sodium succinate, 10–30 mg/kg intravenously and mannitol 2 g/kg intravenously over 30 minutes.

Analgesia and Pain Management

Chapter
10

Robert R. Paddleford

I. Physiology of pain
  A. Definition of pain
    1. Pain is a perception. Unless there is higher central nervous system (CNS) center recognition of a noxious stimulus, no response or adaptation will occur.
    2. Nociception is the neural response to a noxious stimuli. Pain is the subjective interpretation of nociceptive input.
    3. Physiologic pain causes the animal to move away from potential tissue-damaging stimuli. This pain is a protective response.
    4. Pathologic pain is associated with surgery or disease processes that produce organ or tissue damage.
      a. The pathologic pain can be acute or chronic.
      b. It can be somatic or visceral in origin.
      c. It can have varying degrees of severity.
  B. Nociceptors are stimulated when exposed to a noxious or painful stimulus.
    1. The pain pathway is a three-neuron chain.
      a. The first-order neuron originates in the periphery and projects to the spinal cord.
      b. The second-order neuron ascends the spinal cord.
      c. The third-order neuron projects into the brain.
    2. Nociceptors are found in both deep and superficial tissues
    3. Nociceptors are raw nerve endings attached to afferent nerve fibers. They cannot discretely discriminate the source of stimulation.
    4. Nociceptors are found in skin, peritoneum, pleura, periosteum, subchondral bone, joint capsules, muscles, tendons, blood vessels, and some viscera.
    5. Nociceptors respond to mechanical, thermal, and chemical stimuli and are classified as follows:
      a. High-threshold mechanoreceptors respond to pressure.
      b. Low-threshold mechanothermal receptors respond to heat and pressure and are associated with A-delta nerve fibers.
      c. Polymodal receptors respond to mechanical, thermal, and chemical stimuli and are associated with C nerve fibers.
    6. Chemical stimuli can be exogenous or endogenous. Endogenous chemical stimuli include bradykinin, kalidin, acid, leukotrienes, prostaglandins, proteolytic enzymes, potassium, histamines, and serotonin.
    7. Each nociceptor has a detection threshold potential.
      a. This threshold potential must be exceeded before an impulse travels from the peripheral receptor site to the CNS.

   b. The pain-detection threshold is approximately the same for both humans and animals.

C. Physiology of pain transmission

1. A-delta or C nerve fibers carry the nerve impulse from the periphery to the dorsal or ventral spinal root and then to the dorsal horn of the spinal cord after the nociceptor threshold potential has been exceeded.

2. A-delta nerve fibers
   a. These are the so-called "fast" fibers.
   b. They are responsible for the first acute, fast, sharp pain associated with injury.
   c. Their receptive area is very discrete.
   d. They enable the animal to localize the pain to the site of the stimulus.

3. C nerve fibers
   a. These are the so-called "slow" fibers.
   b. They are responsible for the second, dull, aching, burning, throbbing pain associated with injury.
   c. Their receptive area is large.
   d. C fibers limit the localization of the site of stimulus to general body areas.

4. Somatic pain
   a. Somatic pain is conducted by both A-delta and C fibers.
   b. Somatic pain is discretely localizable.

5. Visceral pain
   a. Visceral pain results from broad stimulation of visceral nerve endings.
   b. Visceral pain is conducted by type C nerve fibers only, which carry only dull, nonlocalizable pain sensations.
   c. Focal tissue damage (needle puncture, cutting with a scalpel) does not cause much stimulation.
   d. Visceral pain results mostly from broad stimulation of nerve endings by ischemia, smooth-muscle spasm of hollow organs or ducts, or distension (stretching) of viscera and ligaments.

6. Parietal surfaces
   a. Parietal surfaces of the thorax and abdomen and retroperitoneal organs (kidneys) are richly supplied by A-delta (fast) and C (slow) nerve fibers.
   b. Thus, nociceptive stimulation of parietal surfaces can result in both sharp, focal pain and dull, diffuse, nonlocalizable pain.

7. A-beta nerve fibers
   a. These nerve fibers exhibit lower stimulation thresholds than A-delta and C nerve fibers do.
   b. They transmit innocuous tactile sensations such as vibration, tickling, pricking or tingling.
   c. A-beta fibers constitute the ascending pathways that "close the gate" at the central transmission cell in the dorsal horn of the spinal cord.
   d. Stimulating A-beta nerve fibers seems to diminish A-delta and C nerve fiber nociceptor input.

8. Pain tolerance

    a. Although the pain-detection threshold is similar among species, pain tolerance varies widely among both individuals and species.

    b. Pain tolerance is greatly affected by difference in motivation and by the patient's background.

    c. Pain tolerance is highly susceptible to placebo effects.

9. Hyperalgesia

    a. This phenomenon occurs when a nociceptor is stimulated and then responds to subsequent noxious stimuli more vigorously and at a lower pain-detection threshold.

    b. Primary hyperalgesia occurs as the result of the direct effect of inflammatory mediators on the nociceptor in the injured area.

    c. Secondary hyperalgesia occurs in the surrounding uninjured tissue. It is thought to result from the spread of sensitization of nociceptors from neurons with diffuse collateral branches, one of which innervates the injury site. It may also be associated with central sensitization.

    d. The significance of hyperalgesia is that it allows low-level stimuli to produce pain by activating A-delta and C nerve fibers.

10. Central sensitization

    a. This is an activity-dependent increase in the excitability of spinal neurons.

    b. It appears that once the dorsal spinal horn receives massive nociceptive impulses, the postsynaptic ascending spinal neurons become hypersensitized to subsequent stimuli.

    c. Consequently, the magnitude and duration of response to additional noxious stimuli will increase. So will the response to low-threshold stimuli such as A-beta mechanoreceptors.

    d. Therefore, A-beta nerve fiber stimulation, which would normally be a subthreshold stimulus, becomes a suprathreshold stimulus that can trigger the hypersensitized ascending spinal neurons and cause pathologic pain.

    e. Central sensitization may be significant clinically in that it may be important to treat pain prior to its onset (preemptive analgesia) so that this phenomenon does not occur.

II. Assessment and recognition of pain

  A. General comments

    1. Limitations in the human recognition of pain in animal species results from the absence of verbal communication that expresses pain perception.

    2. Absence of this communication link is a fundamental reason why pain is interpreted in an inconsistent manner in animals.

    3. Animals *do* perceive pain, but their expression of that pain is nonverbal. Therefore, behavioral or physiologic responses must be interpreted to assess pain in animals.

    4. Keep in mind that many animals are unwilling or unable to show behavioral responses to pain. Therefore, if an animal has had surgery or has some disease process that causes pain, it may be beneficial to treat it for pain regardless of its behavioral response.

    5. It can be *extremely* difficult to assess pain in animals.

  B. Physiologic signs of pain

    1. The physiologic changes observed with pain are often due to catecholamine release and activation of the sympathetic nervous system.

    2. Cardiopulmonary changes
       a. Increased heart rate
       b. Increased blood pressure
       c. Cardiac dysrhythmias
       d. Increased respiratory rate
       e. Shallow breathing
       f. Pale mucous membranes as a result of catecholamine-mediated vaso-constriction.
    3. Other physiologic signs
       a. Dilated pupils
       b. Salivation
       c. Hyperglycemia

C. Behavioral signs of pain
    1. Because behavioral signs of pain can be *extremely* variable among patients, each patient must be evaluated on an individual basis.
    2. Remember that some patients are unwilling or unable to show classic behavioral responses to pain.
    3. What may be pain-related behavioral signs in one patient may be completely opposite or missing in another patient.
    4. Behavioral signs of pain
       a. Vocalization—crying, howling, barking, growling, purring
       b. Silence
       c. Guarding of the painful site
       d. Changes in facial expression
       e. Self-mutilation
       f. Muscle rigidity or weakness
       g. Restlessness
       h. Reluctance to move
       i. Behavioral changes (e.g., a gentle animal becomes aggressive, a social animal becomes timid)
       j. Dullness—unresponsive when touched or handled
       k. Loss of appetite or marked decrease in food or water intake
       l. Failure to groom

D. Degree of pain
    1. Mild pain
       a. Mild pain is usually a nuisance-type pain that is easily tolerated.
       b. Mild pain does not usually cause behavioral changes.
       c. The animal may resent manipulation and examination of the involved area; however, the area is not particularly painful when not being stimulated.
    2. Moderate pain
       a. Moderate pain usually occurs when an animal has a disease or has undergone a surgical procedure that would cause pain in humans.
       b. Usually the animal's behavior, appetite, or activity is abnormal.
       c. Signs of moderate pain may include some of the following:
          (1) Decrease or loss of appetite
          (2) Weight loss
          (3) Restlessness or inability to sleep

       (4) Fearfulness or aggressiveness

       (5) "Staring off into space"

       (6) Restlessness causing frequent changes of position

       (7) Assumption of abnormal positions or postures

       (8) Reluctance to move

       (9) Guarding of painful area

       (10) Anxious facial expression

       (11) Crying out or acting aggressively when touched

       (12) Vocalization

    d. Moderate pain is probably the most common degree of pain that is treated.

3. Severe pain

    a. This is pain that is intolerable.

    b. The animal usually exhibits unprovoked vocalizing (howling, crying, screaming).

    c. The animal may throw itself about the cage (this must be differentiated from a "rough" anesthesia recovery or CNS disease).

    d. Severe pain may cause self-mutilation.

III. Pain management

A. General comments

  1. Reasons for treating pain

    a. To make the patient feel better (humane reasons)

    b. To decrease the deleterious physiologic changes that accompany pain

  2. When discomfort is great enough or prolonged enough to alter normal behavior or activity, an individual is said to be suffering from pain that should be treated.

  3. It may not be possible to eliminate all pain.

  4. The goal of pain management is not necessarily to eliminate all pain but to reduce or eliminate *pathologic* pain associated with injury or surgery.

  5. Control of pain for the first 12–24 hours postoperatively seems to be important.

  6. It may be difficult to adequately assess pain in some patients. If it is not clear whether an animal is experiencing undue pain or whether analgesics are needed, it may be appropriate to administer an analgesic or analgesics and observe the response.

  7. A patient that is pain-free, or at least pain-tolerant, will be quiet and calm. Such patients will often sleep.

B. Nonpharmacologic approaches to pain control

  1. Keep the patient clean and dry.

    a. Do not allow the patient to lie in feces or urine.

    b. Place the patient on a grate if possible.

  2. Keep the patient warm.

    a. Warm-water-circulating blankets or regular cloth blankets can be used.

    b. Never put the patient directly on the warm-water-circulating blanket. Place a towel or regular cloth blanket between the water blanket and the patient.

    c. *Never* use electrical heating pads.

3. Keep the patient in a room with a moderate temperature (65–75°F) and a moderate humidity (30–70%).
4. Provide a well-padded place for the patient to sleep.
5. The patient's surroundings should be pleasant and *quiet*.
   a. Avoid loud, sudden noises.
   b. Avoid startling the patient.
   c. Low, soothing background music may be beneficial.
6. Provide human contact to reassure the patient that everything is all right.
   a. Speak in a soothing voice.
   b. Gently touching or petting the patient may help.
7. Acupressure, acupuncture, massage, manipulations, and other mechanisms have been used to stimulate A-beta nerve fibers.
   a. A-beta nerve fibers transmit innocuous tactile sensations such as vibration, tickling, pricking, or tingling.
   b. Stimulating A-beta nerve fibers seems to diminish A-delta and C nerve fiber nociceptor input.
   c. Rubbing the patient's head or ears or petting the patient can stimulate A-beta nerve fibers.
C. Pharmacologic approaches to postoperative pain control
   1. The pharmacologic approach to pain control has become more of a "balanced" approach.
      a. Use multiple drugs for maximal effects.
      b. Use multiple drugs that modulate pain at various sites.
   2. Local anesthetics, nonsteroidal antiinflammatory drugs (NSAIDs) and opioids are the primary agents used either alone or in combination to provide postoperative pain relief in dogs and cats.
   3. Other drugs such as phenothiazine tranquilizers, benzodiazepine tranquilizers, and alpha-2 agonists have been used in combination with opioids to enhance the opioids' effects.
      a. Phenothiazine tranquilizers do not have analgesic properties but will strongly enhance the analgesic properties of an opioid even when the phenothiazine is used in extremely small doses.
      b. Benzodiazepine tranquilizers may have some mild analgesic properties and will enhance the analgesic properties of opioids.
      c. Alpha-2 agonists have analgesic properties. Caution must be used when they are combined with opioids because of the alpha-2 agonists' cardiopulmonary effects.
D. Pharmacologic approach to postoperative pain control with local anesthetics
   1. Local anesthetic agents can be used to help manage peri- as well as postoperative pain.
   2. Local anesthetics can be used in a variety of ways.
      a. Infiltration of a surgical site or "splash blocks"
      b. Direct nerve blocks
      c. Regional infiltration
      d. Intra-articular infiltration
      e. Epidurals
   3. Numerous local anesthetics are available. The two more commonly used in veterinary anesthesia are lidocaine and bupivacaine.
   4. Lidocaine

  a. Lidocaine has a rapid onset of action (5–10 minutes).

  b. It is relatively short-acting (1–2 hours).

  c. It stings when injected into an awake patient.

    (1) The discomfort to the patient can be decreased by mixing one part sodium bicarbonate (1 mEq/L) with 9 parts of 1–2% lidocaine.

    (2) The sodium bicarbonate also reduces the latency period of the lidocaine.

  d. The dose of lidocaine for surgical-site infiltration, "splash blocks," direct nerve blocks, regional infiltration or intra-articular infiltration should not exceed 4–7 mg/kg (2–3 mg/lb).

    (1) A dose of 11 mg/kg (5 mg/lb) can cause toxic side effects.

    (2) Toxic side effects can include restlessness, muscle tremors, seizures, cardiopulmonary depression, coma, and death.

5. Bupivacaine

  a. Bupivacaine has a longer onset of action than lidocaine (20 minutes).

  b. It has a longer duration of action than lidocaine (4–6 hours).

  c. The dose for bupivacaine for surgical-site infiltration, direct nerve blocks, regional infiltration, or intra-articular infiltration should not exceed 2.2 mg/kg (1 mg/lb).

    (1) A dose of 4–5 mg/kg (2–2.5 mg/lb) can produce toxic side effects.

    (2) The toxic side effects are similar to those of lidocaine.

6. Local infiltration of a surgical site

  a. Lidocaine can be infiltrated at the surgical site to help prevent pain associated with intravenous catheterization, aspiration of body cavities, and minor surgeries of the skin.

  b. Lidocaine can be wiped onto the skin prior to catheter placement to help provide analgesia to the skin. One should wait 3–4 minutes before placing the catheter to allow time for the lidocaine to deaden the areas.

7. Surgical-site infiltration or "splash blocks"

  a. Lidocaine (shorter acting) or bupivacaine (longer acting) can be placed or "splashed" into a surgical site to provide postsurgical analgesia.

  b. Local anesthetics can be used in the surgical site following lateral ear resections or ablations, dewclaw removal, onychectomy, and ear cropping.

  c. Local anesthetics can be infused or dripped along surgical incision sites at the time of closure to provide analgesia postoperatively.

  d. Local anesthetics can be infused in and around fracture-repair sites to provide analgesia postoperatively.

  e. Always keep in mind the toxic dose levels, and be sure to not exceed the recommended doses.

  f. Ideally, the local anesthetic should remain in contact with the tissue for 15–20 minutes before it is flushed or blotted away. For this reason, it is better to wait to infuse or drip the postsurgical local anesthetic into the surgical site after the surgical field is dry and no additional blotting of the tissues is needed.

8. Direct nerve infiltration

  a. When amputating a limb, infuse bupivacaine into each nerve before cutting it. It is better to wait several minutes following infiltrating the nerve before cutting it.

  b. Intercostal nerve blocks using bupivacaine should be done prior to closing a thoracotomy incision.

9. Intrapleural infiltration

  a. Bupivacaine can be infused directly through the chest tube following thoracotomy to provide intrapleural analgesia.

  b. An initial dose of 2.2 mg/kg (1 mg/lb) can be used.

  c. Bupivacaine can be repeated every 4–6 hours; however, the cumulative daily dose should not exceed 8 mg/kg (4 mg/lb) on the first day and 4 mg/kg (2 mg/lb) on subsequent days.

  d. Remember, the total dose of bupivacaine for the intercostal nerve block and the initial dose of bupivacaine through the chest tube should not exceed 2.2 mg/kg (1 mg/lb).

10. Intra-articular blocks

  a. Bupivacaine can be infused into a joint following surgery.

  b. The analgesic effects can last up to 24 hours.

  c. The long duration of effect most likely occurs because bupivacaine is so slowly removed from a joint.

  d. Bupivacaine has been used following stifle and shoulder joint surgery, but it can be used in any joint.

  e. The dose should not exceed 2.2 mg/kg (1 mg/lb).

11. Epidurals are discussed under a separate heading in this chapter.

E. Pharmacologic approach to postoperative pain control with nonsteroidal antiinflammatory drugs

1. Nonsteroidal antiinflammatory drugs (NSAIDs) have been traditionally used for chronic pain management.

2. Interest has increased in the use of these drugs for acute postoperative pain.

  a. Some of the newer NSAIDs may be more effective analgesics than some of the older NSAIDs.

  b. Some of the newer NSAIDs have decreased renal and gastrointestinal toxicity.

  c. Some NSAIDs are now available in injectable form.

3. Mechanism of action

  a. NSAID-mediated analgesia has been thought to be entirely the result of the anti-inflammatory effect of these drugs at the site of tissue injury. However, evidence now suggests these drugs may also have significant central analgesic effects. The central effects may be independent of the inhibition of prostaglandin formation.

  b. NSAIDs are inhibitors of cyclooxygenase, which is the enzyme necessary to convert arachidonic acid into prostanoids (thromboxanes, prostacyclin, and prostaglandins).

  c. Prostanoids are mediators of inflammation.

    (1) They amplify nociceptive input and transmission to the spinal cord from peripheral nerves.

    (2) They also affect spinal nociceptive processing by causing the firing of central neurons and by enhancing neurotransmitter release from primary spinal sensory afferents.

  d. Cyclooxygenase has two isomers.

    (1) Cyclooxygenase 1 is the nonregulated form that maintains

physiologic function such as the modulation of renal blood flow and the synthesis of gastric mucous.

(2) Cyclooxygenase 2 is the cytokine-induced form that is activated in injured or inflamed tissue and leads to prostaglandin production.

(3) Cyclooxygenase 2 is thought to be involved in the pain response and hyperalgesia that follow tissue injury.

e. Some NSAIDs inhibit cyclooxygenase and lipoxygenase activity.

(1) Lipoxygenase uses arachidonic acid to produce the leukotriene inflammatory mediators.

(2) Leukotrienes have been implicated in the production of NSAID ulcer formation.

f. NSAIDs vary in their ability to inhibit cyclooxygenase 1 and 2.

(1) This variation in inhibition of cyclooxygenase accounts for their variation in potency and in their potential for toxic side effects.

(2) Some of the newer NSAIDs being developed have more than a thousand-fold specificity for cyclooxygenase 2 over cyclooxygenase 1.

(3) NSAIDs with a high specificity for cyclooxygenase 2 will have enhanced analgesia.

(4) NSAIDs with a low specificity for cyclooxygenase 1 should have decreased toxic side effects.

4. NSAID toxicity

a. Adverse side effects from toxicity of NSAIDs include ulcers of the gastrointestinal tract, renal dysfunction, and hemorrhaging caused by platelet function inhibition.

b. Dogs and cats seem more susceptible than humans to these adverse side effects.

c. Not all NSAIDs are equal in their ability to produce toxic side effects.

d. The ability of the NSAIDs to produce toxic side effects has probably limited their use for acute postoperative pain control; however, with some of the newer NSAIDs, the incidence of toxic side effects may be reduced.

5. Specific NSAIDs (Table 10–1)

a. Flunixin meglumine (Banamine)

(1) Flunixin is available as an injectable.

(2) It has been used in both dogs and cats.

(3) It has been used for acute postsurgical pain.

(4) A major concern with flunixin is its toxic side effects, which include *nephrotoxicity, gastric ulcer formation,* increased alanine aminotransferase production, and an ability to cause hemorrhage.

(5) Patients receiving flunixin should be well-hydrated and receiving intravenous fluids and ulcer prophylaxis (see section E7 on contraindications to NSAID use).

b. Carprofen (Rimadyl)

(1) Carprofen is available as a solution for injection, as rectal suppositories, as a paste, and in tablet form (currently it is available only in tablet form in the United States).

(2) Carprofen has been approved for oral and injectable use in dogs

Table 10–1. Nonsteroidal Antiinflammatory Drugs Used in
the Dog and Cat

Drug	Indication	Dose/Route (mg/lb)		Dose Interval
Flunixin meglumine	Surgical pain	Dog:	0.5 IV, IM, SC	Daily
		Cat:	0.125 SC	One dose, can be repeated in 12–24 hours
Carprofen	Surgical pain	Dog:	1–2 IV, IM, SC	Initially
		Dog:	1 PO, IV, IM, SC	Repeat in 12 hours following initial dose if needed
		Cat:	1–2 SC	Give as a one-time dose only
				Do not repeat dose
	Chronic pain	Dog *only*:	1 PO	Repeat every 12 hours
Ketoprofen	Surgical pain	Dog:	1 IV, IM, SC	Initially
		Cat:	1 SC	Initially
		Dog/cat:	0.5	Subsequent daily doses
	Chronic pain	Dog/cat:	1 PO	Initial dose
		Dog/cat:	0.5 PO	Subsequent daily dose
Ketorolac	Surgical pain	Dog:	0.15–.25 IV, IM	Every 8–12 hours for 1–2 treatments
		Cat:	0.125 IM	Every 8–12 hours for 1–2 treatments

Note: Any patient receiving NSAIDs should be closely monitored for signs of gastrointestinal ulceration or bleeding as well as renal dysfunction.

and injectable use in cats in Europe. At the time of this writing, it is approved only for *oral* administration in the *dog* in the United States.

(3) The mean half-life of carprofen in dogs is 8 hours.

(4) Carprofen's principal mode of action appears to be by mechanisms other than cyclooxygenase or lipoxygenase inhibition.

(5) Carprofen has been reported to be a good analgesic for postoperative soft-tissue and orthopedic pain as well as for pain associated with degenerative joint disease.

(6) Toxicity following carprofen use seems to be minimal, suggesting it does not have major cyclooxygenase 1 inhibition. Isolated, anecdotal reports exist, however, of renal toxicity and gastric ulcer formation following its use (see section E7 on contraindications to NSAID use).

c. Ketoprofen

(1) Ketoprofen is available as a solution for injection and in tablet form.

(2) It has been recommended for chronic pain as well as postoperative pain in both dogs and cats.

(3) It has been widely used in dogs and cats in Europe and has recently been approved for use in dogs and cats in Canada.

(4) Its half-life in dogs and cats appears to be 2–3 hours.

(5) It is a strong inhibitor of cyclooxygenase, and it has significant inhibitory effects on the lipoxygenase pathway.

(6) It has been associated with hemorrhage, renal dysfunction, and gastrointestinal ulcer formation following its use (see section E7 on contraindications to NSAID use).

(7) It should be used with *extreme caution* where surgical hemor-

rhage will be a problem (e.g., patients undergoing laparotomy, hemilaminectomy or laminectomy, rhinotomy, highly vascular tumor excision).

   d. Ketorolac

      (1) Ketorolac is available as an injectable solution and in tablet form.

      (2) It is widely used in human patients with moderate to severe pain. Ketorolac is comparable to morphine in efficacy.

      (3) It *has not* been approved for use in the dog and cat.

      (4) Its duration of effect is 8–12 hours depending on the patient and degree of pain.

      (5) It has produced gastric ulcers and renal insufficiency in human and veterinary patients. These results are especially likely in geriatric, hypovolemic, and hypotensive patients.

      (6) It has a strong potential to cause gastric ulcers; therefore, the use of ulcer prophylaxis is advised.

      (7) It should be used for only one or two treatments in ill patients.

      (8) In healthy, normotensive, normovolemic patients, it should not be given for longer than 3 days.

6. Clinical use of NSAIDs

   a. NSAIDs seem best suited for treating postoperative orthopedic pain in normotensive, normovolemic, well-hydrated patients.

   b. The dog or cat should be of young to middle age with the following status:

      (1) Normal renal function

      (2) No hemostatic abnormalities

      (3) No evidence of or predisposition to gastrointestinal ulceration

      (4) Not currently receiving aspirin or corticosteroids

   c. NSAIDs can and have been used in combination with opioids to provide analgesia postoperatively for soft-tissue and orthopedic pain.

   d. Carprofen has been administered before surgery to provide postoperative analgesia.

   e. NSAIDs have been used in patients with pain caused by soft-tissue swelling, trauma, bone tumors, and meningitis.

      (1) These patients may be more sensitive to NSAID toxicity; therefore, the NSAID dose may need to be reduced.

      (2) Only one or two doses should be given.

   f. NSAIDs have been used in patients with dental pain; however, they should be used with caution after extractions when bleeding may be a problem.

7. Contraindications to NSAID use

   a. NSAIDs should be used with *extreme caution* for postoperative pain management in geriatric patients.

      (1) Use lower doses for geriatric patients than other patients.

      (2) Make sure the geriatric patient has no evidence of gastric ulcers.

      (3) Make sure there is no evidence of renal dysfunction.

      (4) The geriatric patient should be well-hydrated and receiving intravenous fluids.

   b. If NSAIDs are used in a trauma patient, the patient should be stable, with no evidence of hemorrhage.

(1) The patient should be normotensive and should be receiving fluids.

(2) NSAIDs should *not* be given to trauma patients immediately on presentation.

c. NSAIDs should not be used in patients with hemorrhage (epistaxis, head trauma, intra-abdominal bleeding, intrathoracic bleeding).

d. NSAIDs are contraindicated in patients with renal insufficiency.

e. They should not be used in patients that are dehydrated, hypotensive, or in any condition associated with a low or decreased circulating volume (such as ascites or congestive heart failure).

f. NSAIDs should not be used in patients with thrombocytopenia.

g. They are contraindicated in patients with von Willebrand disease.

h. They are contraindicated in patients with evidence of gastric ulceration or any gastrointestinal dysfunction.

i. They are contraindicated in patients with liver disease.

j. They should not be used when a patient is receiving aspirin or corticosteroids concurrently.

k. They should not be used in patients with intervertebral disk disease.

(1) These patients often have received corticosteroids.

(2) Hemilaminectomy or laminectomy may cause bleeding in a noncompressible area.

l. NSAIDs may cause patients with pulmonary disease, including asthma, to deteriorate.

(1) Most NSAIDs inhibit prostaglandins and prostacyclin, which can cause tracheal and bronchial muscle relaxation.

(2) Carprofen, however, is one NSAID that does not inhibit prostaglandin production and therefore might be used in these patients.

8. Ulcer prophylaxis and treatment

a. See Table 10–2.

b. Sucralfate

(1) Sucralfate is available as a suspension of 1 g per 5 ml or as tablets of 1 g.

Table 10–2. Drugs Used for Ulcer Prophylaxis and Treatment in the Dog and Cat

Drug	Indications	Dose/Route/Dose Frequency	
Sucralfate	Gastric ulcer prophylaxis	Dog: Cat:	0.5–1.0 g PO every 8 hours 0.25 g PO every 8–12 hours
	Hemorrhaging ulcer	Dog: Dog:	1–2 g PO initially 0.5–1.0 g PO, repeat every hour for 3 treatments, taper off to a dose every 4 hours and then every 8 hours for 7 days
Ranitidine	Ulcer prophylaxis	Dog: Cat:	0.5–1.0 mg/lb PO; 0.25–.5 mg/lb IV every 12 hours 1.5 mg/lb PO; 1.0 mg/lb IV every 12 hours
Omeprazol	Gastric ulcers	Dogs <10 lbs and cats: Dogs >10 lbs:	0.3 mg/lb PO once a day 20 mg PO once a day

(2) It provides a protective barrier against gastric acid by binding to mucosal defects and ulcerations.

(3) It also indirectly stimulates local prostaglandin production.

(4) It may be advisable to use sucralfate in patients that are more prone to gastric erosions and ulcers from NSAID use. Examples of these patients would include stressed patients, postsurgical patients, and healthy geriatric patients.

(5) Sucralfate suspension can be effective in controlling gastric ulcer hemorrhage.

(6) Sucralfate should be given 1 hour before meals.

(7) It can delay absorption of other oral medications. Therefore, other oral medications should be given at least 1 hour prior to or 2 hours after the administration of sucralfate.

(8) The only reported side effect of sucralfate is constipation.

c. Ranitidine

(1) Ranitidine is a histamine-2 receptor antagonist.

(2) It is available as an injectable solution, as tablets, and as a syrup.

(3) It may be protective against duodenal ulcers.

(4) It inhibits gastric volume secretion and hydrogen ion concentration.

(5) It is more potent and has a longer duration of action than cimetidine. Unlike cimetidine, it does not inhibit hepatic microsomal enzymes.

d. Omeprazole

(1) Omeprazole is a proton pump inhibitor and a potent gastric acid secretion inhibitor.

(2) It is available in 20 mg capsules.

(3) Omeprazole is recommended for the treatment of gastric ulcers and erosions but not as a prophylaxis.

9. With the development of newer NSAIDs that are less toxic and more potent, the use of these drugs for acute postoperative pain control and chronic pain control will increase.

10. Any patient receiving NSAIDs should be closely monitored for signs of the following:

a. Hemorrhaging

b. Renal dysfunction

c. Gastrointestinal ulceration and bleeding (melena, "coffee ground" vomitus)

F. Pharmacologic approaches to postoperative pain control with opioids

1. Opioid analgesics include all drugs that mimic the actions of endogenous peptides responsible for modulating nociception or pain recognition.

2. Opioids bind at specific receptor sites centrally in the brain and spinal cord and peripherally at receptors on nerve terminals in inflamed tissue.

a. Opioids affect impulse processing and transmission at multiple levels of the CNS.

b. Opioids interfere with calcium influx into select target neurons, thus decreasing neurotransmitter release.

c. The presynaptic inhibition of excitatory neurotransmitter release may involve the following:

        (1) Acetylcholine

        (2) Norepinephrine

        (3) 5-Hydroxytryptamine

        (4) Glutamic acid

        (5) Dopamine

        (6) Substance P

        (7) Other mediators

    d. Inhibition of substance P may be responsible for the depression of transmission of impulses in certain central relays.

    e. The opioids react with specific receptor sites in the hindbrain and forebrain. The thalamus and cerebral cortex have a high density of opioid receptors.

    f. The opioid analgesics activate the central receptors that inhibit pain-signal transmission to higher centers. This inhibition blocks the perception of the painful stimulus.

    g. Opioids also modulate at the spinal cord level.

    h. It has been determined that peripherally located opioid receptors are in synovial tissue, the myenteric plexis of the gastrointestinal tract, the heart, the kidneys, and the adrenal glands. Other organs may also contain opioid receptors.

3. Opioid receptors

    a. At least four specific opioid receptors exist, each with subgroups.

    b. Each specific opioid receptor produces distinct responses.

    c. The differences observed among opioid analgesics are primarily due to differences in receptor binding patterns and their affinity for specific receptors.

    d. The most important receptors for antinociception or pain modulation are the mu and kappa opioid receptors. Clinically useful opioids act at one or both of these receptors.

4. Opioid agonists are still the most effective drugs available for moderate to severe postoperative pain.

    a. They can produce highly effective, dose-dependent analgesia and sedation.

    b. They tend not to affect somatosensory function.

5. Opioid agonists

    a. Opioid agonists are drugs that bind at all opioid receptors and produce the full spectrum of opioid effects.

    b. They produce analgesia as well as respiratory depression, sedation, and addiction.

    c. The opioid agonists include morphine, hydromorphine, codeine, oxymorphone, meperidine, fentanyl, alfentanil, sufentanil, carfentanil, etorphine, and methadone.

    d. These drugs differ in their duration of action, side effects, and potency.

    e. Although several of these opioids are more potent than morphine, morphine is still one of the most effective opioid agonists.

    f. Opioid agonists can be safely used in cats.

        (1) Cats are more likely to have excitatory effects from opioid-agonist administration.

        (2) Excitation in the cat is more likely when high doses are used.

(3) Low-dose acepromazine may help attenuate the excitement.

(4) Oxymorphone may be less likely than morphine to produce excitement in the cat.

6. Opioid agonist-antagonists

   a. These opioids act as kappa-receptor agonists but are mu-receptor antagonists.

   b. These opioids include butorphanol, pentazocine, and nalbuphine.

   c. Opioid agonist-antagonists are effective for mild to moderate pain and have minimal serious side effects.

   d. In general, opioid agonist-antagonists have a lower therapeutic ceiling than opioid agonists. Their duration of effect may also be shorter.

   e. For severe pain, opioid agonists are preferred to opioid agonist-antagonists.

   f. Opioid agonist-antagonists produce unreliable sedation in healthy animals.

      (1) Sedation is more predictable in animals already depressed by disease or anesthesia and surgery.

      (2) Additional sedation can be achieved by combining an agonist-antagonist with low-dose acepromazine.

7. Partial opioid agonists

   a. The main drug in this group is buprenorphine.

   b. It binds at the mu receptors but only partially activates them.

   c. It is one of the longer acting opioid analgesics. Its duration of effect is in the 4–8 hour range.

8. Parenteral routes of administration

   a. See Table 10–3 for doses and dose intervals.

   b. Parenteral injection is most often used to control immediate postoperative pain.

   c. Intravenous, subcutaneous, or intramuscular routes can be used (refer to Table 10–3).

   d. Intravenous administration will produce the quickest levels of analgesia.

      (1) Small boluses of opioid can be given until the desired effect is reached.

Table 10–3. Common Parenteral Opioid Analgesics in the Dog and Cat

Drug	Dose (mg/lb)	Route	Dose Interval (hours)
Morphine	Dog: 0.05–.25	IV	1–4
	Dog: 0.05–.25 mg/lb/hr	IV	Continuous infusion
	Dog: 0.25–0.5	IM, SC	2–6
	Cat: 0.025–.05	IM, SC	2–4
Oxymorphone	Dog: 0.01–.1	IV, IM, SC	2–4
	Cat: 0.01–.025	IV	2–4
	Cat: 0.01–.05	IM, SC	2–4
Fentanyl	Dog: 0.0025–.02	IV	0.5–1
Butorphanol	Dog: 0.1–.5	IV, IM, SC	1–4
	Cat: 0.05–.4	IV, IM, SC	1–6
Nalbuphine	Dog: 0.05–.5	IV, IM	1–6
Buprenorphine	Dog: 0.0025–.01	IV, IM	4–8
	Cat: 0.0025–.005	IV, IM	4–8

Table 10–4. Oral Opioid Analgesics in the Dog and Cat

Drug	Dose (mg/lb)		Dose Interval (hours)
Morphine	Dog:	0.15–1.5	4–8
	Cat:	0.05–.5	4–8
Morphine sustained-release	Dog:	0.5–2.5	8–12
Codeine	Dog:	0.5–2.0	4–8
Codeine with acetaminophen*	Dog:	0.5–1.0†	6–8
Butorphanol	Dog/cat:	0.1–.5	4–6
Pentazocine	Dog:	1.0–5.0	4–6

*Toxic to cats
†Dose is in mg/lb of codeine

> (2) Intravenous morphine should be given slowly to decrease the incidence of histamine release in the dog.
>
> (3) Morphine should probably be given only intramuscularly or subcutaneously in the cat.

9. Oral routes of administration

    a. See Table 10–4 for doses and dose intervals.

    b. Many opioids are available as oral preparations.

    c. Oral opioid administration can be an effective means of providing analgesia following surgery; however, the bioavailability of most oral opioids is only 20–30%.

    d. Codeine seems to be better absorbed orally than other opioids.

        (1) Codeine's bioavailability is 60%.

        (2) Codeine with acetaminophen is *toxic* to cats.

    e. The starting dose of oral opioids is often empirical and must be adjusted on an individual patient basis.

    f. Available preparations

        (1) Morphine tablets (15, 30 mg)

        (2) Morphine elixir (4, 20 mg/ml)

        (3) Morphine suppositories (5, 10, 20, 30 mg)

        (4) Morphine sustained-release tablets (15, 30, 60, 100 mg)

        (5) Codeine tablets (15, 30, 60 mg)

        (6) Codeine with acetaminophen tablets (60 mg codeine with 300 mg acetaminophen)

        (7) Butorphanol tablets (1, 5, 10 mg)

        (8) Pentazocine tablets (50 mg)

10. Transdermal routes of administration

    a. Fentanyl is a highly lipid-soluble opioid; thus it can be absorbed through the skin.

    b. Fentanyl transdermal patches have been developed for use in human patients to help control chronic pain.

    c. Fentanyl patches have been used successfully in dogs and cats for pain management.

        (1) These patches have *not* been approved for use in the dog and cat.

        (2) The manufacturer of the patches, Janssen Pharmaceutica, is concerned about accidental human exposure, especially in children, to patches placed on dogs and cats.

(3) For this reason, we use these patches only on hospitalized patients in the vast majority of cases.

(4) If fentanyl patches are applied to patients sent home, the owners must clearly be warned of the following:

    (i) These patches are *not* approved for veterinary use.

    (ii) The possibility of accidental human absorption of the fentanyl exists if the patch comes off and is handled.

d. The advantage of fentanyl patches is that they provide continuous steady-state analgesia for 3–5 days.

(1) In the dog, fentanyl plasma concentrations peak within 24 hours after application of the patch and remain stable for up to 3 days.

(2) In the cat, fentanyl plasma concentrations peak as early as 4–8 hours and remain stable for up to 5 days.

e. Ideally, the fentanyl patch should be applied to the patient 12–24 hours prior to the surgery. Even applying the patch a few hours prior to the surgery seems to be of benefit.

f. If there is pain breakthrough immediately postoperatively, supplemental doses of an opioid agonist such as morphine or oxymorphone may need to be given parenterally to "top off" the fentanyl patch.

g. Placement of the patch

(1) Place the patch on the dorsum of the neck.

(2) The area should be clipped and cleaned.

(3) The area must be *absolutely* dry before the patch is placed.

(4) There *must* be good skin contact for the patch to be effective.

(5) Use a snug (not tight) bandage to hold the patch in place.

(6) Label the bandage so that everyone knows a fentanyl patch is underneath.

h. If prolonged analgesic therapy is needed, the spent patch is removed, and a new patch is applied beside the site of the old patch.

(1) The fentanyl depot at the original site will continue to provide fentanyl for several hours while the new patch saturates the tissues underneath.

(2) This allows for steady-state plasma levels to be maintained.

i. Dose recommendations

(1) Fentanyl patches are dosed by their release rate, i.e., micrograms/hour. Four sizes are available: 25 μg/hr, 50 μg/hr, 75 μg/hr, and 100 μg/hr.

(2) For patients weighing less than 10 lbs (5 kg), fold a 25 μg/hr patch in half so that only half of the patch is in contact with the skin. *Never* cut a patch in half as this alters the release rate.

(3) For patients weighing 10–20 lbs (5–10 kg), use a 25 μg/hr patch.

(4) For patients weighing 20–40 lbs (10–20 kg), use a 50 μg/hr patch.

(5) For patients weighing 40–60 lbs (20–30 kg), use a 75 μg/hr patch.

(6) For patients weighing more than 60 lbs (>30 kg), use a 100 μg/hr patch.

j. Adverse side effects of fentanyl patches

(1) Minimal sedation may occur, although clinically significant sedation is uncommon.

        (2) Mild ataxia may occur.

        (3) Occasional dysphoria occurs.

   k. Absolute or relative contraindications to fentanyl patches

        (1) Hypersensitivity to fentanyl or adhesives

        (2) Central hypoventilation

        (3) Increased or suspected increased intracranial pressure

        (4) Hepatic or renal dysfunction

        (5) Fever (an increased body temperature can increase the patch release rate and thus raise the serum fentanyl concentration)

   l. Precautions and concerns

        (1) High per-patch cost

           (i) For short-term use of only a few hours, the cost is high.

           (ii) For long term use of 3–5 days, the cost is low.

        (2) Damage, removal, or eating of the patch by the patient

           (i) Placing the patch on the dorsum of the neck and putting a bandage over the patch helps prevent this.

        (3) Accidental exposure of humans to the fentanyl in the patch or abuse of the patch by humans

           (i) Use the patch primarily for hospitalized patients to prevent human exposure.

        (4) Suboptimal drug delivery owing to poor skin contact

        (5) Unexpectedly high plasma fentanyl concentrations, causing marked sedation, narcosis, or inappetence

           (i) High body temperature can cause an increased release rate.

           (ii) Too large a patch can result in an overdose for a particular patient.

  m. Fentanyl transdermal patches can be an effective way to provide several days of analgesia following surgery or trauma.

11. Epidural routes of administration

   a. Epidural or spinal administration of morphine has been used in humans as well as animals to relieve pain following surgery.

   b. Epidural morphine has been used to relieve somatic or visceral pain as far forward as the neck.

   c. Advantages

        (1) Epidural morphine administration can produce profound and long-lasting (6–24 hours) analgesia that is not associated with sensory, sympathetic, or motor blockade.

        (2) The analgesia is produced without sedation or marked respiratory depression.

        (3) Patients demonstrate normal locomotor function.

        (4) When administered as part of the general anesthesia regimen, the dose of inhalant anesthetic can be reduced by 30–40%.

   d. Disadvantages

        (1) Epidural morphine is an invasive technique.

        (2) Aseptic technique *must* be used.

        (3) Onset of action takes 30–60 minutes.

        (4) In some patients, especially ones that are obese, it may be difficult to locate landmarks or enter the epidural space.

(5) Sometimes the epidural morphine does not provide the desired level of analgesia.

e. Complications

(1) Occasional postadministration pruritus is seen.

(2) Anecdotal reports exist of hair color changing over the epidural injection site.

(3) Nausea, vomiting, urinary tract retention, and respiratory depression have been reported in human patients.

(4) Subarachnoid space puncture (cerebrospinal fluid is obtained) has been associated with a higher incidence of pruritus, urinary retention, and respiratory depression.

(5) Infection can occur.

(6) Analgesia may be ineffective.

f. Technique

(1) The injection is made at the lumbosacral space.

(2) The site is prepared for surgery. Sterile gloves should be worn.

(3) The iliac crests are palpated, and an imaginary line is drawn between them.

(4) The lumbosacral space is palpated just caudal to this imaginary line on the dorsal midline.

(5) A spinal needle is inserted perpendicular to the skin, directly on midline, and advanced.

(6) A "pop" will be felt as the needle penetrates the intervertebral (flaval) ligament.

(7) The stylet is removed from the spinal needle, and a test dose of air (0.5–2 mls) is injected to test for resistance.

(8) If there is no resistance, the syringe with the morphine solution is attached to the needle and injected.

(9) If cerebrospinal fluid is obtained, the needle is in the subarachnoid space and should be withdrawn. Then the procedure should be started from the beginning.

(10) In small patients a 22 gauge, $1^{1}/_{2}$ inch spinal needle is used. In medium size patients a 20-gauge, $1^{1}/_{2}$-inch spinal needle is used. In large patients a 20-gauge, $2^{1}/_{2}$-inch or $3^{1}/_{2}$-inch spinal needle is used.

g. Dose of morphine

(1) Ideally, preservative-free morphine should be used.

(2) Morphine 0.05 mg/lb (0.1 mg/kg) is diluted in 0.1 ml/lb (0.2 ml/kg) of sterile saline.

(3) A tuberculin syringe can be used for the morphine.

(4) The morphine can then be transferred with a small needle to the larger syringe containing the correct volume of saline. Inject the morphine through the tip of the saline-containing syringe.

h. Contraindications for epidurals

(1) Local infection

(2) Preexisting neurologic dysfunction

(3) Obesity sufficient to cause difficulty in performing the technique

i. The morphine epidural should be done after the patient is anesthetized and prior to the surgical procedure.

IV. Principles of postoperative pain management

    A. Prevent or limit pain.

    B. Use analgesics preemptively to control pain.

    C. Do not wait until behavioral changes are observed to diagnose pain.

    D. Do not ignore patient behavior that is indicative of pain.

    E. Unrelieved pain should never be used as a method of restraint; an animal that is pain-free will lie quietly and sleep.

    F. Do not stop analgesic therapy abruptly; doses should be gradually tapered.

    G. Remember that pain is only one of many stressful things that a hospitalized patient will endure.

Suggested Readings

Bonica JJ: General considerations of chronic pain, in Bonica JJ (ed): The Management of Pain. Philadelphia: Lea & Febiger, 1990, pp. 180–196.

Cross SA: Pathophysiology of pain. Mayo Clin Proc 69:375–383, 1994.

Dahl JB, Kehlet H: The value of preemptive analgesia in the treatment of postoperative pain. Br J Anaesth 70:434–439, 1993.

Dohoo S, Tasker RAR, Donald A: Pharmacokinetics of parenteral and oral sustained-release morphine sulphate in dogs. J Vet Pharmacol Ther 17:426–433, 1994.

Hanson B: Management of postoperative pain in dogs and cats. Proceedings of Symposium on Predictable Pain Management, North American Veterinary Conference, Trenton, NJ, Veterinary Learning Systems, pp. 13–20, 1996.

Hanson B: Analgesic therapy in critically ill animals. Proceedings of Symposium on Predictable Pain Management, North American Veterinary Conference, Trenton, NJ, Veterinary Learning Systems, pp. 27–30, 1996.

Hanson B: Epidural anesthesia and analgesia. Proceedings of Symposium on Predictable Pain Management, North American Veterinary Conference, Trenton, NJ, Veterinary Learning Systems, pp. 49–55, 1996.

Hansen BD: Analgesic therapy. Compend Contin Educ Pract Vet 16:868–875, 1994.

Hansen B, Hardie E: Prescription and use of analgesics in dogs and cats in a veterinary teaching hospital: 258 cases (1983–1989). JAVMA 202:1485–1494, 1993.

Hardie EM: Chronic pain. Proceedings of Symposium on Predictable Pain Management, North American Veterinary Conference, Trenton, NJ, Veterinary Learning Systems, pp. 21–26, 1996.

Jenkins WL: Pharmacologic aspects of analgesic drugs in animals: An overview. JAVMA 191:1231, 1987.

Johnston SA: Physiology, mechanisms and identification of pain. Proceedings of Symposium on Predictable Pain Management, North American Veterinary Conference, Trenton, NJ, Veterinary Learning Systems, pp. 5–12, 1996.

Lascelles BD, Butterworth SJ, Waterman AE: Postoperative analgesic and sedative effects of carprofen and pethidine in dogs. Vet Rec 134(8):189–191, 1994.

Nolan A, Reid J: Comparison of the postoperative analgesic and sedative effects of carprofen and papaveretum in the dog. Vet Rec 133(10):240–242, 1993.

Sackman JE: Pain: Its perception and alleviation in dogs and cats. Part I. The physiology of pain. Compend Contin Educ Pract Vet 13:71–75, 1991.

Short CE, Van Poznak A (eds): Animal Pain. New York: Churchill Livingstone, 1992.

Thompson SE, Johnson JM: Analgesia in dogs after intercostal thoracotomy. A comparison of morphine, selective intercostal nerve block, and interpleural regional analgesia with bupivacaine. Vet Surg 20:73–77, 1991.

Thurmon JC, Tranquilli WJ, Benson GJ: Perioperative pain and distress, in Thurmon JC, Tranquilli WJ, Benson GJ (eds): Lumb & Jones' Veterinary Anesthesia, 3rd ed. Baltimore: Williams & Wilkins, 1996.

Valverde A, Dyson DH, McDonell WN, Pascoe PJ: Use of epidural morphine in the dog for pain relief. Vet Comp Orthop Trauma 2:55–58, 1989.

Werner BE, Taboada J: Use of analgesics in feline medicine. Compend Contin Educ Pract Vet 16:493–499, 1994.

Williams L: Postoperative analgesia. 1993 Surgical Forum Proceedings, San Francisco, pp. 425–427.

Fluid, Electrolyte, and Acid-Base Balance: Maintenance in the Perioperative Period

Chapter **11**

Steve C. Haskins

MAJOR FLUID COMPARTMENTS OF THE BODY

I. Extracellular fluid
   A. Intravascular
   B. Interstitial
II. Intracellular fluid
III. Each compartment is separated by semipermeable membranes that are freely permeable to water.

Colloids and Crystalloids: Their Effect on Water Distribution

I. The distribution of water across vascular and cellular membranes is determined by the osmotic gradients on each side of the respective membrane.
   A. In order for a solute to be osmotically effective, it must be maintained in higher concentrations on one side of the membrane.
II. Colloids
   A. Large colloidal molecules, principally albumin, are not freely permeable across the vascular membrane.
      1. Higher concentrations normally exist in the vascular fluid compartment than in the interstitium.
      2. Colloids are responsible for the osmotic "holding power" of fluids within the vascular fluid compartment.
      3. Hypoproteinemia may be associated with hypovolemia and with subcutaneous edema and ascites.
      4. Diseases that increase capillary permeability to albumin decrease transvascular albumin concentrations. They promote hypovolemia and interstitial fluid accumulations.
   B. Colloid oncotic pressure is measured with a colloid oncometer.
      1. Units of measure are millimeters of mercury.
      2. Values for normal animals are in the 20–25 mm Hg range.
      3. A colloid oncometer is blind to the concentration of crystalloids (sodium and so forth).
   C. Colloid oncotic pressure (COP) can be calculated from total protein or albumin/globulin measurements in one of two ways:

1. COP = 2.1 tp + 0.16 tp^2 + 0.009 tp^3 (where tp = total protein concentration)
2. COP = 2.8 a + 0.18 a^2 + 0.012 a^3 (where a = albumin concentration) + 1.6 g + 0.15 g^2 + 0.006 g^3 (where g = globulin concentration)

D. Treatment guidelines:

	Total Protein (g/dl)	Albumin (G/dl)	Colloid Oncotic Pressure (mm Hg)
Normal	>6.0	>2.5	>20
Low but acceptable	>3.5	>1.5	>15
Low and treatable	<3.5	<1.5	<15
Low and life-threatening!	<2.5	<1.0	<10

III. Crystalloids

A. Extracellular sodium concentrations are maintained high by the sodium-potassium-ATPase pump in the cellular membrane.

1. Sodium and its related anions (predominantly chloride and bicarbonate) are primarily responsible for the osmotic retention of water in the extracellular fluid compartment.
2. An acute decrease in extracellular sodium concentration (and osmolality) results in the flux of fluids into the intracellular fluid compartment (intracellular edema; water intoxication).
3. An acute increase in extracellular sodium concentration (and osmolality) results in the flux of fluids out of the intracellular fluid compartment (intracellular dehydration).
4. Compensation for these osmolality changes that occur during the preoperative normalization of extracellular sodium concentrations warrants some special considerations (see section on hypernatremia).

B. Osmolality (Osm) is measured by freezing-point depression in an osmometer.

1. Colloid concentrations cannot change enough to affect this measurement.

   a. This methodology is blind to the concentration of colloids.
2. The unit of measure is mOsm/kg.
3. Values for normal animals are in the range of 290–310 mOsm/kg.
4. Osmolality is mostly determined by sodium (and its related anion) concentration:

$$Osm_c = 2 \times Na^+ + 10$$

This equation accounts for the normal contributions of glucose and blood urea nitrogen (BUN).

   a. If the glucose and BUN are measured, their contributions to the osmolality can be calculated:

$$Osm_c = (2 \times Na^+) + [glucose\ (mg/dl)/18] + [BUN\ (mg/dl)/2.8]$$

 5. Hyponatremia is the only cause of hypo-osmolality; but many causes of hyperosmolality exist.

   a. "Effective" osmols (osmols that change the freezing-point depression *and* affect transcellular fluid flux)

     (1) Hypernatremia

     (2) Hyperglycemia

     (3) Hypermannitolemia

     (4) Ketoacidosis

     (5) Lactic acidosis

     (6) Phosphate and sulfate acidosis (oliguric renal failure)

   b. "Ineffective" osmols (osmols that change the freezing-point depression and *do not* affect transcellular fluid flux)

     (1) Elevated blood urea nitrogen (it changes the freezing-point depression acutely)

     (2) Ethylene glycol intoxication

     (3) Ethanol/methanol intoxication

 6. The difference between the measured osmolality and the calculated osmolality is an indirect measure of the accumulation of these normally unmeasured osmols.

   a. The normal difference is 10–15 mOsm/kg.

IV. Summary

Terminology	Osmolality	Colloid Oncotic Pressure
Units of Measure	mOsm/kg	mm Hg
Method of Measure	Freezing-point depression	Pressure change associated with a fluid flux across a semipermeable membrane
Solute	Crystalloids	Colloids
Physiologic Importance	Transcellular fluid flux	Transvascular fluid flux

The Nature of Naturally Occurring Fluid Losses

 I. Naturally occurring fluid losses can be divided into general categories.

  A. Purely isotonic extracellular fluid loss occurs with abnormal accumulations of fluids within a body cavity or a newly created tissue space.

    1. These pockets of fluid are in electrolyte equilibrium with the extracellular fluid compartment and therefore will have the same electrolyte concentrations.

    2. These pockets of fluid have variable amounts of albumin.

  B. Fluids that are lost via vomiting, diarrhea, or diuresis generally have a sodium concentration that is variably lower than that of the extracellular fluid compartment.

    1. Animals suffering these losses are usually hypernatremic.

Type of Fluid Loss	Consequence
Whole blood	Hypovolemia
Albumin—glomerulonephritis, enteritis, increased capillary permeability	Hypovolemia, interstitial edema
Isotonic crystalloids—abnormal accumulation in a body cavity	Extracellular volume depletion
"Subisotonic" hypotonic crystalloids—vomiting, diarrhea, diuresis	Mostly extracellular and some intracellular volume depletion
Pure water losses—insensible (lungs and skin)	Total body water depletion

How to Tell If a Patient Is Dehydrated

I. Traditionally, skin turgor has been used to assess the magnitude of the dehydration.
   A. Lift the skin into a fold and determine how fast it returns to its resting position.
      1. When the animal is 5% (of its body weight) dehydrated, the skinfold returns slowly.
      2. When the animal is 12% dehydrated, the skin remains in the fold after it is released.
      3. Intermediate values are interpolated.
   B. The skin turgor sign is highly variable and somewhat unreliable.
      1. It should always be evaluated at the same location (over the thorax), with the patient in the same position (recumbent), by the same evaluator.
      2. Emaciated patients exhibit decreased skin turgor even when they are not dehydrated.
      3. Obese patients may be very dehydrated yet not exhibit any decrease in skin turgor.
II. Compensatory changes in response to dehydration
   A. High specific gravity in urine
   B. Low sodium concentration in urine
III. Changes consistent with the loss of extracellular fluids
   A. Elevated packed cell volume, hyperproteinemia, hypernatremia
   B. Concentration parameters are not volume parameters and do not, per se, define dehydration.
      1. They are only consistent with it.
      2. They define the type of fluid loss rather than the volume.
      3. They serve as a guide to the type of fluid that should be used for therapy.
IV. History of fluid loss or lack of fluid intake
   A. If clinical signs are not clear, but patient has a history of fluid loss, it might be wise to assume dehydration.
      1. Anesthetic induction in these patients can unmask a serious hypovolemia resulting in severe hypotension.
      2. A preinduction fluid load is indicated.

How to Tell If an Animal Is Hypovolemic

I. All animals that are dehydrated are, by definition, hypovolemic.

    A. A decrease in skin turgor is specifically a sign of an interstitial volume deficit.

        1. Interstitial fluids are crystalloid by nature.

        2. Crystalloid fluids are freely permeable across the vascular endothelium.

        3. Crystalloid fluid losses come from both the interstitial and vascular fluid compartments.

II. Compensatory changes for hypovolemia

    A. Tachycardia

    B. Vasoconstriction

        1. Pale color

        2. Prolonged capillary refill time

        3. Cool appendages

III. Consequences of hypovolemia

    A. Weak pulse quality

    B. Low central venous pressure

    C. Oliguria

    D. Metabolic acidosis

    E. High blood lactate

    F. Low venous oxygen

ABNORMALITIES OF COMMON BLOOD COMPONENTS AND ELECTROLYTES

Anemia

I. Hemoglobin is the major player in the oxygen-content game.

    A. The product of oxygen content and cardiac output is oxygen delivery.

    B. The critical level of hemoglobin for any given patient depends a great deal on the ability of the cardiac output to compensatorily increase.

        1. Anesthetics are myocardial depressants.

        2. Packed cell volume needs to be at least 20–25% during anesthesia.

II. Polycythemia increases blood viscosity and decreases cardiac output and tissue perfusion when the packed cell volume exceeds 60–70%.

Hypoproteinemia

I. Protein, specifically albumin, is the major osmotic force holding fluid within the vascular fluid compartment.

    A. Colloid therapy should be instituted in the following cases:

        1. Total protein is less than 3.5 g/dl.

        2. Albumin concentration is less than 1.5 g/dl.

        3. Colloid oncotic pressure is below 15 mm Hg.

II. Hyperproteinemia increases blood viscosity and decreases cardiac output and tissue perfusion.

Coagulopathies

I. Plasma should be administered if coagulation factors are depleted to the point that the animal suffers a hemorrhagic diathesis (or, in some cases, thrombosis).
   A. See section on plasma

Hyperkalemia

I. Hyperkalemia causes membrane hypopolarization, which may result in ventricular extrasystoles, ventricular fibrillation, or asystole if it becomes very severe (over 7–9 mEq/L).
II. Hyperkalemia also increases potassium permeability, which augments the repolarization phases of the electrocardiograph (EKG):
   A. EKG shows tall, tented, narrow T waves.
III. Hyperkalemia diminishes the depolarization phases.
   A. EKG shows the following:
      1. Small P waves
      2. Prolonged PR intervals
      3. Bradycardia
      4. Widened QRS complexes
      5. Blending of the QRS and T waves (a sinusoidal pattern)
      6. Ventricular fibrillation or asystole
IV. Hyperkalemia may also be associated with the following:
   A. Peripheral muscle weakness
   B. Decreased contractility and weak pulse quality
V. The plasma potassium measurement defines the plasma potassium concentration.
   A. The EKG changes define whether or not the animal is having any electrical problems from the potassium imbalance.
   B. Considerable individual variation exists.
      1. Severe hyperkalemia with a fairly normal EKG suggests that the animal's condition is not life-threatening.
      2. Moderate hyperkalemia associated with severe EKG changes suggests a life-threatening emergency.
VI. Causes of hyperkalemia
   A. *Oliguric/anuric renal disease*
   B. *Postrenal obstruction or perforation*
   C. *Hypoadrenocorticism*
   D. *Iatrogenic causes*
   E. Rhabdomyolysis
   F. Metabolic (inorganic)/respiratory acidosis
   G. Periodic familial hyperkalemia
   H. Potassium also may be falsely elevated owing to hemolysis if there is a delay in blood sample analysis (only in the Akita dog) or to platelet or white cell degradation (only in patients with severe thrombocytosis or leukocytosis).
   I. Extracellular redistribution: hypoinsulinemia, beta$_2$-adrenergic blockade, familial periodic hyperkalemic paralysis
   J. Tissue damage or catabolism: trauma, burns, rewarming and washout of ischemic tissues, severe exercise, succinylcholine
VII. Treatment
   A. Non-life-threatening hyperkalemia
      1. Treat the underlying disease process.

B. Life-threatening hyperkalemia
   1. Calcium (0.2 ml of 10% calcium chloride or 0.6 ml of 10% calcium gluconate per kilogram of body weight, administered intravenously)
      a. A dramatic, short-lived (10–20 minutes) effect
   2. Insulin (0.1–.25 units of regular insulin per kilogram of body weight, administered as an intravenous bolus) and glucose (0.5–1.5 g/kg, respectively, administered as an intravenous infusion over 2 hours)
      a. Monitor for hypoglycemia.
   3. Bicarbonate will cause the intracellular redistribution of potassium if it is going to be administered for acidosis.
      a. Be aware of this effect of therapy in hypokalemic patients.
   4. Beta$_2$-agonist activity will also cause the intracellular redistribution of potassium but will have a narrow therapeutic margin.
      a. Specific beta$_2$ drugs (terbutaline) are associated with tachycardia and hypotension.
      b. General beta$_1$ and beta$_2$ drugs (epinephrine, dopamine) are associated with tachycardia, arrhythmias, and hypertension.
      c. Be aware of this effect of therapy in hypokalemic patients.

Hypokalemia

I. Hypokalemia causes membrane hyperpolarization (electrical paralysis) and decreases potassium permeability (diminishes repolarization processes and enhances depolarization processes).
II. Hypokalemia is associated with general muscle weakness (skeletal, gastrointestinal, and myocardial) and may be associated with EKG changes opposite to those of hyperkalemia.
   A. Changes in hypokalemia are not as characteristic as they are in hyperkalemia.
      1. Flattened T waves, U waves (a positive deflection following the T wave)
      2. Elevated P waves, increased R wave amplitudes, and depressed ST segments.
   B. Hypokalemia is also associated with CNS depression and an impaired ability of the renal nephrons to concentrate urine.
III. Causes of hypokalemia
   A. *Insufficient intake:* anorexia; maintenance fluids with low potassium concentrations
   B. Excessive losses
      1. *Vomiting, diarrhea, diuresis*
      2. Dialysis with potassium-free fluids
   C. Hypermineralocorticism
      1. *Appropriate: dehydration*
      2. Inappropriate: Cushing disease
   D. Hypochloremia
   E. Diuretic therapy
      1. Carbonic anhydrase inhibitors
   F. Renal tubular acidosis (proximal and distal)
   G. Carbenicillin and some other penicillin derivatives
      1. Renal tubular sodium reabsorption with a nonreabsorbable anion

H. Intracellular redistribution: insulin and glucose, bicarbonate, beta$_2$-agonists, metabolic alkalosis (hydrogen loss or bicarbonate retention), familial periodic hypokalemic paralysis

IV. A severely hypokalemic patient needs to be potassium loaded.

    A. Potassium can be administered at rates up to 0.5 mEq/kg per hour.

        1. Higher infusion rates must be monitored continuously.

        2. The concentration of potassium in the fluid may vary between 10 mEq/L and 50 mEq/L or higher.

Hypernatremia

I. Hypernatremia initially causes intracellular dehydration.

    A. The central nervous system (CNS) first manifests signs (depressed mentation).

    B. In time (a day or so) the intracellular fluid (ICF) compartment increases its osmolality to offset the extracellular fluid (ECF) osmolality.

    C. Rapid restoration of the sodium imbalance at this time may cause serious water intoxication.

II. Hypernatremia may be associated with hypovolemia and dehydration, normovolemia, or hypervolemia and edema.

    A. Dehydration, hypovolemia

        1. Water loss in excess of sodium

            a. Vomiting, diarrhea

            b. Osmotic diuresis

            c. Enhanced insensible losses: fever

        2. Insufficient free water intake

            a. Inaccessibility

            b. Primary hypodipsia

            c. Iatrogenic

    B. Normovolemia

        1. Diabetes insipidus

        2. Reset osmostat

        3. Iatrogenic: administration of replacement solutions for maintenance needs

    C. Edema, hypervolemia

        1. Excessive sodium intake

        2. Hypertonic sodium chloride or sodium bicarbonate administration

        3. Cation exchange resins

        4. Hyperadrenocorticism

III. Most hypernatremia will self-correct (assuming reasonable renal function) after effective treatment of the underlying problem.

    A. Start fluid therapy with a neutral sodium concentration fluid such as an ECF replacement solution like lactated Ringer's solution.

    B. The kidney will normalize the sodium concentration.

IV. Moderate to severe hypernatremia is corrected by water administration.

    A. When the sodium concentration is moderately or severely elevated (>165 mEq/L), the sodium concentration should be lowered slowly.

        1. The sodium concentration should be lowered no faster than 1–2 mEq per hour.

2. Volume deficits are initially corrected with a solution with a sodium concentration that is only slightly lower than that of the ECF.

3. Water can then be administered at a rate of 3.5 ml of 5% dextrose in water per kilogram of body weight per hour to lower the sodium concentration at the prescribed rate.

Hyponatremia

I. Hyponatremia initially causes intracellular edema.
   A. The CNS first manifests signs (depressed mentation).
   B. In time (a day or so) the ICF compartment decreases its osmolality to offset the ECF osmolality.
   C. Rapid restoration of the sodium imbalance at this time may cause central pontine necrolysis.

II. Hyponatremia may be associated with dehydration and hypovolemia, normovolemia, or edema and hypervolemia.
   A. Dehydration and hypovolemia
      1. Appropriate antidiuretic hormone (ADH) secretion
         a. Ineffective circulating volume
      2. Compensated end-stage renal disease
      3. Natriuretic diuretics
      4. Hypoadrenocorticism
      5. Vomiting associated with water drinking
   B. Normovolemia
      1. Inappropriate ADH secretion
      2. Hypothalamic disease
      3. Pulmonary disease
      4. Major surgery aftermath
      5. Vasopressin therapy
      6. Primary polydipsia
      7. Reset osmostat
   C. Edema and hypervolemia
      1. Heart failure, cirrhosis
      2. Iatrogenic causes
   D. False hyponatremia
      1. Hyperglycemia
      2. Hyperlipemia
      3. Hyperproteinemia

III. Most hyponatremia is corrected by effective treatment of the underlying problem.
   A. Start fluid therapy with a neutral sodium concentration fluid such as an ECF replacement solution like lactated Ringer's solution.

IV. Rapid therapy of moderate to severe hyponatremia with hypertonic saline may cause central pontine myelinolysis.
   A. When the sodium concentration is moderately (or more) decreased (<125 mEq/L), it should be raised slowly.
      1. The sodium concentration should be raised no faster than 1–2 mEq per hour with hypertonic saline.

Metabolic Acidosis

I. The metabolic component is composed of all of the nonrespiratory acidotic processes in the body.
II. The bicarbonate concentration is commonly used as an index of the metabolic contribution to the pH balance.
   A. Values in normal animals are in the range of 20–27 mEq/L.
   B. The greater the decrease is in bicarbonate concentration, the greater the magnitude of the acidosis.
   C. As virtually all of the carbon dioxide in a blood sample is carried in the form of bicarbonate, it is appropriate to use the total carbon dioxide (CO_2) measurement as a reasonable representation of HCO_3^-.
   D. Quantitatively, however, bicarbonate concentration may not accurately estimate the true magnitude of the metabolic acidosis.
      1. It is not independent of changes in CO_2.

Bicarbonate	Carbon Dioxide
21	20
24	40
27	80

      2. The magnitude of change in HCO_3^- underestimates the quantitative magnitude of the acid load because of the other buffer systems.
III. Base excess/deficit is the titratable acidity of a whole blood sample equilibrated to a P_{CO_2} of 40 mm Hg and 100% oxygenated hemoglobin.
   A. Normal values are 0 ± 4 mM/L.
   B. *Actual* base excess/deficit is derived from in vitro experiments.
   C. *Standard* base excess/deficit is an in vivo adjustment derived from calculations to account for interstitial dilution of the acid load.
IV. An elevated anion gap is caused by the accumulation of unmeasured anions.
   A. The common anions are those of organic acids such as lactic and pyruvic acids, ketoacids, sulfuric and phosphoric acids, and proteins.
   B. Anion gap is calculated as sodium − (chloride + bicarbonate).
   C. The normal gap is about 10–20 mEq/L.
V. These assessments of the metabolic contribution to the acid-base balance represent an overview of all of the metabolic processes—both acidotic and alkalotic—that are progressing at the same time, not all of which have been traditionally considered acids or bases.
   A. A new approach (Stewart's) helps identify some of these components.
      1. Metabolic acidosis/alkalosis may be caused by the following:
         a. Free water abnormalities (dilutional acidosis and contraction alkalosis)
            (1) Hyponatremia represents an acidotic effect, and vice versa.
         b. Disproportionate changes in chloride
            (1) Hyperchloremia represents an acidotic effect, and vice versa.
         c. Changes in albumin (a nonvolatile weak acid)
            (1) Hyperproteinemia represents an acidotic effect, and vice versa.
         d. Other unmeasured anions

2. Unmeasured Anion Concentration = Base Deficit − (Δ Free Water + Δ Chloride + Δ Albumin). Keep track of the plus and minus signs; they are

$$\Delta \text{ Free Water} = 0.25 \text{ (Na}^+ - \text{Normal Na}^+)$$

(Normal Na$^+$ for dogs is 146 and for cats is 156.)

$$\Delta \text{ Chloride} = \text{normal Cl}^- - \text{Corrected Cl}^-$$

(Normal Cl$^-$ for dogs is 110 and for cats is 120.)
Corrected Cl$^-$ = Measured Cl$^-$ × 146/Na$^+$ for Dogs
× 156/Na$^+$ for Cats

$$\Delta \text{ Albumin} = 3.7 \times (3.1 - \text{Measured Albumin})$$

(If albumin is not available, use total protein: 3.0 × 6.8 − Measured Total Protein)

B. Phosphate is also a weak acid, and high concentrations can contribute to a metabolic acidosis, but no formulas are available to quantitate the magnitude of its contribution.
1. Normal phosphate is very low, so hypophosphatemia does not cause metabolic alkalosis.
C. Metabolic acidosis in the critically ill patient is often due to aberrations in free water, chloride, and albumin rather than in the unmeasured anions of lactic acid, ketoacids, and sulfuric and phosphoric acids as is commonly presumed.
1. This approach will provide a broader perspective of the metabolic derangements.
   a. Metabolic acidosis resulting from hyponatremia, hyperchloremia, or hyperproteinemia should not be treated with an alkalinizing agent.
   b. A coexistent metabolic alkalosis resulting from hypoalbuminemia, for instance, will offset the metabolic acidosis resulting from lactic acid.

VI. Lactate as a measure of the magnitude of the lactic acidosis
A. Lactic acidosis is most commonly associated with inadequate tissue oxygenation (type A).
1. Anaerobic glycolysis produces lactate, adenosine triphosphate (ATP), and water. Hydrolysis of ATP releases H$^+$.
B. Normal blood lactate is below 1.5 mM/L.
1. Above 2.0 mM/L is elevated.
2. The magnitude of the elevation is positively correlated with the magnitude of the underlying problem and the lactic acidosis.
C. Lactate concentration is a position statement rather than a prognostic indicator.
1. Very high levels indicate a severe underlying disease process.
2. Severe underlying disease conditions are usually associated with poorer outcomes.
3. High blood lactate does not *define* the poor outcome; the disease does.
D. Lactate may not truly represent the magnitude of the poor tissue oxygenation.
1. Other causes of high blood lactate are possible.

2. Global measurements may not represent local tissue perfusion/oxygen-ation defects because of local blood flow maldistributions and arteriovenous shunts.

VII. Causes of metabolic acidosis

    A. With a normal anion gap

        1. Gastrointestinal loss of bicarbonate

            a. Diarrhea

            b. Vomiting with reflux from the duodenum

        2. Renal loss of bicarbonate

            a. Proximal tubular acidosis

            b. Carbonic anhydrase inhibitors

        3. Renal hydrogen retention

            a. Distal tubular acidosis

            b. Hypomineralocorticism

        4. Intravenous nutrition

        5. Ammonium chloride administration

        6. Compensation for respiratory alkalosis

        7. Dilutional acidosis (large-volume saline administration)

    B. With an elevated anion gap

        1. Lactic and pyruvic acidosis

        2. Ketoacidosis

        3. Phosphate and sulfate acidosis (oliguric renal failure)

        4. Ethylene glycol intoxication

        5. Ethanol or methanol intoxication

        6. Salicylate poisoning

        7. Extensive rhabdomyolysis

VIII. The treatment of metabolic acidosis is primarily aimed at correction of the underlying disease process.

    A. If the metabolic acidosis is severe, the patient may benefit from alkalinization therapy to initially support its pH until the underlying disease process can be stabilized.

        1. If the metabolic acidosis is relatively easy to treat, as is the case for diabetic ketoacidosis or moderate hypovolemic shock, alkalinizing therapy should be conservative.

        2. If the metabolic acidosis is difficult to treat, as is the case for severe hypovolemic shock or septic shock, alkalinizing therapy should be relatively aggressive.

    B. Alkalinization therapy should be considered if the patient's pH is below 7.2, if the base deficit is greater than 10 mEq/L, or if the bicarbonate concentration is below 14 mEq/L.

IX. Alkalinizing agents

    A. Sodium bicarbonate has traditionally been used to treat metabolic acidosis.

        1. It normally works very well.

        2. The administration of sodium bicarbonate generates carbon dioxide (via carbonic acid).

            a. Animals with normal respiratory responsiveness and capability will eliminate this carbon dioxide in very short order.

            b. If they do not, however, because of medullary or ventilatory compromise, carbon dioxide rapidly diffuses into the ICF compartment and into the cerebrospinal fluid.

      c. Once inside, it re-equilibrates (via carbonic acid), generating an excess of hydrogen ion.

      d. Intracellular acidosis may be associated with myocardial and CNS depression.

   3. Sodium bicarbonate administration increases plasma sodium concentration and osmolality.

   4. Hypertonic solutions have been implicated in promoting systemic vasodilation.

   5. The dose (mEq) of bicarbonate to administer can be calculated as follows:

      a. Multiply the base, or bicarbonate deficit, by 0.3 by the body weight (BW) in kilograms ($0.3 \times BW$ is a slight overestimate of the ECF volume).

      b. Another guideline estimate is 1–5 mEq/kg of body weight for a mild to severe metabolic acidosis.

   6. Sodium bicarbonate should not be administered any faster than it can be redistributed from the vascular fluid compartment to the interstitial fluid compartment (20–30 minutes).

      a. If administered as an intravenous bolus, it can cause severe hypotension and death.

B. Tromethamine (Tham)(Abbott) is an organic amine buffer that binds directly with hydrogen ion.

$$(CH_2OH)_3C-NH_2 + HA \rightleftharpoons (CH_2OH)_3C-NH_3{}^+ + A^-$$

   1. Tromethamine thus diminishes carbon dioxide via the carbonic acid system.

   2. The unionized portion of tromethamine (about 30%) is freely diffusible into the cell.

      a. More rapid intracellular buffering (compared with that of sodium bicarbonate) occurs.

   3. Tromethamine is also an osmotic diuretic.

   4 It is a very alkaline solution (a 0.3 M solution has a pH of 10.6) and is irritating to tissues and small veins.

      a. It should be administered via large veins or with significant dilution.

   5. The dosage is calculated by this formula: Base Deficit $\times$ 0.4 $\times$ Body Weight (kg).

C. Carbicarb is a combination of 0.33 M solution of sodium carbonate and a 0.33 M solution of sodium bicarbonate (International Medications Systems Ltd., South El Monte, CA).

   1. It has a reduced carbon dioxide–generating tendency.

D. Tromethamine may offer some advantages over sodium bicarbonate, but the wholesale abandonment of sodium bicarbonate seems unwarranted. Sodium bicarbonate has not been clearly demonstrated to lack efficacy, nor have the alternative agents been clearly demonstrated to be superior.

Metabolic Alkalosis

I. Metabolic acidosis may be caused by the following:

  A. Gastric losses

    1. Vomiting due to a pyloric obstruction

    2. Gastric suctioning

  B. Diuretics
  C. Hypermineralocorticism
  D. Hypochloremia
  E. Hypokalemia
  F. Compensation for respiratory acidosis
  G. Excessive alkalinization therapy
  H. Contraction alkalosis (hypernatremia)
  I. Hypoproteinemia
  J. Carbenicillin and other penicillin derivatives
  K. Citrate and ketone metabolism
II. Therapy is directed at the underlying cause.

PERIOPERATIVE FLUID THERAPY

  I. Preoperative fluid therapy should be directed at normalizing circulating blood
     volume and correcting some or all of the dehydration and electrolyte abnor-
     malities.
     A. This is normally accomplished by combinations of crystalloids, artificial
        colloids, plasma, and red blood cells.
     B. Animals that are freshly traumatized and actively bleeding can be worsened
        by aggressive fluid therapy.
        1. Resuscitation should be adequate to move the animal out of its life-
           threatening situation but not so aggressive as to worsen the bleeding.
 II. Intraoperative fluid therapy is directed at maintaining circulating blood volume
     while also maintaining packed cell volume and colloid concentrations.
     A. This is normally accomplished by combinations of crystalloids, artificial
        colloids, plasma, and red blood cells.
III. Postoperative fluid therapy is directed at maintaining circulating blood vol-
     ume, packed cell volume, and colloid concentrations while continuing to
     correct any residual dehydration and electrolyte abnormalities.

Crystalloids

  I. Solutions with approximately normal sodium concentrations are categorized
     as isotonic ECF replacement solutions.
     A. These solutions can be administered in large volumes without causing
        alterations in sodium concentration or transcellular fluid balance.
     B. ECF solutions can generally be subdivided into those fluids that contain
        a "bicarbonate-like" anion (bicarbonate, lactate, gluconate, or acetate) and
        those that do not.
        1. The bicarbonate-like anion prevents the dilutional acidosis induced by
           fluids without such anions (saline, Ringer's).
        2. As the anion is metabolized, a hydrogen ion is dragged along with it
           (and thereby comes the alkalinizing effect).
 II. During the operative period in a normal patient, the ECF replacement solu-
     tion is administered at a rate of 10 ml/kg per hour.
     A. This dose should be increased to 20 ml/kg per hour if the animal is
        slightly hypotensive or dehydrated or if it is desirable to maximize visceral
        tissue perfusion.
     B. The dose should be decreased to 5 ml/kg per hour if the animal is slightly

hypertensive or edematous, if it has marginal heart function, or if it has pulmonary or cerebral edema.

   C. It may be necessary to administer bolus doses of 10 ml/kg if the animal becomes moderately hypotensive.

     1. It may be necessary to repeat several dosages in order to achieve adequate blood volume restoration.

     2. It may be necessary to administer as much as one blood volume or more.

       a. The dog has a blood volume of approximately 80–90 ml/kg.

       b. The cat has a smaller blood volume (50–55 ml/kg) and should receive a proportionately smaller dose of fluids.

III. Only about 25–30% of an isotonic crystalloid fluid remains within the vascular fluid compartment 30 minutes following its administration.

   A. The remainder readily diffuses across the endothelial membrane and is redistributed into the interstitial fluid compartment.

   B. The volume restoration achieved by crystalloid fluids may be fleeting.

     1. If hypotension recurs, further fluid administration, perhaps in the form of colloids or whole blood, is indicated.

IV. Excessive hemodilution is a common limitation to crystalloid fluid administration.

   A. Excessive hemodilution is defined as one of the following:

     1. Packed cell volume below 15–25%

     2. Total protein below 3.5 g/dl or albumin below 1.5 g/dl

Hypertonic Saline

I. Hypertonic saline provides better volume expansion and higher cardiac output, blood pressure, and tissue perfusion, with much lower infusion volumes, than isotonic ECF solutions.

   A. Indications

     1. When the time needed to achieve the necessary volume restoration is lacking

     2. In larger animals, when it is difficult to administer large volumes of fluids

     3. In ambulatory practices, when the transport of large volumes of fluids is impractical

II. Hypertonic saline also causes prominent vasodilation.

   A. This vasodilation may be associated with some lowering of arterial blood pressure

III. The deleterious effects of hypertonic saline include the following:

   A. Hypernatremia, hyperchloremia, and hyperosmolality

   B. Hypokalemia and a decrease in bicarbonate concentration

IV. The commonly recommended dose of 7.5% hypertonic saline is 4–6 ml/kg.

Artificial Colloids

I. Artificial colloids are indicated in the following cases:

   A. The total protein is below 3.5 g/dl, albumin is below 1.5 g/dl, or the colloid oncotic pressure is below 15 mm Hg (or is likely to be reduced below this level with crystalloid therapy).

   B. Edema develops prior to adequate blood volume restoration.

   C. Longer lasting blood volume support is needed.

D. The patient does not appear to be responding appropriately to the crystalloid fluid infusion.

E. Neither platelets, coagulation precursors, nor red blood cells are needed.

II. Colloids, although more expensive than crystalloids on a per-bottle cost, provide better blood volume expansion with less interstitial expansion than crystalloids.

A. They are quite cost-effective on a "per-effect" basis.

III. Commercial colloidal solutions are iso-osmotic and hyperoncotic in the bottle.

A. Colloids of less than m.w. 50,000 are rapidly excreted in the urine and exhibit a short duration of action (2–4 hours).

IV. Characteristics of common colloid solutions

Colloid	m.w.* (range)	m.w.* (wt ave†)	m.w.* (n ave‡)	COP (mm Hg)	Osmolality (mOsm/L)	Volume (+10 min*)	Expansion (+3–4 hrs§)
Albumin 5%	66–69	69	69	24	290		
Plasma	66–400	119	88	22	285	67	29
Dextran 40	10–80	40	26		310	81	33
Dextran 70	15–160	70	41	62	310	76	40
Hetastarch	10–1000	450	69	32	310	71	42
Pentastarch	150–350	264	35		310		
Gelatins	5–100	35	6		310	70	19
Saline	23–35	29	29	0	310	60	<10

*In daltons
†Simple numeric weight of all molecular weights
‡Numeric weighted average
§Expressed as a percentage of the volume administered

Dextran 70

I. Dextrans are mixtures of polysaccharides produced by the bacteria *Leuconostoc mesenteroides* or lactobacilli grown on sucrose media.

A. Molecular weights of less than 50,000 are rapidly filtered at the glomerulus.

B. Molecular weights of more than 50,000 are widely distributed in the body and are metabolized by dextrinases.

II. Dextran 40 is seldom used for blood volume expansion for the following reasons:

A. Its numeric molecular weighted average is very small, and its duration of action is short—only 1.5–3 hours.

B. It has been associated with renal failure.

1. It is rapidly filtered by the glomerulus and may be associated with an osmotic diuresis.

2. In states of active tubular reabsorption of sodium and water, the dextran is concentrated in the tubular lumen, increasing the viscosity of the filtrate and plugging the tubule.

III. Dextrans produce a dose-related defect in hemostasis that is greater than the defect resulting from simple dilution.
   A. Activated partial thromboplastin time (aPTT) is prolonged owing to a reduction in factor VIII activity.
   B. Bleeding time is prolonged, and platelet adhesiveness is decreased owing to inhibition of the vWF:Ag activity.
   C. Although it is not expected that even large doses will induce bleeding in normal patients, dextrans should be used conservatively, if at all, in patients with von Willebrand disease.
   D. Dextran 70, by virtue of this effect, may be therapeutic for the hypercoagulable phase of disseminated intravascular coagulation.

Hetastarch

   I. Hetastarch is a modified amylopectin, a branched glucose polymer.
   A. Hydroxylation makes hetastarch more resistant to degradation by serum amylase.
   B. Its half-life depends on the degree of hydroxylation and on molecular size.
   C. Starches are metabolized by plasma and interstitial alpha-amylase.
  II. Hetastarch may also cause bleeding tendencies.
   A. Little evidence exists to support the contention that hetastarch is less likely to cause a hemorrhagic diathesis.
 III. Pentastarch has a smaller, more homogeneous particle size with less hydroxyethyl substitution than hetastarch.
  IV. Hetastarch is commonly presumed to have a considerably longer half-life than dextran 70 owing to its larger sized molecules.
   A. The decay curves of plasma volume enhancement with hetastarch and dextran 70 are, however, remarkably similar.

Plasma

   I. Albumin constitutes 50% of the total plasma protein and 80% of the plasma colloid oncotic pressure.
   A. The ECF has approximately 5 g albumin per kilogram of body weight.
      1. The intravascular space has 40%.
      2. The interstitial space has 60%.
   B. The plasma albumin concentration is about 2.5–3.5 g/dl.
      1. Interstitial albumin concentration is about 1–1.5 g/dl.
  II. Albumin maintains intravascular colloid oncotic pressure.
   A. Each gram of albumin osmotically holds 13–18 ml of fluid.
 III. Albumin is strongly negatively charged and is an important carrier of certain drugs, hormones, metals, and enzymes, as well as certain chemicals and toxins such as cations, anions, toxic oxygen radicals, and toxic inflammatory substances.
  IV. Plasma also contains coagulation factors.
   A. Fresh plasma, of course, contains all coagulation factors and therefore is good for the treatment of all coagulation disorders, including thrombocytopenia and disseminated intravascular coagulation.
      1. Fresh plasma should be used within 6 hours after taking it from the donor.

B. Storage causes the loss of certain coagulation factors.
  1. Freezing destroys the platelets.
     a. Fresh frozen plasma would not be good for the treatment of thrombocytopenia or disseminated intravascular coagulation.
  2. Refrigerator storage is associated with the loss of both platelets and labile coagulation factors of V, VIII, and von Willebrand factor.
     a. This product would not be good for the treatment of hemophilia A or von Willebrand disease, but it could still be used for the stabile factors for vitamin K-antagonist rodenticide-induced bleeding.
  3. Bench-top storage at room temperature for longer than 6 hours or frozen storage for longer than 1 year is also associated with the loss of both platelets and labile coagulation factors of V, VIII, and von Willebrand factor.

Whole Blood

I. Oxygen delivery is the product of blood oxygen content and cardiac output.
  A. Hemoglobin is the major determinant of oxygen content.
  B. Notwithstanding hypoxemia, hemoglobin concentration and cardiac output are the major determinants of oxygen delivery.
    1. Relatively lower hemoglobin concentrations could be well-tolerated if the cardiac output were able to increase to supranormal values.
    2. In situations where cardiac output is likely to be decreased (while the patient is receiving any anesthetic, or is in a condition of sepsis), relatively higher hemoglobin concentrations are necessary to assure adequate oxygen delivery.
II. A red blood cell (RBC) transfusion is indicated in the following situations:
  A. The hemoglobin concentration is below 5–8 g/dl.
  B. The packed cell volume (PCV) is below 15–25%.
  C. Further crystalloid fluid therapy is likely to reduce levels to those specified in items A and B.
III. The amount of whole blood to administer can be estimated several ways:
  A. An amount of 2 ml/kg (1 ml/lb) is associated with about 1% change in the measured PCV.
  B. An amount of 10 ml/kg and 30 ml/kg in the dog, or 5 ml/kg and 20 ml/kg in the cat, represents a small or large transfusion, respectively.
  C. The formulae in items A and B should be halved if packed cells are being used.
  D. The calculated volume is usually rounded up to the nearest whole unit of blood.
IV. Dogs exhibit a very low incidence of weakly reacting, naturally occurring alloantibodies.
  A. Random, first-time canine blood transfusions are seldom associated with a transfusion reaction.
  B. Although all erythrocytic antigens incite an antibody response, canine erythrocytic antigens DEA 1.1 and DEA 1.2, and to a lesser extent DEA 7, induce a strong antibody response.
    1. Clinically significant transfusion reactions are much more likely to occur following a second transfusion of unmatched blood.
    2. Potential donors should be typed and found negative for DEA 1.1, DEA 1.2, and DEA 7.

C. In vitro cross-matching is generally recommended, even if the donors are typed, to check out the intended transfusion if either of the following applies:

1. The recipient has received a previous transfusion.

2. The recipient suffers immune-mediated hemolytic anemia.

V. The two commonly identified red cell antigens in the domestic cat are A and B.

A. The domestic shorthair "mongrel" cat is virtually always Type A.

1. Type A cats have low titers of naturally occurring anti-B antibodies.

2. Transfusion of Type B blood into Type A cats has been associated with a mean RBC survival time of 2 days and minor transfusion reactions.

B. Type B populations are more likely to occur in feline breeds such as Scottish Fold, Berman, Himalayan, Abyssinian, Somali, Persian, Cornish and Devon Rex, and British shorthair (30–70%).

1. Type B cats have high titers of strong, naturally occurring anti-A antibodies.

2. Transfusion of Type A blood into Type B cats has been associated with a mean RBC survival time of 1 hour and marked transfusion reactions.

C. Typing the blood of donor cats may be useful, but it would also be necessary to know the blood type of the recipient to make sure the transfusion was properly matched.

1. In the absence of known blood types, in vitro cross-matching may be important in cats in general and is a "must do" in the above mentioned specialty breeds of cats.

VI. The rate of whole blood and plasma administration should be conservative, especially in the beginning, so as to minimize the clinical manifestations of transfusion or foreign protein histamine-mediated reactions.

A. Immunologic transfusion reactions may be manifested by the following:

1. Fever

2. Restlessness

3. Hemoglobinemia or hemoglobinuria

4. Wheezing or dyspnea

5. Urticaria

6. Hypotension or acute collapse

B. Additional adverse effects of blood transfusion include the following:

1. Pulmonary emboli from platelet, white cell, or red cell clumps in the transfused blood

2. Hypothermia if cold blood is administered

3. Hypocalcemia if large quantities of citrate are administered

4. Heparinization if large quantities of heparin are administered

5. Acidosis if large quantities of the citrate anticoagulants are administered

VII. Autotransfusion of whole blood should be considered if the animal is bleeding excessively into the pleural or peritoneal cavity and an exogenous source of whole blood is not readily available.

A. The blood should be gently aspirated, anticoagulated, and filtered when administered.

Anesthetic Considerations in Patients with Preexisting Problems or Conditions

Robert R. Paddleford

The successful outcome of a patient's anesthetic experience depends on the correct selection of anesthetic agents and techniques, the skill of the anesthesiologist, and the anesthesiologist's knowledge of the pathophysiologic conditions in the patient and their potential effects on the anesthetic management.

I. Pediatric Patients
  A. Definitions
    1. *Neonate (newborn)*: a puppy or kitten up to 2 weeks of age
    2. *Infant*: a puppy or kitten 2 – 6 weeks of age
    3. *Pediatric patient*: a puppy or kitten 6 – 12 weeks of age
  B. Surgery in the pediatric patient may be either of an elective nature or of an emergency nature.
    1. Types of elective surgery
      a. Tail and dewclaw removal
      b. Ear trimming
    2. Types of emergency surgery or procedures
      a. Fractures and dislocations
      b. Congenital defects
        (1) Patent ductus arteriosus
        (2) Persistent right aortic arch
        (3) Peritoneal-pericardial diaphragmatic hernia
        (4) Megaesophagus
        (5) Elongated soft palate, stenotic nares, or everting laryngeal saccules in brachycephalic breeds
        (6) Entropion and ectropion
      c. Intestinal problems, primarily intussusceptions
      d. Ruptured urinary bladders
  C. Physiologic differences between pediatric patients and adult patients
    1. Respiratory system
      a. The young dog's or cat's respiratory system has one third less alveolar area than the adult's and less alveolar surfactant.

  b. Gas flow resistance and chest wall compliance are greater in the pediatric patient.

  c. Pediatric patients have increased respiratory rates and minute volumes.

   (1) The minute volume may be as much as twice that of an adult.

   (2) The decreased alveolar surface area and increased metabolic rate of pediatric patients require the increased minute volume.

  d. Pediatric chemoreceptors are less sensitive than adult chemoreceptors and have a decreased response to high Pa_{CO_2} levels and low Pa_{O_2} levels.

  e. Pediatric patients have up to twice the oxygen consumption of adults.

 2. Cardiovascular system

  a. The pediatric patient's myocardium is less able to increase its force of contraction and is less compliant than the adult's. Its sympathetic innervation is incomplete.

   (1) Therefore, cardiac output is largely rate-dependent.

   (2) Bradycardia in the pediatric patient can greatly decrease the cardiac output.

  b. The pediatric patient has decreased pulmonary vascular resistance.

  c. Hypotension may be more of a problem because of poor vasomotor control and decreased baroreceptor sensitivity.

  d. Pediatric patients have lower red cell counts, hemoglobin levels, packed cell volumes, and arterial oxygen levels (Table 12–1).

  e. They have decreased plasma protein–binding capabilities.

  f. Distribution of cardiac output to the vessel-rich group of organs is greater and more rapid in the pediatric patient.

 3. Liver and kidneys

  a. The pediatric patient has an immature hepatic microsomal enzyme system and therefore a decreased biodegredation rate for drugs.

  b. Renal function may be dimished in the pediatric patient.

   (1) This is especially true when dehydration is present. With 5% dehydration there is oliguria, and with 15% dehydration there is anuria.

   (2) Pediatric patients do not concentrate urine as well as adults.

Table 12–1. Average Pediatric Physiologic Values for the Dog

Value	Newborn	2 weeks	6 weeks	Adult
Heart rate	160–200	180–210	180–200	80–130
Respiratory rate	40	40	20–30	10–20
Tidal volume (ml/kg)	2–3	2–3	2–3	2–3
Arterial blood pressure (torr)	60/40	80/50	90/60	120/70
Pa_{CO_2} (torr)	33	—	—	38
Pa_{O_2} (torr)	60–80	—	—	80–100
pH	7.45	—	—	7.4
Plasma H_{CO_3} (mEq/L)	14–20	—	—	18–24
Blood volume (% body weight)	—	8.5	—	8
Hemoglobin (g%)	17	10	10	15
Packed cell volume	55	27–32	28–35	46
Erythrocytes (millions)	6	3.2	4.9	8

From Robinson EP: Anesthesia of the pediatric patient. Presented at the 32nd Gaines Symposium on Small Animal Pediatrics and published in *The Compendium*, vol. 5, no. 12, December 1983, pp. 1004–1011.

         (3) Pediatric patients have increased sodium losses.

    4. Fluid and electrolyte balance

       a. The pediatric patient has lower intracellular fluid reserves and a higher body-water turnover.

         (1) In the newborn, 80% of body weight is total body water versus 60% in the adult.

         (2) In the newborn, 40% of the body weight is extracellular water versus 25% in the adult.

       b. Pediatric patients are more prone to hypoglycemia and hypocalcemia.

    5. Thermoregulation

       a. Pediatric patients are prone to hypothermia.

       b. They have a large ratio of surface area to volume.

       c. They have an immature thermoregulation system and a decreased ability to shiver.

       d. They have less insulating subcutaneous fat.

D. Anesthetic considerations

    1. Weigh the patient *accurately*, and use simple anesthetic techniques.

    2. The small size of the patient may lead to difficulty with intubation, intravenous catheter placement, and monitoring.

    3. Preanesthetic and anesthetic agents that must undergo hepatic biodegradation may have longer-lasting effects in the pediatric patient.

    4. The effects of injectable anesthetic agents may be more profound in the pediatric patient because of the following:

       a. Greater percentage of total body water and extracellular water

       b. Decreased protein binding

       c. Decreased percentage of body fat

       d. More rapid distribution of cardiac output to vessel-rich organs

    5. Because of increased minute ventilation, pediatric patients may respond more quickly to concentration changes of the inhalant anesthetics.

    6. Bradycardia may greatly decrease cardiac output in the pediatric patient.

    7. Pediatric patients are more prone to hypotension.

E. Preanesthetic medications

    1. Anticholinergics

       a. Puppies and kittens younger than 14 days may have little response to atropine or glycopyrrolate because of immature vagal innervation.

       b. Because cardiac output in the pediatric patient is largely rate-dependent, atropine or glycopyrrolate should be used in the preanesthetic regimen.

    2. Tranquilizers, sedatives, hypnotics

       a. All of these drugs depend on hepatic biodegradation and therefore may have prolonged effects in the pediatric patient.

       b. Phenothiazine-derivative tranquilizers

         (1) Hypotension and prolonged central nervous system (CNS) depression may be produced.

         (2) Phenothiazine tranquilizers tend to potentiate hypothermia as

a result of the depression of the thermoregulation center and the peripheral vasodilation they produce.

    (3) Low-dose acepromazine (0.05 mg/lb intramuscularly) has been used successfully in these patients, especially older pediatric patients. The total dose should not exceed 0.5 mg.

  c. Benzodiazepine-derivative tranquilizers

    (1) Diazepam (Valium) has been safely used in pediatric patients at a dose of 0.1–0.2 mg/lb intramuscularly.

    (2) Diazepam has minimal cardiopulmonary depressant effects.

  d. Alpha-2 agonists

    (1) Xylazine and medetomidine should be used with *extreme* care in the pediatric patient because of their tendency to cause cardiovascular depression (bradycardia and atrioventricular heart blocks).

    (2) Prolonged sedation may also occur.

3. Narcotic analgesics

  a. Narcotic analgesics have minimal direct cardiovascular depressant effects.

  b. They may cause sinus bradycardia; therefore, atropine at a dose of 0.02 mg/lb intramuscularly should be given prior to their administration.

  c. Oxymorphone HCI (Numorphan) at a dose of 0.05–.1 mg/lb intramuscularly or meperidine HCI (Demerol) at a dose of 2 mg/lb intramuscularly can be used in the puppy.

  d. Butorphanol at a dose of 0.1–.2 mg/lb intramuscularly or intravenously has been used in puppies and kittens.

  e. The response of kittens to narcotics is more unpredictable.

  f. Respiration should be monitored closely as the narcotics may cause marked respiratory depression. Means should be available to intubate and ventilate the patient with 100% oxygen if necessary.

  g. The effects of the narcotics can be readily antagonized with naloxone (Narcan).

4. Neuroleptanalgesics

  a. Various narcotic-tranquilizer combinations have been used in puppies and kittens, including oxymorphone-acepromazine, oxymorphone-diazepam, meperidine-diazepam, meperidine-acepromazine, butorphanol-acepromazine, and butophanol-diazepam.

  b. This clinician prefers butorphanol at a dose of 0.2 mg/lb intramuscularly and diazepam at a dose of 0.2 mg/lb intramuscularly. Atropine is also given at a dose of 0.02 mg/lb intramuscularly.

  c. Diazepam *cannot* be mixed in the syringe with the narcotics or atropine. It will cause precipitation.

F. Injectable general anesthetics

1. Barbiturates

  a. Pentobarbital (a short-acting barbiturate) depends on hepatic biodegradation to terminate its anesthetic effects. Therefore, its effects are prolonged by the decreased hepatic microsomal enzymes, and its use is not recommended.

  b. Ultra-short-acting barbiturates can be used for short procedures and anesthetic inductions.

    (1) Dilute the ultra-short-acting barbiturate to 1–2% to allow for administration in small increments.

        (2) Ultra-short-acting barbiturates have a more pronounced effect at a given dose in the pediatric patient because pediatric patients tend to have a lower percentage of body fat than adults as well as decreased plasma protein–binding capability.

        (3) Because arousal from thiopental depends on its redistribution to fat, the lowest possible dose should be used.

    c. Barbiturates are potent respiratory depressants, so respiration must be watched closely.

  2. Dissociative agents

    a. Ketamine HCl and tiletamine (Telazol) have been used in both puppies and kittens.

    b. The dissociative agents are excreted predominately unchanged via the kidneys in the cat, whereas hepatic biodegradation is the primary route of detoxification in the dog.

    c. Both intravenous and intramuscular administration have been used, with doses on the lower end of the range being recommended.

    d. Dissociative agents tend to maintain cardiac output and blood pressure.

    e. Large doses can cause apneustic ventilation and respiratory depression.

    f. Atropine or glycopyrrolate should be used to decrease salivation.

    g. Acepromazine or diazepam is usually used in combination with ketamine to provide better muscle relaxation, decrease the incidence of delirium, and provide for a smoother induction and recovery.

  3. Propofol (Diprivan, Rapinovet)

    a. Cardiovascular and pulmonary effects of propofol are similar to those of thiopental.

    b. Propofol can cause respiratory depression or apnea. The initial calculated dose should be administered over 60–90 seconds or until the desired level of anesthesia is reached.

    c. Puppies have good conjugation enzyme activities and therefore should be able to metabolize propofol efficiently.

G. Inhalant general anesthetics

  1. Inhalant anesthetic agents are probably the preferred general anesthetic agents for the pediatric patient.

  2. Methoxyflurane, halothane, isoflurane, sevoflurane, and nitrous oxide have all been used in pediatric patients.

  3. The minimum alveolar concentration of the inhalant anesthetic agents seems to be higher in children than in adult humans, but this does not seem to be the case in puppies and kittens. Concentrations used in the adult dog and cat appear suitable for puppies and kittens.

  4. Induction of anesthesia can be accomplished with the inhalants by means of a mask or chamber.

  5. Because of the small size of most pediatric patients, a non-rebreathing delivery system (Ayre's T-piece, Norman Elbow, Magill, or Bain coaxial delivery system) should be used. These systems decrease both mechanical dead space and resistance to ventilation.

  6. Primary bronchial intubation can occur because of the small size of pediatric patients. Endotracheal tubes should be cut off at a proper length to prevent this problem.

H. Other considerations

1. Fluid maintenance
   a. Pediatric patients do not tolerate overinfusion of fluids.
   b. A pediatric minidrip infusion set (60 drops/ml) and a burette should be used to administer fluids. Pumps for fluid administration can be very beneficial in treating the pediatric patient.
   c. Various types of fluids can be used in the pediatric patient; however, dextrose-containing, balanced-electrolyte solutions are preferred.
      (1) The dextrose will help to prevent hypoglycemia.
      (2) The fluids are administered at a rate of 2–5 ml/lb per hour for maintenance during anesthesia. This rate may be increased or decreased depending on the patient's status.
   d. Plasma or whole blood replacement should be considered if blood loss from hemorrhage exceeds 10% of the estimated blood volume.
   e. Oral fluids should be allowed up to 1 hour prior to anesthesia, and they should be offered as soon as possible after recovery from anesthesia.
2. Body temperature
   a. Every effort should be made to minimize decreases in body temperature.
   b. Efforts may include the use of warm prep solutions, warm intravenous fluids, warm towels on the surgery table, circulating-warm-water heating blankets in surgery and recovery, and warm irrigation fluids.
   c. Hypothermia can lead to cardiopulmonary depression and prolonged recoveries.
3. The cardiopulmonary system should be closely monitored.

II. Geriatric patients
   A. It is often difficult to define a geriatric patient simply on the basis of chronologic age.
      1. Some younger patients have organ systems typical of a geriatric patient, whereas some geriatric patients have organ systems typical of a younger patient.
      2. Some researchers have suggested that a patient be considered as aged, or geriatric, when it has reached 75–80% of its life expectancy.
      3. Ultimately each patient must be evaluated as an individual and not simply as a "geriatric" patient.
   B. General considerations
      1. The geriatric patient is likely to have more underlying diseases than a younger patient.
      2. The geriatric patient has less functional organ reserve than a younger patient.
         a. This decreased organ reserve has been termed "elderly normal."
         b. This decreased reserve may not be apparent until the animal is stressed by disease, hospitalization, anesthesia, or surgery, at which time overt organ failure may occur.
   C. Physiologic changes associated with aging
      1. Most of the knowledge regarding physiologic changes associated with aging have been derived from human studies but much of it may be applicable to the geriatric dog and cat as well.
      2. Cardiovascular system
         a. Geriatric patients have a decreased cardiac reserve compared with

younger patients and may have difficulty compensating for cardio-vascular changes that occur during anesthesia.

b. Geriatric patients show a decrease in the following:
   (1) Baroreceptor activity
   (2) Blood volume
   (3) Cardiac output
   (4) Blood pressure
   (5) Circulation time

c. Geriatric patients have vagotonia.

d. In addition, geriatric patients may suffer from progressive and degenerative myocardial disease.
   (1) Myocardial disease is usually associated with chronic valvular disease.
   (2) Myocardial disease can lead to an increased myocardial work-load and increased myocardial oxygen consumption and de-mand. The result is to make the myocardium extremely sensi-tive to hypoxemia.

d. The decreased cardiovascular function capabilities of geriatric pa-tients make them very susceptible to anesthetic-induced cardiovas-cular depression and hypotension.

3. Respiratory system

a. Respiratory function progressively diminishes as a patient ages.

b. Physical changes occur in the geriatric patient's lungs and chest wall.

c. Geriatric patients show a decrease in the following:
   (1) Lung elasticity
   (2) Closing volume
   (3) Vital capacity
   (4) Respiratory rate, tidal volume, and thus minute volume
   (5) Oxygen consumption
   (6) Carbon dioxide production
   (7) Maximal diffusion capacity for oxygen
   (8) Capillary blood volume
   (9) Protective airway reflexes

d. Geriatric patients show an increase in the following:
   (1) Anatomic dead space
   (2) Residual volume
   (3) Functional residual capacity
   (4) Residual volume/total lung capacity

e. All of the preceding changes are considered a normal part of the aging process.

f. These changes in the respiratory system are significant in the following ways:
   (1) Even mild to moderate respiratory depression resulting from anesthesia may produce marked hypoxemia and hypercarbia.
   (2) Any pathologic disease of the respiratory system (e.g., pneumo-nia, edema, pulmonary fibrosis, emphysema) will be greatly exacerbated in the geriatric patient.

4. Renal system

a. The kidney is the major effective organ in fluid and electrolyte balance.

b. Renal function may be greatly impaired in the geriatric patient.

c. In human beings, and therefore possibly in animals, the following normal aging changes occur in the kidneys:

    (1) Decreased renal blood flow

    (2) Decreased glomerular filtration rate

    (3) Decreased concentrating ability

    (4) Nephron degeneration

    (5) Increased blood urea nitrogen levels

    (6) A redistribution of blood flow from the cortex to the medulla owing to renal cortical vascular deterioration

    (7) Decreased distal tubular function resulting in a decreased ability to handle acid excretion

    (8) An increase in the urine volume necessary for excretion of the obligatory solute load

d. The functional renal reserve is diminished in geriatric patients making them more susceptible to the decrease in renal function caused by anesthesia.

e. Geriatric patients are much less tolerant of body-water deficits or the excessive administration of fluid.

f. The plasma half-life of drugs dependent on renal excretion is increased in the geriatric patient.

5. Liver

a. The aging process results in a reduction in the functional state of the microsomal enzyme systems of the liver.

b. This reduction is present even when the standard biochemical function tests are normal.

c. Geriatric patients often have a decreased hepatic blood flow, most likely the result of a decreased cardiac output.

d. The plasma half-life of drugs dependent on hepatic biodegradation is often increased in the geriatric patient.

6. Central nervous system (CNS)

a. In human beings, and therefore possibly in animals, aging is associated with a reduction in brain weight that is most likely a result of individual neuron degeneration.

b. Myelin sheaths also degenerate, resulting in an increased effect of local anesthetics.

c. Strong evidence exists that neurotransmitters change with age.

    (1) Destruction of neurotransmitters increases, and production decreases.

    (2) The reduction in neurotransmitter function may be a result of the decreased quantity of neurotransmitters or perhaps of a change in the receptors themselves.

d. The effects of the neuromuscular blocking agents may be prolonged in geriatric patients.

e. Thermoregulatory center function is decreased in geriatric patients, making them more susceptible to hypothermia produced by anesthesia.

7. Endocrine system

      a. Adrenal glands

         (1) Although aging does not appear to alter ACTH-stimulated plasma cortisol levels, there are reports that human geriatric patients may not have the adrenal gland reserves necessary to adequately protect them during stress from anesthesia and surgery.

         (2) Renin and aldostorone, hormones that are necessary for water, sodium, and potassium balance as well as blood pressure control, are attenuated in geriatric human patients when stressed.

         (3) Hyperadrenocorticism may be seen in older dogs.

         (4) Geriatric patients on chemotherapy may develop iatrogenic mineralocorticoid deficiencies and thus marked electrolyte imbalance.

      b. Pancreas

         (1) Glucose tolerance decreases with age.

         (2) Diabetes mellitus may be a problem in the geriatric patient.

      c. Thyroid glands

         (1) Hypothyroidism is reported to be the most common endocrine disease in the dog.

         (2) Hypothyroidism can occur in the geriatric patient.

      d. Pituitary glands

         (1) Antidiuretic hormone increases with aging as a result of increased resistance of the distal renal tubules to its effects.

         (2) This increase leads to impaired renal concentrating ability.

  8. Autonomic nervous system

      a. The autonomic nervous system loses some of its ability to respond to stress as human being age.

      b. The reduced response to stress appears to be most marked in the sympathetic nervous system.

      c. Despite this reduced response, there appears to be an enhanced response to iatrogenic epinephrine and norepinephrine. Thus, one might conclude that even though the output of the autonomic nervous system output is decreased, perhaps the receptors are more sensitive.

  9. Geriatric patients may be obese.

      a. Relative overdoses of injectable drugs, especially general anesthetics, may occur.

      b. Obesity often impairs a patient's ability to adequately ventilate under sedation or general anesthesia.

      c. Assisted or controlled ventilation is often necessary for obese patients.

D. Pharmacodynamic changes

  1. Geriatric patients have decreased cardiovascular and respiratory reserves. Associated with these decreased reserves are decreased hepatic and renal function and decreased volumes of intravascular and total body water. These factors may alter the pharmacodynamic characteristics of a drug.

  2. Decreased metabolic rates in the geratric patient may prolong a drug's action.

  3. Decreased plasma proteins in the geriatric patient will increase the bioavailability of drugs.

4. A decrease exists in the numbers as well as the functional characteristics of the receptors in the geriatric CNS.

5. Elimination of drugs through the kidneys is prolonged owing to diminished renal function.

6. All of the preceding factors often lead to a decreased anesthetic requirement in the geriatric patient and a prolonged recovery time from anesthesia.

7. One must also be aware that geriatric patients usually have a decreased cardiac output, which will delay the onset of action of preanesthetic and anesthetic agents. This delay may be interpreted as an inadequate dose of preanesthetic or anesthetic drugs. If so, more may be given, resulting in an overdose.

E. Anesthetic considerations

1. Preanesthetic examination

   a. A thorough and complete history should be taken from the owner, with special emphasis on the following:

      (1) Present medical or surgical problems

      (2) Current medications

      (3) Previous medical or surgical problems

      (4) Previous anesthesia experience

   b. A complete preanesthetic physical examination should be performed and a complete laboratory profile obtained, with special emphasis on renal and hepatic function.

   c. Special attention should be directed toward the cardiovascular and pulmonary systems and should include an electrocardiogram (EKG) and thoracic radiographs.

2. Preanesthetic medications

   a. The preanesthetic medication used in a particular geriatric patient will depend on that particular patient's physical condition, the amount of sedation required, and the experience of the veterinarian.

   b. Whatever agent is used, a decrease in the normal dose by one third to one half should be considered.

   c. Low-dose acepromazine (0.05 mg/lb intramuscularly with a maximum dose of 1.5 mg) can be very effective.

      (1) Be aware that hypotension may develop.

      (2) Acepromazine should not be used in patients with a history of seizures.

      (3) Acepromazine has minimal respiratory depressant effects and minimal direct myocardial depressant effects.

   d. Diazepam at a dose of 0.1–.2 mg/lb intramuscularly may be another useful tranquilizer, especially when used in combination with a narcotic.

      (1) Diazepam has minimal cardiopulmonary depressant effects.

      (2) It is very useful in patients with seizures.

      (3) It can be combined with butorphanol for an effective neurolept-analgesic in the geratric patient. A dose of 0.1–.2 mg/lb intramuscularly of butorphanol can be used.

   e. Alpha-2 agonists (xylazine, medetomidine) must be used only with *extreme* caution in the geriatric patient.

      (1) The alpha-2 agonists' marked cardiovascular depressant effects

may limit their use in the geriatric patient. An anticholinergic should be considered when alpha-2 agonists are used.

(2) In addition, respiratory depression may be significant.

f. Narcotic analgesics

(1) Narcotic analgesics are often used in geriatric patients because they produce minimal direct myocardial depression, although they may slow the heart rate as a result of increased vagal tone.

(2) Marked respiratory depression may occur.

(3) Their effects can be readily reversed by narcotic antagonists.

(4) Morphine, oxymorphone (Numorphan), fentanyl, butorphanol, and meperidine (Demerol) have all been used in geriatric patients, alone and in combination with tranquilizers.

(5) The low end of the dose range of a narcotic analgesic should be considered for the geriatric patient.

g. Anticholinergics

(1) The indiscriminate use of atropine or glycopyrrolate should be avoided in the geriatric patient.

(2) This is to prevent an unwanted and potentially dangerous sinus tachycardia from occurring.

(3) If sinus bradycardia does occur, atropine can be given, to effect, intravenously.

(4) If vagotonic drugs such as narcotics or alpha-2 agonists are to be used, then an anticholinergic may be warranted.

h. Neuroleptanalgesics

(1) Various combinations of tranquilizers have been used in combination with narcotics in geriatric patients (Table 12–2).

(2) Neuroleptanalgesics used in combination with local anesthetics may be all that is needed for minor surgical or diagnostic procedures.

3. Injectable anesthetic agents

a. Injectable anesthetic agents can be used in geriatric patients but should be used with care because of the often altered hemodynamics and decreased plasma protein–binding and metabolism in these patients.

b. Ultra-short-acting barbiturates can be used to induce anesthesia and for short surgical procedures.

(1) The lowest possible doses necessary for the procedure should be used.

(2) In addition, respiratory function must be watched closely because of the marked respiratory depression that can be produced by the barbiturate.

c. Ketamine has been used intravenously at a dose of 1–2 mg/lb to induce anesthesia.

(1) Ketamine tends to be supportive of the cardiovascular system, although it may cause depression if the patient has preexisting cardiovascular disease.

(2) It may also cause seizures, especially in dogs, and for this reason is often combined with diazepam.

(3) Larger intramuscular doses of ketamine have been used in both the dog and cat but may produce prolonged recoveries in the

dog (owing to decreased hepatic function) and in the cat (owing to decreased renal function).

   d. Tiletamine (Telazol) has been used intravenously at a dose of 1 mg/lb to induce anesthesia.

     (1) Its effects are similar to those of ketamine.

     (2) Larger intramuscular doses may produce a prolonged recovery similar to that of ketamine.

   e. Propofol (Diprivan, Rapinovet)

     (1) Propofol has been used to induce anesthesia and to maintain anesthesia in the geriatric patient.

     (2) Renal or hepatic dysfunction do not seem to prolong its effects.

     (3) *Watch* ventilation. Propofol is a respiratory depressant. Be prepared to provide supplemental oxygen or possibly intubate and ventilate the patient.

  4. Inhalant anesthetic agents

   a. Inhalant anesthetic agents are probably the anesthetics of choice in the geriatric patient, especially for procedures lasting longer than 10–15 minutes and for procedures in very debilitated patients.

   b. Halothane, methoxyflurane, isoflurane, and sevoflurane can all be used either with or without nitrous oxide.

   c. Isoflurane is preferred because of the high cardiac index and rapid induction and recovery times associated with it.

   d. Mask induction may be the preferred method to induce anesthesia.

  5. Miscellaneous considerations

   a. Geriatric patients should be preoxygenated for 2–4 minutes prior to anesthetic induction to help prevent hypoxemia from developing during induction.

   b. If a general anesthetic is to be used, the patient should be intubated.

   c. Close attention must be paid to cardiovascular and respiratory parameters.

   d. If necessary, the patient's ventilation should be assisted or controlled.

   e. Adequate fluid replacement should be given to prevent a renal crisis and maintain a proper hemodynamic state.

   f. Be prepared to prevent or treat hypothermia.

III. Patients with cardiovascular dysfunction

  A. General comments

   1. The anesthetic management of a patient with cardiovascular dysfunction can be very challenging, as most preanesthetic and anesthetic agents capable of CNS depression are also capable of producing cardiovascular depression.

   2. Patients with cardiovascular dysfunction may be more prone to fluid overload.

   3. Cardiac dysrhythmias may be more of a problem in these patients.

   4. Extremes in heart rate may cause severe problems, including heart failure.

   5. Patients with cardiovascular dysfunction may lack sufficient cardiac reserve to respond to the potential cardiovascular depression caused by the preanesthetic and anesthetic agents.

  B. Cardiovascular physiology

1. The function of the myocardial cell is to rhythmically contract and relax with other myofibers so that the heart will act as a pump.
2. The contraction of the heart muscle depends on the amount of free calcium ions available around the myofibril.
3. Part of the contractile-dependent calcium originates from superficial sites on cell membranes. It is in equilibrium with extracellular calcium and therefore can be affected by drugs that do not penetrate the myocardial cell.
4. The basic contractile unit of heart muscle is the sarcomere, which is composed of interdigitating protein filaments referred to as actin and myosin.
5. Muscle shortening develops in the myocardial muscle when the actin and myosin filaments are activated.
6. This activation is regulated by tropomyosin and troposin.
7. Tropomyosin prevents the interaction of actin and myosin during diastole. When tropomyosin is no longer at its blocking position, systole is initiated.
8. The availability of ionized calcium in the area of the troponin-tropomyosin protein unit acts as an immediate catalyst for the contraction-relaxation cycle.
9. Few clinically used drugs affect the actin-myosin proteins; however, many drugs can alter the availability of calcium for activation of the contractile process.
   a. Digitalis increases calcium movement to the troponin-tropomyosin protein unit and thus increases contractile strength.
   b. Barbiturates and inhalant agents seem to disrupt calcium movements and thus reduce contractile strength.
10. Myocardial intracellular acidosis also inhibits the binding of calcium to the troponin-tropomyosin unit causing a decreased myocardial contractile strength.
    a. Disease conditions or drugs that can produce metabolic or respiratory acidosis may decrease myocardial contractile strength.
    b. Many of the preanesthetic and anesthetic agents can produce respiratory and metabolic acidosis.
11. Blood pressure is determined by the peripheral vascular resistance multiplied by the cardiac output. Cardiac output is determined by the heart rate multiplied by stroke volume.
    a. Drugs that alter any or all of these parameters can greatly affect blood pressure and cardiovascular function.
    b. Preanesthetic and anesthetic agents can alter peripheral resistance (phenothiazine tranquilizers, barbiturates, inhalant agents), heart rate (narcotics, alpha-2 agonists, ketamine, inhalant agents) and stroke volume (inhalant agents).
C. Types of cardiovascular dysfunction that may increase the risk of anesthesia
   1. Diseases causing impaired cardiac output
   2. Congenital heart disease
   3. Hypotension or hypovolemia
   4. Anemia
   5. Heartworms
D. Diseases causing impaired cardiac output
   1. Cardiomyopathies

a. *Hypertrophic cardiomyopathy* is characterized by ventricular hypertrophy, decreased ventricular compliance, and impaired ventricular filling that results in reduced cardiac output. Ventricular performance (pump function) is usually not impaired.

b. *Congestive cardiomyopathy* is characterized by marked ventricular dilation, increased ventricular diastolic volume, and poor ventricular performance. Often congestive heart failure is present.

2. Pericardial disease

a. *Pericardial tamponade* is associated with impaired cardiac output secondary to reduced ventricular filling. Expansion of the cardiac chambers is limited, resulting in decreased ventricular filling, stroke volume, and cardiac output. Pump function is not impaired.

b. *Constrictive pericarditis* is associated with reduced ventricular compliance, decreased ventricular filling, and decreased cardiac output. Pump function is generally not impaired.

3. Valvular heart disease

a. Valvular heart disease is associated with impaired cardiac output, with or without congestive heart failure.

b. *Mitral insufficiency* is probably the most common valvular disease. It is characterized by ventricular hypertrophy and dilation, pulmonary vascular engorgement, and, eventually, right heart failure. Left ventricular pump function and systemic cardiac output are usually maintained until late in the disease.

4. The primary goals in the anesthetic management of patients with disease associated with impaired cardiac output are to avoid the following:

a. Tachycardia

b. Reduced preload

c. Hypovolemia

5. Anesthetic techniques

a. Patients with cardiovascular dysfunction should be preoxygenated prior to induction.

b. If pump function is adequate, the anesthetic choice is not specific for these patients; however, drugs that may produce tachycardia (anticholinergics, dissociative agents) are best avoided. The exception would be patients with congestive cardiomyopathy, in which case an increased heart rate may help increase cardiac output.

c. Narcotics are often used as a preanesthetic medication owing to their minimal effects on the myocardium.

   (1) They can be used in combination with low-dose acepromazine or diazepam.

   (2) Their effects can be antagonized.

   (3) The fact that they slow the heart rate may be beneficial; however, if severe bradycardia occurs, atropine or glycopyrrolate should be given to effect.

d. If only tranquilization is to be considered, then low-dose acepromazine may be given (0.05 mg/lb intramuscularly to a maximum dose of 1.5 mg).

e. Because of their depressant and dysrhythmic effects, alpha-2 agonists should be avoided.

f. Induction of anesthesia can be accomplished using low doses of thiopental or propofol, although a neuroleptanalgesic or mask induction may be the preferred method.

    g. Inhalant anesthetics are the preferred maintenance agent for these patients. Isoflurane with or without nitrous oxide is probably the best choice because of its high cardiac index.

E. Congenital heart disease

    1. The problems encountered in anesthetizing patients with congenital heart disease may be similar to those related to patients with congestive heart failure.

    2. The most common surgically correctable problems are patent ductus arteriosus (PDA) and persistent right aortic arch (PRAA).

    3. PDA

        a. PDA is usually recognized early in life before the patient deteriorates, and it is corrected at that time.

        b. If the patient is normal in other respects, the anesthetic protocol is the same as for a pediatric patient undergoing a thoracotomy.

        c. Surgical manipulation around the heart may cause ectopic beats.

        d. When the PDA is ligated, the alterations caused in blood pressure may cause a reflex slowing of the heart rate. In some instances atropine may be needed to counteract the sinus bradycardia.

        e. Intraoperative hypothermia is often a problem with patients undergoing PDA surgery because of their small size.

    4. PRAA

        a. Like PDA, PRAA is usually recognized early in life and corrected at that time.

        b. If the patient is normal in other respects, the anesthesia protocol is the same as for a pediatric patient undergoing a thoracotomy.

        c. It is important to remember that a patient with PRAA may be suffering from aspiration pneumonia and all the respiratory problems associated with it.

        d. As with PDA, surgical manipulation around the heart may cause ectopic beats.

        e. Intraoperative hypothermia may be a problem in patients with PRAA because of their small size.

F. Hypotension or hypovolemia

    1. Patients with hypotension or hypovolemia should be stabilized with fluids or whole blood prior to anesthesia.

    2. Many preanesthetic and anesthetic drugs are potentially hypotensive; therefore, these drugs can exacerbate preexisting hypotension.

    3. The phenothiazine tranquilizers should be used with caution because of their hypotensive characteristics.

G. Anemia

    1. Anemic patients are of concern from an anesthetic standpoint because the oxygen-carrying capacity of their blood is diminished.

        a. These patients should be preoxygenated prior to anesthetic induction.

        b. Whole blood transfusions should be considered if a dog has a packed cell volume (PCV) of less than 30% or a cat has a PCV of less than 25%.

        c. Patients seem better able to cope with chronic anemia than acute anemia.

       d. Anesthesia itself will often cause a fall in the PCV of 3–5% because of hypotension and fluid compartment shifts.

       e. Whole blood should be available for adminstration both intraoperatively and postoperatively. The rate and total amount of whole blood administered will depend on the status of the particular patient.

   2. Anemic patients may also have decreased plasma protein levels.

       a. Many of the preanesthetic and anesthetic drugs (especially injectable anesthetics) are protein-bound.

       b. Hypoproteinemia will increase the bioactivity of these drugs, causing a more pronounced effect from any given dose.

   3. Anemic patients should have serial PCVs and total plasma protein values recorded during surgery and postoperatively.

   4. Supplemental oxygen may be very beneficial in the preanesthetic as well as postoperative period for anemic patients.

       a. A high inspired oxygen tension will allow more oxygen to be dissolved into the plasma and thus help to counteract the decreased oxygen-carrying capacity caused by low red blood cell numbers.

       b. A mask, nasal catheter, or oxygen cage can be used to deliver 40–100% oxygen to the patient.

  H. Heartworm disease

   1. Heartworm disease in itself does not contraindicate any particular anesthetic regimen or protocol.

   2. Patients with heartworms may be more prone to spontaneous cardiac dysrhythmias while under anesthesia.

   3. Cardiac output may be decreased as a result of the heartworms.

   4. Heartworms may lead to pulmonary dysfunction.

IV. Patients with pulmonary dysfunction

  A. Most preanesthetic and anesthetic agents depress respiratory function; therefore, these agents may further compromise pulmonary function in a patient with preexisting pulmonary problems.

  B. Ventilatory control system

   1. The system is a series of complex feedback loops made up of sensors, controllers, and effectors.

   2. Principal ventilatory receptors or sensors

       a. Peripheral carotid-body chemoreceptors (at the bifurcations of the carotid arteries)

       b. Central chemoreceptors (near the surface on the ventrolateral aspect of the medulla oblongata)

       c. Receptors sensing stretch, irritation, and proprioception in the lungs, airways, and muscles of respiration

   2. The carotid body chemoreceptors are responsive to oxygen and stimulate respiration when hypoxemia is present.

   3. The central chemoreceptors respond to carbon dioxide and stimulate ventilation when hypercarbia (respiratory acidosis) is present.

   4. Increased ventilation resulting from metabolic acidosis may be mediated through either the central or peripheral chemoreceptors.

   5. Major controllers of the ventilatory feedback loop are located in the brain.

       a. Automatic breathing is governed by specialized regions in the brainstem.

b. The cortex controls voluntary and behavioral modifications of ventilation.

c. Respiratory rhythm is controlled by the medulla.

d. Control functions are integrated both centrally (brainstem) and peripherally (spinal cord).

4. The effectors of ventilation are the muscles of respiration and include the intercostal muscles, the diaphragm, and the muscles of the upper airways.

C. Effects of preanesthetic and anesthetic drugs on ventilatory control

1. Drugs depress or stimulate ventilation by acting directly or indirectly on one or more of the elements of the ventilatory control system.

2. Anticholinergics

a. Atropine and glycopyrrolate decrease airway resistance by causing direct dilation of the airways.

b. Atropine also increases respiratory dead space because it dilates the larger bronchi.

3. Phenothiazine tranquilizers

a. At therapeutic doses the effects of the phenothiazine tranquilizers on ventilation are negligible, although large doses can depress ventilation.

b. They may produce a decrease in rate, but this is usually compensated for by an increase in tidal volume.

c. They do not delay the central respiratory center response (threshold) to increases in arterial carbon dioxide, although the maximum ventilatory response (sensitivity) may be decreased.

4. Alpha-2 agonists (xylazine, medetomidine)

a. Alpha-2 agonists have variable effects on the respiratory system.

b. In some patients little or no respiratory depression occurs, whereas in other patients *marked* decreases in respiratory rate and tidal volume may occur.

5. Benzodiazepine tranquilizers (diazepam, midazolam)

a. These tranquilizers produce minimal respiratory depression at therapeutic doses, although midazolam has been reported to produce respiratory depression.

b. Diazepam and midazolam can decrease the ventilatory response to increased carbon dioxide levels.

6. Narcotic analgesics

a. Narcotics are potentially potent respiratory depressants.

b. The depression is drug-and dose-dependent and may occur at doses that do not produce marked CNS depression or analgesia.

c. Narcotics directly depress the pontine and medullary centers, causing a decrease in respiratory rate and tidal volume.

d. They produce a delayed response (altered threshold) and a decreased response (altered sensitivity) to increases in arterial carbon dioxide.

e. The panting observed in some dogs following narcotic administration may be due to an initial stimulation of the respiratory centers or to alteration of the thermoregulation center.

7. Barbiturates

a. Barbiturates are potent respiratory depressants.

b. At anesthetizing doses, they depress the respiratory centers of the brain.

c. They can depress both the respiratory rate and tidal volume and thus minute ventilation.

d. They produce a delayed response (altered threshold) and a decreased response (altered sensitivity) to increases in arterial carbon dioxide.

e. They also depress the carotid-aortic chemoreceptors.

8. Dissociative agents (ketamine, tiletamine)

a. Dissociative agents are one of the few anesthetics that may have a dual effect on ventilation.

b. They may influence ventilation at two or more anatomic sites, causing stimulation at one site and depression at another.

c. They produce apneustic ventilation (i.e., a ventilatory pattern characterized by a prolonged pause after inspiration).

d. Dissociative agents often decrease the respiratory rate.

e. In general, dissociative agents do not affect blood gases; however, in some patients, they may produce marked hypoxemia and hypercarbia, especially when other CNS depressant drugs are combined with them or when they are used in high doses.

f. Pharyngeal and laryngeal reflexes are not depressed, although they may be activated only with stimulation. As a result, patient may be more prone to laryngospasm, bronchospasm, and coughing.

g. Dissociative agents increase salivation and respiratory secretions.

(1) Salivation may increase to the point of aspiration and respiratory obstruction.

(2) For this reason, the use of an anticholinergic in combination with ketamine or tiletamine (Telazol) may be needed.

9. Propofol (Diprivan, Rapinovet)

a. Propofol is a *potent* respiratory depressant.

b. Its depressant effects rapidly reverse when it is discontinued.

c. Propofol's respiratory depressant effects can be attenuated by administering the initial calculated dose over 60–90 seconds or until the desired level of anesthesia is reached.

10. Etomidate (Amidate)

a. At theraputic doses, etomidate produces minimal respiratory depression.

b. With excessive doses, respiratory depression can occur.

11. Inhalant anesthetics

a. Methoxyflurane, halothane, isoflurane, and sevoflurane depress ventilation by decreasing tidal volume.

b. These anesthetics may produce a decrease in respiratory rate.

c. They increase the level of arterial carbon dioxide at which spontaneous ventilation ceases, that is, the "apneic threshold." The degree of elevation of the apneic threshold is directly related to the depth of anesthesia.

d. They reduce the slope of the carbon dioxide response curve. They produce a delayed response (altered threshold) and a decreased response (altered sensitivity) to increases in arterial carbon dioxide.

e. They depress the ventilatory responses to hypoxemia. In addition, the interaction between hypoxemia and hypercarbia in stimulating ventilation is greatly attenuated or eliminated by moderate concentrations of these agents.

    f. Nitrous oxide possesses some respiratory depressant properties, but they are minimal.

D. Anesthetic considerations

    1. Patients with pulmonary dysfunction may lack the ability to properly expand the lungs (extrapulmonary dysfunction) or may have impaired oxygen–carbon dioxide transfer across the alveolar membranes (intrapulmonary dysfunction).

    2. Examples of extrapulmonary dysfunction

        a. Diaphragmatic hernia

        b. Pneumothorax

        c. Hydrothorax

        d. Space-occupying lesions of the thorax

        e. Flail chest

        f. Any condition that restricts chest wall expansion

    3. Examples of intrapulmonary dysfunction

        a. Pneumonia

        b. Pulmonary edema

        c. Intrapulmonary hemorrhage (contusions)

        d. Atelectasis

        e. Interstitial disease

        f. Upper airway, tracheal, or bronchial obstruction

    4. Preanesthetic evaluation of the respiratory patient

        a. Any patient with respiratory dysfunction must be thoroughly examined prior to anesthesia.

        b. An extensive physical examination of the thorax, including auscultation, should be performed.

        c. Thoracic radiographs should be taken.

        d. As EKG should be performed.

        e. Arterial blood gases should be analyzed when possible.

        f. A baseline complete blood count (CB), electrolyte panel, and organ chemistry panel should be obtained.

        g. Patients with respiratory dysfunction can be classified in one of four ways:

          (1) Category I: Dyspnea does not occur even with exertion.

          (2) Category II: Dyspnea occurs with moderate exertion.

          (3) Category III: Dyspnea occurs with mild exertion.

          (4) Category IV: Dyspnea occurs while the patient is at rest.

        h. Patients in Categories III and IV definitely have a high anesthetic risk.

    5. General considerations

        a. If possible, surgery and anesthesia should be postponed in patients with pneumonia, pulmonary edema, lung contusions, atelectasis, pneumothorax, and hydrothorax to allow time for these problems to improve.

        b. A thoracocentesis should be done in patients with moderate to severe pneumothorax or hydrothorax prior to anesthesia. In some cases a chest tube may need to be placed prior to surgery.

    c. Patients with respiratory dysfunction should be preoxygenated with 100% oxygen a minimum of 5–7 minutes prior to anesthetic induction. A mask or oxygen chamber can be used.

    d. Supplemental oxygen should be available both preoperatively and postoperatively.

6. Anesthetic considerations

    a. Mild preanesthetic sedation may be necessary to allow the patient to be handled without causing stress and exacerbating respiratory dysfunction.

    b. If preanesthetic medication is needed, those drugs with minimal respiratory depression should be considered, such as the following:

      (1) Acepromazine 0.05–.1 mg/lb intramuscularly to a maximum total dose of 1.0 mg

      (2) Diazepam (Valium) 0.1–.2 mg/lb intramuscularly to a maximum total dose of 10 mg

      (3) Diazepam (same dose as preceding) or acepromazine (same dose as preceding) plus butorphanol 0.1–.2 mg/lb intramuscularly or intravenously to a maximum total dose of 20 mg

    c. Rapid induction of anesthesia may be needed to gain quick control of the airway to allow for positive pressure ventilation.

      (1) A rapid mask induction using isoflurane or sevoflurane may be used; however, because of the patient's inability to ventilate properly, this technique may result in delayed anesthetic induction and hence in struggling by the patient.

      (2) Rapid anesthetic induction can be accomplished by administering thiopental or propofol to effect or by administering 1–2 mg/lb of ketamine intravenously or 1 mg/lb tiletamine (Telazol) intravenously.

      (3) Whichever induction technique is used, rapid and accurate intubation must be accomplished.

    d. Maintenance of anesthesia is best accomplished using an inhalant anesthetic and controlled or positive pressure ventilation.

      (1) Nitrous oxide should be used with care in patients with respiratory dysfunction. It can increase the severity of a pneumothorax. It should be discontinued if cyanosis is evident.

      (2) Even if a patient with respiratory dysfunction seems to have adequate spontaneous ventilation, assisted or controlled ventilation should be provided.

7. Goals in the anesthetic management of the patient with respiratory dysfunction

    a. Preoxygenate the patient.

    b. Establish a patent airway rapidly.

    c. Provide a means for positive pressure ventilation.

    d. Avoid preanesthetics that are potent respiratory depressants.

    e. Provide a means of supplemental oxygen preoperatively and postoperatively.

V. Patients with hepatic dysfunction

    A. The patient with hepatic dysfunction presented for anesthesia can represent an extremely challenging case.

    B. Hepatic physiology

      1. The liver is the largest single organ in the body. It receives approximately 25% of the cardiac output.

2. The liver plays a major role in carbohydrate, protein, and lipid metabolism. It is responsible for detoxification and elimination of endogenous wastes and exogenous drugs.

3. The liver plays a major role in the body's immune system and in maintaining hemostatic mechanisms.

4. The liver has a phenomenal ability to regenerate and a tremendous functional reserve capacity.

   a. Dogs may regenerate up to 70% of their hepatic mass in 10–14 days.

   b. Insulin, thyroxine, glucocorticoids, diet, and age influence this ability to regenerate.

   c. Animals with as little as 10–20% of their liver mass can function well.

   d. The two factors in items "a" and "c" account for why most patients with hepatic dysfunction can tolerate preanesthetic and anesthetic agents so well.

4. Carbohydrate metabolism

   a. The liver plays a major role in the formation, storage, and release of glucose.

   b. Glucose is released from the liver when plasma glucose concentrations are low. The liver stores glucose when the plasma concentrations are high.

   c. Glucose uptake by the liver is not insulin-dependent.

   d. Hypoglycemia is uncommon in patients with hepatic dysfunction. Patients with mild to moderate hepatic disease can maintain a fasting blood glucose within a normal range.

   e. When hypoglycemia occurs with hepatic dysfunction, it is usually associated with acute hepatocellular necrosis or end-stage hepatic disease.

5. Hemostatis

   a. Factors I, II, V, VII, IX, and X are produced in the liver.

   b. The liver synthesizes activators and inhibitors of the fibrinolytic system.

   c. The liver is involved with the catabolism of many coagulants and procoagulants.

   d. Because of the liver's importance in maintaining hemostasis, clotting abnormalities can occur in the patient with hepatic dysfunction.

   e. Clotting problems are more likely to occur in patients with acute hepatic dysfunction than in patients with chronic disease.

   f. Patients with hepatic disease should have coagulation profiles determined prior to surgery.

6. Protein synthesis

   a. With the exception of gamma globulins, 90–95% of plasma protein biosynthesis occurs in the liver.

   b. Patients with hepatic dysfunction may have decreased circulating plasma protein levels.

      (1) These decreased levels are important because many preanesthetic and anesthetic agents are variably protein-bound.

      (2) The protein-bound portion is a nonactive form of the drug.

      (3) As the protein-bound portion is nonactive, a higher concentration of the active form of the drug is allowed and thus a more pronounced effect of the drug on the patient.

    c. The liver is important in the biosynthesis of circulating enzymes, including plasma cholinesterase (pseudocholinesterase).

      (1) In patients with chronic hepatic dysfunction, this enzyme may be reduced.

      (2) Plasma cholinesterase is involved in the biodegradation of ester local anesthetics (procaine, 2-chloroprocaine, tetracaine), succinylcholine, and the hypnotic induction agents etomidate and metomidate.

    d. Chronic liver disease may cause a decrease in albumin levels.

      (1) Albumin is extremely important in maintaining colloid oncotic pressure.

      (2) The colloidal pressure is responsible for maintaining fluid within the intravascular space.

      (3) When albumin levels are less than 2.0 g/dl, the patient is susceptible to movement of fluid from the intravascular space to the extravascular space and thus development of tissue edema.

      (4) Patients with low albumin levels are especially susceptible to fluid overload from the administration of intravenous crystalloid fluids.

7. Drug metabolism

    a. The liver is the most important organ involved in drug biotransformation.

    b. The liver produces drug biotransformation in several ways:

      (1) The hepatocytes first transform lipid-soluble drugs into more polar water-soluble compounds. (Lipid solubility enhances a drug's movement into cells but delays its excretion.)

      (2) Second, the polar water-soluble intermediates are conjugated with an organic acid.

      (3) The biotransformed molecules are usually secreted into the bile.

      (4) Many drugs then undergo an enterohepatic circulation and are eventually eliminated in the urine.

    c. The rate at which the hepatic microsomes metabolize drugs is modified by several factors and is highly variable among species and individuals.

    d. The elimination of drugs with a high hepatic extraction ratio (lidocaine, opioids) is not greatly affected by a decrease in hepatic microsomal enzyme activity. Their elimination is affected more by hepatic blood flow.

    e. Decreased hepatic microsomal enzyme activity will greatly prolong drugs with low extraction ratios (drugs that are slowly metabolized by the liver).

      (1) Drugs with low extraction ratios include diazepam, chlorpromazine, acepromazine, digitoxin, and quinidine.

      (2) These drugs are minimally affected by changes in blood flow.

    f. Effects of hepatic disease on drug biotransformation

      (1) The effects of hepatic disease on drug biotransformation are very unpredictable.

      (2) In general, the more severe the hepatic dysfunction, the more likely it is that drug metabolism will be impaired.

      (3) Acute hepatic dysfunction is more likely than chronic hepatic dysfunction to cause delayed metabolism.

(4) Hepatic blood flow, hepatocellular function, and bile flow all interact during drug metabolism.

(5) Hepatocellular damage will most likely decrease the clearance of drugs with a low extraction ratio.

(6) Decreased hepatic blood flow will reduce the clearance of drugs with a high extraction ratio.

(7) Hypoalbuminemia will exacerbate the pharmacologic effects of a drug because there is less protein binding.

(8) Acquired or congenital portal-systemic shunts and intrahepatic arteriovenous shunting will reduce hepatic drug elimination.

C. Biotransformation of preanesthetic and anesthetic agents

1. Almost all preanesthetic and anesthetic agents undergo direct or indirect hepatic biotransformation.

2. Anticholinergic agents

   a. Atropine undergoes hepatic hydrolysis, with some of the drug being excreted intact by the kidney.

   b. Glycopyrrolate is metabolized by the liver.

3. Tranquilizers, sedatives, hypnotics

   a. Phenothiazine tranquilizers are conjugated in the liver and eliminated as glucuronide salts. Their effects are most likely prolonged in the patient with hepatic dysfunction.

   b. Butyrophenone tranquilizers (droperidol, lemperone, azaperone) are relatively long-acting, with a hepatic metabolic pathway similar to that of the phenothiazine tranquillizers.

   c. Benzodiazepine tranquilizers (diazepam and midazolam) are conjugated by the liver. The half-life of these drugs is increased in patients with acute and chronic hepatic dysfunction. Specific antagonists are available for benzodiazepine tranquilizers.

   d. Alpha-2 agonists (xylazine, medetomidine) are conjugated by the liver. Some of the intact drug as well as its metabolites are eliminated in the urine. Alpha-2 agonists should be used with caution in patients with hepatic dysfunction. Specific antagonists are available for these drugs.

4. Narcotic analgesics

   a. Narcotics are conjugated to glucuronide metabolites in the liver, and the metabolites are eliminated via the kidney.

   b. Because narcotics are biotransformed in the liver, their effects may be prolonged in the patient with hepatic dysfunction.

   c. Narcotic effects can be counteracted by narcotic antagonists; thus, narcotics have potential use in the patient with hepatic dysfunction.

   d. Narcotics also have a high extraction ratio; therefore, a decreased hepatic microsomal enzyme activity may not greatly affect their elimination.

   e. Remember that the clinical effects of narcotic antagonists are usually of shorter duration than the clinical effects of narcotics; therefore, renarcotization may occur, necessitating repeated antagonist administration.

5. Dissociative agents

   a. The cat eliminates the majority of ketamine and tiletamine unchanged through renal excretion.

   b. In the dog, horse, and man, the dissociative agents are demethylated and hydroxylated by the liver prior to excretion. Therefore, hepatic disease may prolong their effects in these species.

6. Barbiturates

a. The oxybarbiturates (phenobarbital, pentobarbital, methohexital) undergo extensive biotransformation in the liver. This biotransformation is responsible for the termination of their anesthetic effects.

b. The thiobarbiturate thiopental also undergoes extensive hepatic biotransformation. The termination of its anesthetic effects is primarily dependent on redistribution from the vessel-rich organs to striated muscle and eventually to the fat of the body. The thiobarbiturates are slowly released from the fat and are then metabolized by the liver.

c. Barbiturates can produce enzyme induction in the liver with repeated administration.

7. Propofol

a. Propofol has both hepatic and extrahepatic routes of metabolism.

b. Hepatic dysfunction does not seem to prolong its effects.

8. Inhalant anesthetic agents

a. Methoxyflurane

(1) Methoxyflurane can reduce hepatic blood flow by 50% owing to vasoconstriction of the hepatic artery and portal vein.

(2) The reduced blood flow appears to be unrelated to anesthetic depth.

(3) As much as 50% of the inspired methoxyflurane can be metabolized in the liver. Potentially nephrotoxic inorganic fluoride ion and oxalic acid are produced.

b. Halothane

(1) Halothane produces a dose-related decrease in hepatic blood flow as a result of a decrease in cardiac output.

(2) Halothane has minimal effects on hepatic vascular resistance.

(3) Surgical concentrations of halothane can decrease hepatic blood flow by up to 40%.

(4) As much as 30% of the inspired halothane may be biotransformed by the liver.

(5) If halothane is biotransformed by oxidative pathways, relatively nontoxic fluoroacetic acid, bromine, and chloride are formed.

(6) If biotransformation occurs by reductive pathways, then intermediate free radical metabolites are formed. These radicals covalently bind with intracellular proteins and phospholipids to cause hepatocellular necrosis. Reductive biotransformation depends on decreased oxygen levels, genetic factors, and concurrent medications.

c. Isoflurane

(1) Isoflurane does not appear to produce a major decrease in hepatic blood flow unless high concentrations or an overdose occurs.

(2) Only about 0.2% of the inspired isoflurane is metabolized by the liver.

d. Sevoflurane

(1) Sevoflurane has no direct hepatic effects.

(2) Only 3% of the inspired concentration is metabolized.

   e. Desflurane
      (1) Desflurane has no direct hepatic effects.
      (2) Only 0.02% of the inspired concentration is metabolized.
   f. Nitrous oxide
      (1) Nitrous oxide does not appear to affect hepatic blood flow or vascular resistance.
      (2) No significant biotransformation of nitrous oxide occurs in the liver.
9. Local anesthetics
   a. All local anesthetics undergo biotransformation prior to elimination.
   b. The ester group of local anesthetics (procaine, 2-chloroprocaine, and tetracaine) are biotransformed by plasma cholinesterase.
   c. The amide group of local anesthetics (lidocaine, mepivacaine, and bupivacaine) are metabolized by the liver to water-soluble metabolites.
10. Neuromuscular blocking agents
   a. Succinylcholine is metabolized by plasma cholinesterase. Its effects are prolonged in patients with hepatic dysfunction.
   b. Gallamine is excreted intact by the kidney and does not undergo any significant hepatic biotransformation.
   c. Pancuronium is partially excreted intact by the kidney and partially conjugated in the liver. Its effects are prolonged in patients with hepatic dysfunction.
   d. Atracurium undergoes extrahepatic metabolism.
D. Anesthetic considerations
   1. Preanesthetic exposure to antiepileptic drugs, corticosteroids, antiparasitics, and exogenous hormones can produce hepatocellular dysfunction that can be exacerbated by the administration of preanesthetic and anesthetic agents.
   2. Hepatic evaluation
      a. Hepatic enzyme evaluation will indicate whether hepatic disease is present but will not aid in assessing the functional integrity of the liver.
      b. If the serum concentrations of alanine aminotransferase (ALT) and alkaline phosphatase (ALP) are normal, it is unlikely there is significant hepatic dysfunction.
      c. Patients with cirrhosis of the liver may have normal enzyme levels even though their liver function is greatly impaired.
      d. If the ALT or ALP levels are abnormally elevated, then the patient may have significant hepatic dysfunction that may or may not alter the response to anesthesia.
         (1) ALT is a specific liver enzyme in the dog and cat. Its magnitude parallels the number of damaged hepatic cells.
         (2) ALP is an inducible enzyme found in the liver, bones, gastrointestinal tract, kidneys, and placenta. It is usually elevated in the young. Steroid use will increase its levels.
   3. Prior to anesthesia, the patient's liver disease should be evaluated as to whether it is acute or chronic and what the predominant hepatic lesion is (hepatocellular, cholestatic, or vascular).
      a. A patient with acute hepatic failure offers the poorest anesthetic risk.

b. A patient with chronic hepatocellular disease that is compensated offers a better anesthetic risk.

4. Patients with chronic compensated hepatocellular disease

   a. Most currently available preanesthetic and anesthetic agents can probably be safely used in these patients.

   b. Ideally, agents that have a short biologic half-life or undergo minimal hepatic biotransformation should be used.

   c. Preanesthetic agents of choice would include midazolam, diazepam, or a low dose of a narcotic analgesic with or without the diazepam or midazolam. Phenothiazine tranquilizers and alpha-2 agonists should be used with caution.

   d. Low-dose thiopental or propofol can be used as injectable general anesthetics. Propofol is probably the prefered agent.

   e. Any of the inhalant anesthetics can probably be used, although isoflurane and sevoflurane are the preferred inhalants.

   f. Local anesthetics can also be used if indicated.

5. Patients with active hepatocellular disease, icterus, or acute hepatic failure

   a. These patients are at high risk and are often debilitated.

   b. They may be depressed and thus require no preanesthetic medications.

   c. If preanesthetics are needed, low-dose diazepam, midazolam, or a low dose of a narcotic (butorphanol or oxymorphone) with or without the midazolam or diazepam may be used.

   d. The preferred method of induction is via mask using a potent inhalant anesthetic with or without nitrous oxide.

      (1) Isoflurane or sevoflurane are the agents of choice.

      (2) Halothane or methoxyflurane may also be used.

      (3) Halothane is probably contraindicated only if the patient has had unexplained icterus following a previous exposure to halothane.

   e. The injectable anesthetic agent of choice would be propofol because of its rapid elimination and extrahepatic breakdown.

6. It is critical that adequate ventilation and oxygenation be maintained in patients with liver dysfunction.

7. Adequate blood pressure must be maintained because hypotension can exacerbate hepatic dysfunction.

8. Renal function should be closely monitored.

9. Fluid and electrolyte balance must be maintained prior to, during, and after anesthesia.

   a. A balanced crystalloid solution such as lactated Ringer's can be used.

   b. A 5% dextrose infusion may be indicated in patients with chronic hepatic disease to maintain serum glucose levels.

10. Hypothermia must be prevented or counteracted.

11. Liver function tests should be monitored closely postoperatively. Remember that anesthetics may cause a transient rise in hepatic enzymes 24–48 hours postoperatively.

12. Regardless of the anesthetic technique used, assume there will be a prolonged recovery time in patients with hepatic dysfunction.

VI. Patients with renal dysfunction

   A. Renal physiology

1. The kidneys are largely responsible for maintaining the volume and composition of the body fluids within normal limits.
2. Seven eighths of the water filtered by the glomeruli are reabsorbed by the proximal renal tubules.
   a. The proportion of the remaining water that is reabsorbed in the distal tubules is under the control of antidiuretic hormone (ADH) released from the pituitary gland.
   b. Most of the inhalant anesthetics cause the release of ADH.
3. The majority of the filtered electrolytes are also reabsorbed in the proximal renal tubules in association with water.
   a. Further electrolyte exchange occurs in the distal tubule under the influence of the adrenocortical hormone aldosterone.
   b. Aldosterone causes retention of sodium and water and excretion of potassium.
4. The kidneys help maintain normal acid-base balance by tubular excretion of hydrogen ions and formation of acid sodium phosphate and ammonium salts.
5. The kidneys also excrete many toxic substances, drugs, and drug metabolites in the urine.
6. The kidneys receive 25% of the cardiac output although they constitute only 0.4% of the body mass.
   a. The kidneys function at a high metabolic rate and are very susceptible to hypoxemia and hypotension.
   b. When renal damage occurs, abnormalities in water and electrolyte balance may be observed.

B. Anesthesia and the kidney
   1. Anesthesia and surgery generally cause an increased activity of the sympathetic nervous system and of the renin-angiotensin system. Both of these factors decrease total renal blood flow and redistribute intrarenal blood flow away from the renal cortex.
   2. General anesthesia may decrease renal blood flow by 40% and the glomerular filtration rate by up to 40%. When the effects of the anesthetics terminate, renal function returns to normal.
   3. Decreased renal function will be enhanced by
      a. Hyovolemia
      b. Hypotension
      c. Hypoxemia
      d. Hypercapnia
      e. Drugs that potentiate or mimic sympathetic tone (i.e., dissociative agents)
      f. Nephrotoxins

C. Specific effects of preanesthetic and anesthetic agents on the kidney
   1. Anticholinergics (atropine, glycopyrrolate) do not significantly affect renal function at therapeutic doses.
   2. Tranquilizers, sedatives, hypnotics
      a. Phenothiazine tranquilizers cause no appreciable changes in real function unless hypotension occurs.
         (1) They can produce hypotension because of peripheral vasodilation.
         (2) This response is somewhat dose-independent.

  (3) The vasodilation may actually improve renal blood flow and increase renal output as long as normal blood volume and blood pressure are maintained.

  (4) The effects of phenothiazine tranquilizers may be prolonged in the uremic patient.

  b. Alpha-2 agonists

  (1) Alpha-2 agonists can cause glucosuria and polyuria of short duration.

  (2) This occurs because alpha-2 agonists produce a pronounced and persistent hyperglycemia by increasing hepatic glucose production and decreasing plasma insulin levels.

  (3) Alpha-2 agonists have no direct effect on the kidney.

  c. Benzodiazepine tranquilizers appear to have no effect on renal function at therapeutic doses.

3. Narcotic analgesics

  a. Narcotics have no direct effect on the kidneys.

  b. Narcotics stimulate ADH release and may produce transient oliguria, especially at high doses.

4. Barbiturates

  a. Barbiturates can decrease renal blood flow and the glomerular filtration rate.

  b. Evidence exists that phenobarbital and pentobarbital inhibit water diuresis by stimulating ADH release.

  c. Uremia will increase a patient's sensitivity to barbiturates.

  (1) Uremia increases the amount of nonionized (active) form of barbiturate in the blood.

  (2) Uremia decreases the amount of protein-bound barbiturate in the blood.

5. Dissociative agents (ketamine, tiletamine)

  a. Dissociative agents appear to have no direct effect on the kidney.

  b. They do increase sympathetic tone, which can cause a transitory decrease in renal blood flow as a result of vasoconstriction.

  c. In the cat, ketamine and tiletamine are excreted virtually intact by the kidney.

6. Propofol

  a. Propofol does not seem to directly affect the kidneys.

  b. Transitory renal function can decrease because of hypotension.

7. Methoxyflurane

  a. Methoxyflurane causes a transient decrease in renal function owing to a decrease in cardiac output, vasoconstriction, and ADH release.

  b. It can produce proximal renal tubular necrosis owing to metabolites.

  (1) Fluoride ion is released during the hepatic biotransformation of methoxyflurane.

  (2) Fluoride ion can produce proximal renal tubular necrosis.

  (3) The tubular damage produces a high-output renal failure 24–72 hours after anesthesia.

  (4) The renal damage is enhanced by prolonged use of methoxyflurane, obesity in the patient, and the use of drugs excreted through the kidney.

        (5) The incidence of proximal renal tubular necrosis in animals following methoxyflurane exposure appears to be very low.

  8. Halothane

    a. Halothane does not have a direct nephrotoxic effect.

    b. Halothane does decrease renal function, primarily because of a decrease in cardiac output, peripheral vasodilation, and ADH release.

  9. Isoflurane, sevoflurane, and desflurane

    a. These inhalants are not nephrotoxic.

    b. Any decrease in renal function produced is most likely due to a decrease in renal blood flow and ADH release.

  10. Nitrous oxide

    a. Nitrous oxide produces no known renal dysfunction.

    b. It will potentiate the release of ADH produced by the other inhalant anesthetics.

D. Anesthetic considerations

  1. Surgery and anesthesia may precipitate renal failure in patients with preexisting renal disease.

  2. In human patients, 10–15% of the postanesthetic complications involve renal dysfunction, a fact that might have significance for animal patients.

  3. Preanesthetic evaluation

    a. A thorough and complete clinical pathologic workup should be done on any patient with suspected renal dysfunction.

    b. Renal function tests (BUN and creatinine) and a urinalysis should be performed for all middle-aged or older patients and all patients with renal disease or dysfunction prior to anesthesia.

    c. Renal function tests will begin to show abnormalities when renal function is decreased 70–75%; therefore, even mild elevations in renal function tests may actually indicate moderate to severe renal disease.

    d. Serial values may be very informative.

  4. Classification of uremia

    a. Prerenal uremia

      (1) This is caused by factors that decrease renal function by decreasing renal perfusion.

      (2) Cardiac disease, shock, dehydration, and hypoadrenalcorticoidism (Addison disease) are examples of causes of prerenal uremia.

      (3) Patients with prerenal uremia have structurally normal kidneys that are initially capable of normal function.

    b. Primary uremia

      (1) This is caused by primary disease of the kidney.

      (2) Infection, ischemia, toxic agents, renal obstruction, congenital anomalies, and neoplasia can all cause primary uremia.

    c. Postrenal uremia

      (1) This is caused by obstruction or rupture of the ureters, bladder, or urethra.

      (2) The kidneys may or may not have normal function.

  5. Patients with moderate to severe renal dysfunction pose an increased risk in anesthesia.

a. Uremic patients are often debilitated.

b. Uremia increases sensitivity and decreases tolerance to essentially all preanesthetic and anesthetic agents.

c. Uremia can impair the ability of the liver to detoxify drugs.

d. Uremic patients may have additional pathologic conditions, including dehydration, hypovolemia, anemia, metabolic acidosis, and hyperkalemia.

e. Uremic patients may be more susceptible to vagal-induced bradycardia and cardiac arrest.

6. Anesthetic protocol

a. An anticholinergic should be given as a premedication.

b. If preanesthetic sedation is needed, a low dose of a phenothiazine tranquilizer, a benzodiazepine tranquilizer, or a narcotic with or without a tranquilizer can be given.

c. Induction can be accomplished with a mask using a potent inhalant anesthetic with or without nitrous oxide, a neuroleptanalgesic technique, or low dose of thiopental or propofol.

(1) Barbiturates should be used with extreme care because the patient's sensitivity may be increased owing to acid-base imbalance.

(2) Because methoxyflurane may cause renal necrosis, it should be used with caution in the patient with primary renal disease.

d. Maintenance of anesthesia can be accomplished with an inhalant anesthetic with or without nitrous oxide.

e. Ketamine or tiletamine (Telazol) should not be used in cats with primary renal disease.

7. Monitoring and support

a. Regardless of the preanesthetic and anesthetic agents used, adequate renal function cannot always be predicted.

b. Proper monitoring of cardiovascular, pulmonary, CNS, and renal parameters must be done.

c. It is critical to maintain good renal blood flow and minimize hypovolemia, hypotension, and hypoxemia during any anesthesia and surgical procedure.

d. Adequate fluid administration is the *most important* factor in the support of renal function.

(1) In the absence of congestive heart failure, pulmonary edema, or anuria, a balanced electrolyte solution should be adminstered at 10 ml/lb per hour (20 mls/kg per hour) to provide a physiologic duresis.

(2) The rate of fluid administration can be increased or decreased depending on the patient's needs.

(3) If fluids do not initiate or maintain urine output, active diuresis using 10% dextrose, mannitol, or furosemide (Lasix) may be needed.

(4) An intravenous infusion of dopamine (2.5–5 mcg/lb per minute) can be used in an attempt to increase cardiac output and vasodilate the renal arteries, thus increasing renal perfusion. If the heart rate increases, then the amount of dopamine being given should be reduced.

e. Close monitoring of the cardiopulmonary and renal systems must be continued following anesthesia or surgery.

       f. Continued fluid support will be needed in the postanesthetic period.

  E. Cats with urethral obstruction

    1. Cats with urethral obstruction are often dehydrated, hyperkalemic, azotemic, acidotic, hyperphosphatemic, and hypothermic.

    2. Hyperkalemia

      a. Severe hyperkalemia may cause bradycardia leading to cardiac arrest.

      b. Cats that are severally depressed and bradycardic are most likely hyperkalemic.

      c. EKG signs of hyperkalemia include bradycardia, flattening or absence of the P wave, prolongation of the QT interval, and peaking of the T wave.

      d. Severe hyperkalemia can be treated with sodium bicarbonate (0.5–1 mEq/lb) intravenously and 5% dextrose in half-strength saline intravenously. This treatment helps force the potassium into the cells.

    3. Anesthesia for urethral catheterization

      a. If the cat is severely depressed, no anesthesia may be needed.

      b. Preanesthetic sedation is usually not needed.

        (1) If a preanesthetic sedative is needed, then diazepam, midazolam, or a narcotic with or without the diazepam or midazolam can be used.

        (2) Do not use alpha-2 agonists as they can potentiate bradycardia and ventricular dysrhythmias.

      c. If anesthetia is needed, then ketamine, thiopental, or propofol may be given intravenously to effect. Always use the lowest dose possible.

      d. A mask induction using halothane, isoflurane, or sevoflurane with or without nitrous oxide may also be used.

      e. An anticholinergic agent should be given prior to anesthesia to prevent bradycardia.

    4. Anesthesia for perineal urethrostomy

      a. Perineal urethrostomy should not be performed until the urethral obstruction is relieved and the cat has been returned to a normal physiologic state and is stable.

      b. If the cat is stabilized prior to surgery, it does not offer a particular anesthetic challenge, so most preanesthetic and anesthetic agents may be safely used.

      c. If a catheter cannot be passed or a cystocentesis cannot be done, an emergency perineal urethrostomy may be needed.

        (1) This cat will most likely be unstable and have metabolic derangements.

        (2) Preanesthetic considerations and anesthetic induction would be the same as described for urethral catheterization.

        (3) Maintenance of anesthesia can be accomplished with an inhalant agent.

        (4) *Extreme* care must be used as the patient will be more sensitive to preanesthetic and anesthetic agents.

VII. Patients with neurologic dysfunction

  A. The patient with a history of seizures

    1. The use of phenothiazine tranquilizers and ketamine are contraindicated in a patient with seizures.

      a. Phenothiazine tranquilizers lower the seizure threshold and may precipitate a seizure.

      b. Ketamine stimulates the CNS and can cause seizures, especially in the dog.

  2. Diazepam or midazolam, with or without a narcotic, can be used for preanesthetic sedation.

  3. Pentobarbital (1–2 mg/lb) intramuscularly can also be used as a premedicant.

  4. Thiopental, propofol, and the inhalant anesthetic agents can all be used in the patient with a history of seizures.

B. The patient with organic disease of the CNS

  1. These patients may have preexisting CNS depression because of their CNS disease.

  2. They may be more sensitive to the depressant effects of preanesthetic and anesthetic agents.

  3. If preanesthetic sedation is needed, diazepam or midazolam, with or without a narcotic, can be used.

  4. Induction of anesthesia can be accomplished with thiopental or propofol given to effect or by use of an inhalant anesthetic given via mask.

  5. Avoid the use of ketamine or tiletamine (Telazol), as this may precipitate a seizure and may increase intracranial pressure.

  6. Maintenance of anesthesia can be accomplished with inhalant anesthetics.

  7. Close monitoring of cardiopulmonary function is critical. Assisted or controlled ventilation may be needed to support pulmonary function and to decrease intracranial pressure.

C. The patient with head trauma

  1. A patient with head trauma should be thoroughly evaluated and stabilized prior to anesthesia.

  2. These patients may have depressed consciousness, cardiopulmonary depression, or increased intracranial pressure.

  3. Increased intracranial pressure

      a. The increased intracranial pressure should be lowered prior to anesthesia.

      b. Mannitol (0.5–1 gm/lb) intravenously can be given to lower the pressure.

      c. Furosemide and corticosteroids can also be used to reduce cerebral edema and inflammation.

      d. Hyperventilation can be used to decrease intracranial pressure.

        (1) The patient must be intubated.

        (2) Hyperventilation decreases the arterial carbon dioxide levels and thus causes cerebrovascular vasoconstriction.

        (3) The vasoconstriction will reduce cerebral blood flow and thus intracranial pressure.

  4. If the patient is comatose or semicomatose, additional anesthetics may not be needed. Even without additional anesthetics, the patient may need to be intubated and hyperventilated with oxygen to decrease the intracranial pressure.

  5. If the patient needs sedation or anesthesia for a procedure, the following drugs can be used:

      a. An antichoinergic should be given to counteract bradycardia.

    b. Preanesthetic sedation can be accomplished using diazepam or a diazepam-butorphanol combination.

       (1) Diazepam produces minimal cardiopulmonary depression.

       (2) Diazepam is useful in controlling post–head trauma seizures.

       (3) Butorphanol is useful for its analgesic properties and because it has a ceiling effect on ventilatory depression.

    c. Thiopental or propofol given to effect can be used to induce anesthesia or as the primary agent for short procedures. Monitor ventilation closely.

    d. Ketamine and other dissociative agents should probably be avoided.

    e. Anesthesia for long procedures can be maintained with any of the potent inhalant anesthetics.

       (1) Inhalant anesthetics can increase intracranial pressure owing to respiratory depression; therefore, the patient should be hyperventilated to help prevent this.

       (2) Nitrous oxide can be used in combination with any of the other inhalant agents.

  6. Patients with head trauma may be more prone to the cardiopulmonary depressant effects of preanesthetic and anesthetic agents; therefore, cardiopulmonary parameters must be closely and continually monitored.

D. The patient scheduled for a myelogram

  1. The choice of preanesthetic and anesthetic agents for this patient will depend on the physical status of the patient.

  2. The choice of preanesthetic and anesthetic agents is often not as critical as an awareness of the potential complications that a myelogram can cause.

  3. Complications during a myelogram

    a. Patients may develop respiratory depression or arrest during or shortly after the injection of contrast media.

       (1) The depression or arrest may last from a few seconds to 10–15 minutes.

       (2) Controlled ventilation is necessary during this time.

       (3) It is usually not necessary to adjust the inhalant anesthetic concentration as the depression or apnea is due to the contrast media and not the anesthetic.

    b. Patients may also develop cardiovascular depression.

       (1) Severe sinus bradycardia can develop during the injection of contrast media.

       (2) Intravenous atropine should be given to counteract the severe bradycardia.

       (3) In rare instances cardiac arrest may occur, in which case cardiopulmonary resuscitation must be instituted immediately.

    c. Some patients may have an increase in the respiratory rate or heart rate just before the rate decreases. It is imperative that the anesthetist distinguish the cause of this increased rate. It may be too light a plane of anesthesia, or it may be the initial stimulatory effect of the contrast media.

  4. Post-myelogram complications

    a. As the patient awakens from the anesthesia, seizures may be caused by the contrast media.

b. Seizures can be controlled with diazepam or midazolam. Repeated doses may be necessary.

c. If diazepam or midazolam does not control the seizures, pentobarbital or phenobarbital may be needed.

5. Anesthetic protocol

a. Patients should be premedicated with atropine to help counteract the sinus bradycardia that may be caused by the myelogram.

b. A tranquilizer, narcotic, or neuroleptanalgesic can be used for preanesthetic sedation.

(1) The use of phenothiazine tranquilizers is controversial. They probably should be avoided in the patient scheduled for a myelogram. This is especially true if a "high" myelogram (cervical myelogram) is to be done.

(2) A combination of diazepam or midazolam with butorphanol can be used for preanesthetic sedation.

c. Thiopental, propofol, or an inhalant anesthetic via mask can be used for induction.

d. Any of the potent inhalant anesthetic agents can be used for maintenance.

6. Adjunct therapy

a. Corticosteroids can be given to help decrease CNS inflammation from the contrast media.

b. The use of 5% dextrose in lactated Ringer's solution given at a rate of 10 mls/lb per hour may decrease the incidence and severity of postmyelogram seizures caused by metrizamide. These seizures occur because metrizamide interferes with glucose uptake by the CNS.

VIII. Anesthetic management of the cesarean section

A. Anesthetic goals for the cesarean section

1. Deliver viable youngsters with the least amount of depression.

2. Produce the least amount of depression in the mother.

3. Return the mother and youngsters to their own environment as quickly as possible.

B. Physiologic changes during parturition

1. Pulmonary system

a. The mother may have an increased respiratory rate because of pain and discomfort.

b. There is usually a decreased tidal volume owing to anterior displacement of the abdominal viscera by the gravid uterus. This displacement puts pressure on the diaphragm and prevents maximal expansion of the thoracic cavity.

c. Respiratory acidosis may occur as a result of decreased tidal volume.

2. Cardiovascular system

a. Usually heart rate is increased because of pain and catecholamine release.

b. Cardiac output may increase because of the increased heart rate and the increased blood volume that results from uterine contracture and release of blood into the peripheral circulation.

c. The increased cardiac output will increase blood pressure.

d. Venous return to the heart may be decreased when the patient is placed on her back.

        (1) This decreased venous return results from compression of the vena cava by the gravid uterus.

        (2) The decreased venous return will then produce a decreased cardiac output and possible fall in blood pressure.

    e. Usually a delayed capillary refill time and an increased venous distensibility result from hormonal changes at the time of parturition. This condition may cause a delay in the uptake of drugs given intramuscularly or subcutaneously.

  3. Gastrointestinal system

    a. Usually gastric acidity is increased and gastric muscular tone is decreased.

    b. The decreased gastric muscular tone and the physical pressure of the gravid uterus pushing against the other abdominal viscera will delay gastric emptying.

C. General considerations

  1. Twice the blood loss may occur with a cesarean section as with normal parturition resulting in blood volume loss and hypotension.

  2. All preanesthetic and anesthetic agents cross the placenta to some degree and therefore can affect the newborn.

    a. Placental transfer of drugs depends on

        (1) Lipid solubility

        (2) Molecular size

        (3) Degree of protein binding

        (4) Concentration gradient across the membrane

    b. The drugs used in anesthesia tend to be highly lipid-soluble and of small molecular size and therefore readily cross the placenta.

    c. Drugs that are highly protein-bound do not cross the placenta as rapidly.

    d. Neuromuscular blocking agents are about the only drugs that may be used in anesthesia that do not readily cross the placenta. They do not readily cross because of their large molecular size.

  3. Pregnant animals are more prone to vomiting and possible aspiration during and after anesthesia.

    a. This is due to the decreased gastric muscular tone and increased gastric acidity.

    b. The preanesthetic use of metoclopramide (Reglan) and cimetidine (Tagamet) may be indicated.

    c. Metoclopramide

        (1) This is a dopamine antagonist and may sensitize tissues to acetylcholine.

        (2) Its actions can be abolished by anticholinergic drugs.

        (3) Metaclopramide increases gastric motility and emptying without increasing gastric acidity, and it inhibits the chemoreceptor trigger zone.

        (4) The recommended dose is 0.1–.2 mg/lb subcutaneously or intramuscularly.

        (5) Its onset of action is 10–15 minutes after intramuscular injection, with a duration of action of 1–2 hours.

    d. Cimetidine

        (1) This is a histamine H2 receptor antagonist.

(2) It inhibits gastric acid secretion and increases gastric pH.

(3) The recommended dose is 3–5 mg/lb intramuscularly or orally. It should be given intramuscularly in a prospective surgical patient.

(4) Its onset of action is 15–20 minutes after intramuscular injection or 45–60 minutes after oral administration.

(5) Its effects last 2–4 hours.

(6) Cimetidine will prolong the effects of diazepam and lidocaine.

D. Anesthetic techniques for cesarean section

   1. Epidural analgesia

   2. Neuroleptanalgesia and local midline block

   3. General anesthesia

E. Epidural analgesia

   1. This technique involves the injection of a local anesthetic into the epidural space at the lumbosacral junction.

   2. Lidocaine (2%) without epinephrine can be used and will provide analgesia for 1½–2 hours.

   3. Prior to needle placement, the patient should be sedated using a tranquilizer, narcotic, or neuroleptanalgesic.

   4. Needle placement

      a. The skin over the lumbosacral junction must be surgically prepped.

      b. The patient is placed in lateral recumbency or in sternal recumbency with the rear legs extended forward.

      c. The anesthetist palpates the dorsal wings of the ilium, the dorsal process of the seventh lumbar vertebra (L7), and the indentation between L7 and the sacrum.

      d. A spinal needle, bevel facing forward, is inserted directly on and perpendicular to the midline of the patient at the indentation between L7 and the sacrum.

      e. The needle is inserted until it "pops" through the flaval ligament into the epidural space.

      f. The stylet is removed, and the dose of lidocaine is then injected.

   5. Recommended doses of 2% lidocaine without epinephrine

      a. A dose of 1 ml/10 lbs will block approximately to the first lumbar vertebra.

      b. A dose of 1 ml/7.5 lbs will block to approximately the fifth thoracic vertebra.

      c. A block to the first lumbar vertebra is usually adequate for a cesarean section.

      d. The block should take effect within 2–5 minutes and last 1½–2 hours.

      e. The dose of lidocaine may need to be decreased in the obese patient to prevent an excessive dose from being administered.

   6. Advantages of epidural analgesia

      a. It is a relatively inexpensive technique.

      b. It produces minimal depression of the newborn.

      c. Usually depression of the mother is minimal, allowing a rapid return to preanesthetic alertness.

   7. Disadvantages of epidural analgesia

  a. Respiratory depression or arrest can occur if the epidural block advances to the anterior thoracic or cervical area.
  b. Hypotension occurs posterior to the block because of a loss of vascular tone and vasodilation.
  c. Bradycardia can occur with a high block.
  d. Hypothermia can occur as a result of the vascular dilation caused by the lidocaine.
  e. Infection can occur if aseptic technique is not used during needle placement.
  f. Spontaneous movements of the head and front limbs of the mother can occur.
  g. In some patients it is difficult to place the epidural needle.
  h. Cord laceration can occur, especially if the needle is inserted at L5 or above.
  i. If respiratory problems occur, it may not be possible to intubate the mother without the use of a general anesthetic.

F. Neuroleptanalgesics and local midline block
  1. A neuroleptanalgesic is administered to the mother (Table 12–2).
  2. After the neuroleptanalgesic has taken effect, 0.5–1% lidocaine without epinephrine is injected subcutaneously along the incision site.
    a. Dilute 2% lidocaine to 0.5–1% with sterile water or normal saline.
    b. Never exceed a total dose of 5 mg/lb of lidocaine. Doses exceeding this may cause toxicity. Keep the dose of lidocaine in the 2–3 mg/lb range.
    c. Local anesthetic toxicity is characterized by the following:
      (1) Hyperexcitability
      (2) Twitching and spontaneous movements of the extremities
      (3) Cardiovascular depression
      (4) Seizures
      (5) Coma and death
    d. Diazepam or midazolam can be used to control seizures caused by local anesthetic toxicity.
  3. Supplemental oxygen should be provided to the mother by a mask or, if the mother can be intubated, by an endotracheal tube.
    a. This not only benefits the mother but also the youngsters.
    b. Intubation may be facilitated by spraying the vocal folds with 0.5% lidocaine without epinephrine.

Table 12–2. Neuroleptanalgesic Combinations for the Geriatric Dog and Cat

Neuroleptic (Tranquilizer)	Analgesic (Narcotic)
Acetylpromazine 0.05 mg/lb IM or IV, not to exceed a maximum total dose of 1.0 mg	Oxymorphone 0.1 mg/lb IM or IV, not to exceed a maximum total dose of 3 mg
Diazepam 0.1 to 0.2 mg/lb IM or IV, to a maximum total dose of 10 mg	Oxymorphone—same as above
Acetylpromazine—same as above	Meperidine 0.5–2.0 mg/lb IM or IV
Acetylpromazine—same as above	Butorphanol 0.1–0.2 mg/lb IM or IV
Diazepam—same as above	Butorphanol—same as above

  4. Advantages

    a. This can be a fairly inexpensive technique depending on the neuro-leptanalgesic used.

    b. The narcotic can be antagonized in both the mother and newborn.

    c. Less fetal depression may occur than with general anesthetics.

  5. Disadvantages

    a. Narcotics can produce respiratory depression in both the mother and newborn.

    b. The narcotic and tranquilizer will cross the placenta and therefore can affect the fetus.

    c. The neuroleptanalgesic and local anesthetic may not provide adequate sedation and analgesia for the surgery.

G. General anesthesia for cesarean section

  1. Barbiturates

    a. Pentobarbital, a short-acting barbiturate, is not recommended.

    b. An ultra-short-acting barbiturate such as thiopental or methohexital can be used to induce general anesthesia prior to an inhalant anesthetic.

    c. Just enough ultra-short-acting barbiturate is administered to allow for intubation.

    d. An ultra-short-acting barbiturate should not be used as the primary general anesthetic because of the following reasons:

      (1) Fetal depression from the barbiturate can be significant.

      (2) Respiratory depression of the mother may be marked.

      (3) Repeated doses of the barbiturate are usually required to provide adequate anesthesia time. This may cause prolonged anesthetic recovery times in both the mother and the newborn.

  2. Dissociative agents

    a. Ketamine has been the primary dissociative agent used.

    b. Ketamine has been used at a dose of 1–2 mg/lb intravenously to induce general anesthesia prior to an inhalant agent, often in combination with a benzodiazepine tranquilizer.

    c. Spraying the vocal folds with 0.5% lidocaine without epinephrine may facilitate intubation.

    d. Administering ketamine intramuscularly at the higher doses may produce prolonged recoveries of the mother, especially in the cat, and may cause marked depression of the youngsters.

    e. Ketamine may produce seizures in the dog; therefore, it should be used in combination with diazepam.

    f. As with the ultra-short-acting barbiturates, ketamine should be used as an inducing agent and not as a primary agent for cesarean section.

  3. Propofol

    a. Propofol has been used to induce anesthesia prior to administering an inhalant anesthetic.

    b. Propofol has been used for cesarean section surgery.

    c. Fetal depression appears minimal in puppies delivered from mothers anesthetized with propofol because puppies have good conjugation enzyme activity.

    d. Respiratory depression may be significant with propofol.

  4. Inhalant general anesthetics

    a. Any of the potent inhalant anesthetics can be used for cesarean section.

    b. By supplementing with nitrous oxide, the concentration of the potent inhalant can be reduced.

    c. All inhalant anesthetic agents cross the placenta.

    d. A neuroleptanalgesic, ultra-short-acting barbiturate, ketamine, or propofol can be used to induce anesthesia prior to the inhalant agent.

    e. A mask induction using the inhalant agent can also be used.

    f. The lowest concentration needed to perform the cesarean section should be used.

H. Combination of neuroleptanalgesic, local midline block, and inhalant general anesthetic

    1. Nitrous oxide can be used to supplement a neuroleptanalgesic and local midline block.

    2. Low concentrations of halothane, methoxyflurane, isoflurane, or sevoflurane can be used as needed.

    3. The inhalant agent can be administered via mask, but the patient should be intubated if possible.

    4. Advantages

        a. The narcotic can be antagonized in both the mother and youngsters.

        b. Nitrous oxide causes minimal depression of the mother and youngsters.

        c. The neuroleptanalgesic and local midline block will allow one to decrease the amount of potent inhalant anesthetic needed.

I. Adjunct medications

    1. Intravenous fluids should be given to the mother during the cesarean section.

        a. A balanced crystalloid solution should be administered at a rate of 7–10 ml/lb per hour. The rate is adjusted to the patient's needs.

        b. The fluids help counteract the blood loss during the procedure and help maintain cardiovascular volume and stability.

    2. Additional supportive therapy may be needed depending on the specific requirements of the mother.

J. Management of the newborn

    1. The youngsters should be delivered as quickly as possible following the administration of the anesthetic.

    2. Their oral-pharygeal cavities should be cleared of any fluid or secretions.

    3. They should be rubbed vigorously to stimulate breathing and movement.

    4. Supplemental oxygen can be administered via a mask or oxygen chamber.

        a. An anesthetic induction chamber can be lined with towels and a warm-water heating blanket and used as an oxygen chamber.

        b. A 1.5–2.0 mm noncuffed endotracheal tube can be used to intubate youngsters when assisted ventilation is needed.

    5. A narcotic antagonist should be administered to the newborns if a narcotic was used in the anesthetic protocol.

        a. Naloxone is the preferred narcotic antagonist.

      b. Naloxone is readily absorbed from the mucous membranes.

      c. Naloxone is drawn into a tuberculine syringe, and one or two drops are placed under each newborn's tongue.

      d. Naloxone can also be given intramuscularly at a dose of 0.05–.1 ml per puppy or kitten.

      e. Naloxone may be repeated as necessary.

    6. An analeptic such as doxapram (Dopram) can be used to stimulate respiration in newborns.

      a. Doxapram is administered in the same way as naloxone.

      b. The dose of doxapram in the puppy is 1–5 mg and in the kitten 1–2 mg.

      c. If doxapram does not stimulate respiration, intubation should be attempted so that assisted ventilation can be provided.

    7. Atropine may be administered to newborns to counteract bradycardia.

      a. Atropine may be indicated if the newborn's heart rate is less than 80 bpm.

      b. Atropine (0.5 mg/cc) is diluted to 0.25 mg/cc and drawn into a tuberculine syringe.

      c. A dose of 0.02–.025 mg (0.1 cc) is given intramuscularly.

    8. The newborns must be kept warm.

    9. They should be allowed to nurse as soon as the mother has recovered sufficiently from the anesthetic.

IX. Anesthetic considerations in patients with endocrine dysfunction

  A. Diabetes mellitus

    1. Effects of insulin on normal cellular function

      a. Inhibition of glycogenolysis

      b. Inhibition of gluconeogenesis

      c. Inhibition of lipolysis

      d. Stimulation of glucose uptake into cells

      e. Stimulation of potassium transport into cells

      f. Suppression of ketogenesis

    2. Metabolic effects of insulin deficiency

      a. Carbohydrates

        (1) Decreased uptake of glucose, especially in fat and muscle

        (2) Loss of control of hepatic gluconeogenesis

        (3) Hyperglycemia leading to osmotic diuresis

      b. Protein

        (1) Catabolism of muscle for energy

        (2) Inhibition of protein synthesis, resulting in muscle wasting

      c. Fat

        (1) Production of acetylcoenzyme A and ketone bodies for energy

        (2) Inhibition of lipolysis regulation

        (3) Resultant accumulation of ketone bodies with osmotic diuresis and metabolic acidosis

      d. Prolonged hyperglycemia and ketonemia can lead to the following:

        (1) Metabolic acidosis

        (2) Dehydration

        (3) Circulatory collapse

    (4) Renal failure

    (5) Coma and death

3. Diabetes mellitus should be suspected in patients with the following clinical signs:

    a. Recent history of polyuria, polydipsia, weight loss, or rapid onset of cataracts

    b. Presence of dehydration, weakness, collapse, mental dullness, cataracts, hepatomegaly, or muscle wasting

    c. Increased rate and depth of respiration, with a sweet, acetone odor to the breath

4. Diabetes mellitus occurs more frequently in female dogs and male cats.

5. A ketoacidotic crisis may be precipitated by other systemic disorders.

6. Diagnosis of diabetes mellitus

    a. The preceding signs should alert the clinician to the possibility of diabetes mellitus.

    b. The presence of glucose and ketones in the urine is diagnostic.

    c. A resting blood glucose greater than 250 mg/dl with ketonemia is also diagnostic.

    d. Electrolyte and renal function tests may be altered.

    e. Serum alkaline phosphatase may be increased as a result of hepatic fatty infiltration.

7. Anesthetic considerations

    a. The patient with diabetes mellitus should be stabilized and regulated prior to anesthesia.

    b. The anesthetic regimen used in this patient is probably not as critical as is the adjunct support during and after anesthesia and surgery.

    c. The key to the anesthetic management of a diabetic is to use preanesthetic and anesthetic agents that will result in the shortest anesthetic recovery time.

        (1) Drugs that can be antagonized (narcotics) or are readily eliminated from the patient (propofol, inhalant anesthetics) should be considered.

        (2) The goal is to get the patient awake as soon as possible so the patient can resume its normal feeding schedule.

        (3) A satisfactory technique is to use a combination of diazepam-butorphanol or diazepam-oxymorphone as the preanesthetic medication, followed by propofol induction or masked induction using one of the potent, rapid-acting inhalant anesthetic agents (isoflurane or sevoflurane).

        (4) Anesthesia can be maintained for shorter procedures with propofol infusion or an inhalant agent.

        (5) For longer procedures, an inhalant agent should be used.

    d. The procedure should be scheduled early in the morning following the administration of the patient's normal dose of insulin or, if preferred, half the patient's normal dose of insulin.

    e. Preoperative, serial intraoperative, and postoperative blood glucose levels should be determined.

    f. During the procedure, 2.5% or 5% dextrose in a balanced crystalloid solution should be administered to the patient in order to prevent hypoglycemia.

(1) Depending on the blood glucose values, the dextrose drip may need to be continued following the procedure.

(2) A rate of 5–7 ml/lb per hour is usually adequate.

(3) After the patient starts eating, it is probably not necessary to maintain the dextrose drip.

(4) Blood glucose levels should be kept at 200–250 g/dl.

  g. Close monitoring of the patient should be continued after the procedure as the stress of anesthesia and surgery may cause a diabetic to decompensate.

  h. The use of corticosteroids can also cause decompensation in the diabetic and therefore should be used only if absolutely necessary.

B. Hypoadrenocorticism (Addison disease)

  1. As with the diabetic, the patient with hypoadrenocorticism should be stabilized and regulated prior to any anesthesia and surgery.

  2. Hypoadrenocorticism is a deficiency of aldosterone or glucocorticoids resulting from adrenal cortex dysfunction.

  3. Causes of hypoadrenocorticism

    a. Diseases or destruction of adrenal glands

(1) Primary idiopathic hypoadrenocorticism is the most common cause of hypoadrenocorticism in dogs and may be immune-mediated. It is characterized by an acute necrosis of the adrenal cortex.

(2) Systemic mycosis

(3) Metastatic tumors

(4) Hemorrhagic infarction

(5) Amyloidosis of the cortices

(6) Canine distemper

(7) Therapy with O,p'-DDD for hyperadrenocorticism may inadvertently produce a selective deficiency of glucocorticoids owing to destruction of the zona fasciculata.

    b. Decreased corticotropin secretion

(1) Adrenocorticotropic hormone (ACTH) directly controls glucocorticoid secretion and is secreted by the pituitary gland.

(2) Decreased ACTH secretion may develop with diseases or tumors of the pituitary gland or with decreased secretion of corticotropin releasing factor (CRF) owing to hypothalamic lesions.

(3) Prolonged negative feedback from exogenous corticosteroid therapy also results in decreased ACTH secretion and atrophy of the adrenal cortex.

(4) Decreased ACTH secretion usually produces glucocorticoid insufficiency whereas mineralocorticoid secretion often remains normal.

  4. Clinical signs of hypoadrenocorticism

    a. Clinical signs depend on the particular adrenal hormones most affected by the disease.

    b. Aldosterone deficiency

(1) Aldosterone's primary function is to stimulate absorption of sodium in the distal renal tubules and facilitate the excretion of potassium.

(2) Aldosterone deficiency produces hyponatremia and hyperkalemia.

(3) Hyponatremia with concurrent water loss will produce the following:
   (i) Lethargy
   (ii) Nausea
   (iii) Impaired cardiac output
   (iv) Hypovolemia
   (v) Hypotension
   (vi) Impaired renal perfusion

(4) Hyperkalemia will produce the following:
   (i) Muscle weakness
   (ii) Decreased cardiac conduction and excitability
   (iii) Bradycardia

c. Glucocorticoid deficiency
   (1) Cortisol has the following actions:
      (i) Stimulates gluconeogenesis
      (ii) Increases blood glucose
      (iii) Enhances extravascular fluid movement to the intravascular compartment
      (iv) Stabilizes lysosomal membranes
      (v) Counteracts the effects of stress
   (2) Cortisol depletion produces the following:
      (i) Impaired renal excretion of water
      (ii) Impaired energy metabolism
      (iii) Decreased stress tolerance
      (iv) Anorexia
      (v) Vomiting
      (vi) Diarrhea
   (3) Cortisol depletion rarely produces electrolyte imbalances

5. Diagnosis of hypoadrenocorticism
   a. Hypoadrenocorticism should be suspected in any dog with a history of anorexia, vomiting, diarrhea, and lethargy when there are clinical findings of muscle weakness, dehydration, and bradycardia.
   b. Diagnosis is confirmed by electrolyte determinations and cortisol response tests.
      (1) Electrolytes
         (i) Sodium is often less than 135 mEq/L, and potassium may be greater than 5.5 mEq/L.
         (ii) The sodium-to-potassium ratio may be less than 25:1 (normal is 33:1).
      (2) Cortisol tests
         (i) Resting cortisol levels are often less than 10 ng/ml and won't respond to exogenous ACTH stimulation.
         (ii) Plasma cortisol levels are the most accurate method of diagnosing hypoadrenocorticism, but glucocorticoid replacement therapy must be withheld for 2 hours.
   c. Other diagnostic aids

(1) CBC reflects dehydration. Decreased cortisol will cause eosinophilia and lymphocytosis.

(2) BUN may be elevated because of prerenal uremia or renal failure.

(3) EKG may show evidence of hyperkalemia.

6. Anesthetic considerations

a. A patient with hypoadrenocorticism must be stabilized prior to
anesthesia.

b. The treatment objectives are as follows:

(1) Correct the dehydration and treat the hypovolemic shock.

(2) Return renal function to normal.

(3) Correct electrolyte imbalances.

(4) Supply glucocorticoids.

c. The anesthetic regimen used in a patient with hypoadrenocorticism
is probably not as critical as the medical management prior to
anesthesia.

d. Remember that these patients have *decreased stress tolerance.*

e. The key to their anesthetic management is to provide adequate
intravenous fluid volume replacement during and following surgery.

f. In addition, glucocorticoids should be used as part of the anesthetic
regimen.

(1) Preoperatively 1–2 mg/lb of dexamethasone should be given
intravenously or intramuscularly.

(2) Intraoperatively a rapid-acting glucocorticoid such as prednisolone sodium succinate (Solu-Delta-Cortef) 5–10 mg/lb or prednisolone sodium phosphate (Cortisate-20) 5 mg/lb should be
given intravenously and repeated as necessary.

(3) Postoperatively additional glucocorticoids should be given as
needed.

g. The patient with hypoadrenocorticism should be closely monitored
for signs of hypotension and shock.

C. Hypothyroidism

1. A hypothyroid patient often has a decreased metabolic rate.

a. This decreased metabolism can prolong the effects of many preanesthetic and anesthetic agents.

b. Preanesthetic and anesthetic agents should be used in low doses.
They should be agents that require minimal or no metabolism or
that can be readily antagonized.

c. Narcotics, tranquilizers in low doses, propofol, and inhalant agents
are the preferred preanesthetic and anesthetic drugs.

2. A hypothyroid patient is often obese.

a. The obesity may cause ventilatory problems under anesthesia.

b. Assisted or controlled ventilation may be necessary in these patients.

3. A hypothyroid patient may suffer from anemia.

a. The anemia may range from subclinical to severe.

b. If the anemia is severe, whole blood transfusion should be considered prior to anesthesia and surgery.

D. Hyperthyroidism

1. Patients with thyroid adenomas or adenocarcinomas may exhibit evidence of hyperthyroidism.
2. The thyroid tumor may place mechanical pressure on the trachea, causing a partial obstruction and interfering with respiration.
3. The surgical area is highly vascular.
4. Hyperthyroid patients may develop "thyroid storm."
    a. It is precipitated by catecholamine release and excessive thyroid hormone production.
    b. It is characterized by an increased heart rate, increased blood pressure, elevated body temperature, and shock.
5. Hyperthyroid patients often have increased metabolic rates.
    a. Oxygen and glucose demand is increased.
    b. Carbon dioxide production is increased.
6. These patients are more sensitive to hypoxemia.
7. These patients may be more prone to heart failure.
    a. They have an increased heart rate and increased myocardial oxygen consumption.
    b. They are more prone to cardiac dysrhythmias under anesthesia.
    c. They may have cardiomyopathy.
8. Anesthetic considerations
    a. Because of their increased metabolic rate, hyperthyroid patients may rapidly metabolize preanesthetic and anesthetic agents.
    b. Adequate oxygenation must be provided because of the increased oxygen consumption and demands of the patient.
    c. Intubation may be difficult if the tumor is compressing the trachea.
    d. Preanesthetic and anesthetic agents that decrease catecholamine response and myocardial irritability are preferred.
    e. Preanesthetic agents
        (1) A phenothiazine tranquilizer can be used as a preanesthetic in hyperthyroid patients.
        (2) Phenothiazine tranquilizers decrease myocardial irritability.
        (3) They block alpha-adrenergic receptors and thus may help counteract the hypertension.
        (4) A narcotic can be combined with the phenothiazine tranquilizer, because narcotics may slow the heart rate and decrease myocardial oxygen consumption and demand.
    f. Induction can be accomplished with low-dose thiopental, propofol, or an inhalant agent by mask.
    g. Isoflurane is probably the inhalant agent of choice because of its high cardiac index and antidysrhythmic properties.
    h. Ventilation should be assisted or controlled to prevent hypoxemia.
    i. Cardiovascular and respiratory parameters should be monitored closely.
    j. A 5% dextrose drip should be administered to counteract the increased glucose demands.
X. Anesthetic considerations in patients with gastrointestinal dysfunction
    A. The patient with vomiting or diarrhea
        1. The anesthetic regimen used for a patient with vomiting or diarrhea is not as critical as the medical management prior to and during anesthesia.

    2. The anesthetic regimen will depend on the patient's physical status.

    3. Electrolyte imbalances and volume depletion should be corrected prior to anesthesia.

    4. The preanesthetic and postanesthetic use of metoclopramide (Reglan) and cimetadine (Tagamet) may be indicated in vomiting patients.

B. The patient with intestinal obstruction

    1. The anesthetic regimen will be dictated by the patient's physical status.

    2. Adequate fluid and electrolyte therapy should be instituted.

    3. Nitrous oxide should be used with caution.

       a. Nitrous oxide will diffuse into the lumen of the obstructed intestine.

       b. It takes 1–2 hours before any appreciable enlargement of the obstructed intestine occurs from nitrous oxide diffusion.

    4. Patients with proximal intestinal obstruction may have an increased incidence of postsurgical vomiting; therefore, metoclopramide and cimetadine may be indicated preoperatively and postoperatively.

    5. Proper fluid and electrolyte therapy should be continued until the patient can take food orally.

C. The patient with gastric dilation or volvulus

    1. The patient with gastric dilation or volvulus definitely represents an emergency; however, the patient should be stabilized prior to anesthesia and surgery.

    2. Gastric dilation or volvulus can cause the following:

       a. Respiratory depression

       b. Decreased cardiac output

       c. Cardiac dysrhythmias

       d. Hypotension

       e. Hypoxemia

       f. Acid-base imbalance

    3. Prior to anesthesia, the stomach should be decompressed using an orogastric tube or percutaneous needle deflation.

    4. Intravenous fluids should be administered to counteract the decreased cardiac output and hypotension.

    5. The acid-base status of the patient should be determined and treated as needed.

    6. Generally cardiac dysarrhythmias (primarily premature ventricular contractions) occur postoperatively but may occur at any time and should be treated appropriately.

       a. EKG monitoring is essential in dilation-volvulus patients.

       b. Premature ventricular contractions (PVCs) are treated with an intravenous lidocaine bolus of 0.5 – 1 mg/lb followed by infusion of lidocaine at 20 – 30 μg/lb per minute.

       c. The lidocaine infusion is given to effect, increasing or decreasing the dose as needed.

       d. Lidocaine administration should be considered if there are five or more PVCs in a row or ten or more PVCs per minute. Multifocal PVCs *always* indicate the need for treatment.

       e. If the PVCs are refractory to lidocaine, procainamide (3 – 6 mg/lb intramuscularly every 6 – 8 hours) or quinidine (3 – 6 mg/lb orally every 6 hours), or both, may be used in combination with the lidocaine.

f. Refractory dysrhythmias may be caused by electrolyte imbalance, especially potassium and magnesium.

7. If preanesthetic medications are needed in the patient, low-dose acetylpromazine (0.05 mg/lb intramuscularly to a maximum dose of 1 mg) or diazepam (0.1 – .2 mg/lb intramuscularly or intravenously to a maximum dose of 10 mg) may be used in combination with butorphanol (0.1 – .2 mg/lb intramuscularly or intravenously to a maximum dose of 20 mg).

   a. Acetylpromazine and diazepam are antiemetic.

   b. Acetylpromazine may help prevent ventricular dysrhythmias.

8. Induction of anesthesia needs to be rapid so that intubation can be accomplished as quickly as possible.

   a. Following preanesthetic sedation, a low dose of propofol or thiopental may be used to induce anesthesia. Administer just enough so that intubation may be accomplished.

   b. Mask induction using isoflurane has also been used.

9. Anesthesia should be maintained with an inhalant agent.

   a. Isoflurane is the inhalant of choice because of its high cardiac index and antidysrhythmic properties.

   b. The use of nitrous oxide in a patient with gastric dilation-volvulus is controversial.

      (1) Nitrous oxide may cause further distension of the stomach as a result of diffusion into the lumen; however, it will probably take 1–2 hours for a significant problem to occur.

      (2) Nitrous oxide will allow the concentration of the potent inhalant agent to be reduced.

      (3) After the volvulus has been relieved, there should be no problem with adding nitrous oxide to the anesthetic regimen.

      (4) If the patient develops cyanosis, the nitrous oxide should be discontinued.

10. Ventilation should be assisted or controlled to maintain adequate oxygenation.

11. Close monitoring of cardiovascular and respiratory parameters is necessary.

    a. Continuous EKG monitoring is needed to determine if PVCs are occurring.

    b. Blood pressure should be monitored for evidence of hypotension.

    c. If shock develops in the patient, corticosteroids, increased fluid administration, and perhaps colloids are indicated.

    d. Intraoperative PVCs may indicate that treatment with lidocaine is needed.

12. Postoperative care includes intravenous fluid support, maintenance of acid-base balance, and continuous EKG monitoring for the presence of PVCs or other cardiac dysrhythmias.

13. Anesthetic management of the patient with gastric dilation-volvulus includes the following:

    a. Decompress the stomach, and stabilize the patient prior to anesthesia.

    b. Maintain adequate fluid volume replacement.

    c. Use drugs that are sparing of the cardiopulmonary system.

    d. Watch for and treat ventricular dysrhythmias.

XI. Traumatized patients
  A. Prior to anesthesia, the traumatized patient should be thoroughly examined and evaluated and vital signs stabilized.
    1. Intravenous fluid replacement and shock therapy should be instituted as needed.
    2. Any obvious external hemorrhage should be controlled.
    3. Supplemental oxygen therapy should be provided if indicated.
  B. After the patient is stable, thoracic radiographs should be taken to determine if there has been thoracic injury.
    1. Approximately one third of the patients with blunt forelimb or hindlimb trauma have thoracic injury.
    2. The thoracic injuries may be mild to severe and can include the following:
      a. Pulmonary contusions
      b. Emphysematous bulla
      c. Hydrothorax
      d. Pneumothorax
      e. Diaphragmatic hernia
      f. Fractured ribs
    3. If possible, surgery should be postponed on patients with moderate to severe thoracic trauma.
      a. This will allow time for the injuries to subside.
      b. If there is moderate or severe hydrothorax or pneumothorax, thoracentesis or a chest tube may be needed.
    4. The heart needs to be closely monitored for dysrhythmias.
      a. Myocardial contusions may cause ventricular dysrhythmias.
      b. The dysrhythmias will usually occur 12 – 72 hours after trauma.
      c. An EKG should be performed for any patient with an irregular pulse or pulse deficits.
      d. The most common dysrhythmia is PVC.
      e. The PVCs may indicate a need for treatment, depending on their severity and frequency.
  C. The anesthetic regimen for a traumatized patient will depend on the following:
    1. Physical status of patient.
    2. Type of procedure or surgery to be performed.
    3. Length of surgical procedure.
  D. Specific anesthetic considerations will depend on the particular organ system that has been traumatized. (Refer to the various sections in this chapter regarding considerations for the specific organ systems.)
XII. Miscellaneous conditions or problems
  A. Brachycephalic breeds
    1. Brachycephalic breeds represent anesthetic challenges because of their airway problems.
    2. Brachycephalic breeds that can experience airway problems include the English bulldog, Pug, Boston terrier, Pekingese, French bulldog, and Persian cat. Two other breeds with brachycaphalic characteristics are the Shar pei and Chow Chow.
    3. The airway problems most often encountered include the following.
      a. Stenotic nares

      b. Elongated soft palate

      c. Eversion of the lateral saccules

      d. Hypoplastic trachea

  4. The preceding problems may be further exacerbated by preanesthetic and anesthetic agents that lead to a further compromise of ventilation.

  5. Anesthetic management of these patients includes the following:

      a. Use preanesthetic medications that cause minimal respiratory depression.

      b. Preoxygenate the patient prior to anesthetic induction.

      c. Induce anesthesia rapidly so that intubation can be accomplished quickly.

      d. Assist or control ventilation during anesthesia.

      e. Use anesthetic agents that will allow for a quick recovery.

      f. Maintain postanesthesia intubation as long as is feasible.

  6. Low-dose acetylpromazine or diazepam in combination with butorphanol will usually cause only minimal respiratory depression in the preanesthetic period.

  7. Propofol, thiopental, or intravenous ketamine can be used for anesthetic induction.

  8. Any of the potent inhalant anesthetics, with or without nitrous oxide, can be used for anesthetic maintenance, as recovery from their effects is rapid. Isoflurane or sevoflurane are probably preferred because they are associated with the most rapid recovery.

  9. During recovery, someone should be with the patient at all times until the patient has been extubated and is ventilating adequately.

      a. Have supplemental oxygen available in the recovery area.

      b. Leave the endotracheal tube in as long as possible.

      c. Be prepared to reintubate the patient if necessary.

      d. Place the patient on its sternum to make ventilation easier.

      e. If dyspnea develops after extubation, pulling the patient's tongue forward will move the epiglottis forward and may help alleviate the dyspnea.

  10. Brachycephalic breeds seem more prone to regurgitation during induction and recovery from anesthesia.

B. Sight hounds and thin dogs

  1. Sight hounds—Greyhounds, Whippets, Russian wolfhounds (Borzois)—appear to be more sensitive to tranquilizers, sedatives, and barbiturates.

  2. Part of the problem may be that these breeds, as well as any thin dog, do not have significant body fat.

      a. Consequently, the recovery from the effects of drugs that depend on redistribution to body fat will be prolonged.

      b. Thiopental, ketamine, possibly the phenothiazine tranquilizers, and perhaps other drugs depend on redistribution to body fat; therefore, their effects may be prolonged in sight hounds and thin dogs.

  3. In addition, the sight hound's hepatic enzyme system may not be as efficient in detoxifying some of the preanesthetic and anesthetic agents.

  4. In the sight hounds, preanesthetic CNS depressants should be limited to benzodiazepine tranquilizers and narcotic analgesics. If acetylpro-

mazine is used, it should be used in low doses (0.05 mg/lb to a maximum total dose of 1.0 mg/lb).

5. Ultra-short-acting barbiturates can be used for induction.

   a. Methohexital (Brevital) is preferred because recovery from its effects does not depend on redistribution to body fat.

   b. If thiopental (Pentothal) is used, only minimal doses should be administered because recovery from its effects depends on redistribution to body fat.

6. Intravenous ketamine in combination with diazepam has also been used.

7. Propofol may be the injectable anesthetic of choice because of its rapid elimination via hepatic and extrahepatic routes.

8. Any of the inhalant anesthetics can be used in sight hounds or thin patients. Isoflurane or sevoflurane can be used for masked induction and maintenance of anesthesia.

9. Greyhounds may be more prone to malignant hyperthermia than other breeds.

C. Obese patients

1. Two factors should be considered in the obese patient: the percentage of body fat and the condition of the respiratory system.

   a. Percentage of body fat

      (1) Fat makes up a higher percentage of total body mass in the obese patient.

      (2) Fat has a correspondingly lower blood supply than other body-tissue systems.

      (3) Therefore, normally used doses of preanesthetic and injectable anesthetic agents may produce a relative overdose of drug in the highly vascular organs (CNS, heart, lungs, liver, kidneys, etc.). An overdose may occur because although an increased percentage of the body mass is fat, the fat receives a relatively small percentage of the cardiac output.

      (4) It may be advisable to decrease the dose of preanesthetic and injectable anesthetic agents in obese patients to prevent their relative overdose.

   b. Respiratory system

      (1) Obese patients may have difficulty ventilating adequately, especially when sedated or anesthetized.

      (2) The excess abdominal, thoracic, and subcutaneous fat interferes with the ability of the patient to properly expand the thoracic cavity.

      (3) Awake obese patients often have very rapid respiratory rates with a markedly decreased tidal volume and thus a greatly decreased minute ventilation.

      (4) Sedation and anesthesia can greatly compromise an obese patient's already impaired ventilatory capacity.

      (5) In addition, some of the smaller breeds are more prone to tracheal collapse as they become obese.

      (6) Therefore, it is often necessary to provide supplemental oxygen during sedation and assisted or controlled ventilation during anesthesia in the obese patient.

Suggested Readings

Bednarski RM: Anesthetic concerns for patients with cardiomyopathy. Vet Clin North Am Small Anim Pract 22(2):460–464, 1992.

Berry FA: Neonatal anesthesia. In Barash, PG, Cullen BF, Stoelting RK (eds): Clinical Anesthesia. Philadelphia: JB Lippincott, 1989, pp. 1253–1280.

Estabrook SG, Levine EG, Bernstein LH: Gastrointestinal crises in intensive care. Anesthesiol Clin North Am 9:367–391, 1991.

Garvey MS: Fluid and electrolyte balance in critical patients. In Kirby R, Stamp GL (eds): Veterinary Clinics: Critical Care. Philadelphia: WB Saunders, 1989, pp. 1021–1058.

Giesecke AH Jr: Anesthesia for trauma surgery. In Miller RD (ed): Anesthesia. New York: Churchill Livingstone, 1981, pp. 1247–1264.

Gilroy BA: Neuroanesthesiology. In Slatter D (ed): Textbook of Small Animal Surgery. Philadelphia: WB Saunders, 1985.

Grandy JL, Dunlop CI: Anesthesia of pups and kittens. J Am Vet Med Assoc 198:1244–1249, 1991.

Green SA, Harvey RC, Paddleford RR, Sims MH: Anesthesia for selected diseases. In Thurmon JC, Tranquilli WJ, Benson GJ (eds): Veterinary Anesthesia. Baltimore: Williams & Wilkins, 1996, pp. 766–811.

Hackner SG: Emergency management of traumatic pulmonary contusions. Compend Cont Educ 17(5):677–686, 1995.

Haskins SC: Management of septic shock. J Am Vet Med Assoc 200(12): 1915–1924, 1992.

Hellyer PW: Anesthesia for cesarian section. Anesthetic considerations for surgery. In Slatter D (ed): Textbook of Small Animal Surgery, 2nd ed. Philadelphia: WB Saunders, 1991, pp. 2300–2303.

Kovacic J: Management of life-threatening trauma. Vet Clin North Am Small Anim Pract Emerg Med 24(6):1057–1094, 1994.

Ludders JW: Anesthesia for ophthalmic surgery. Anesthetic considerations for surgery. In Slatter D (ed): Slatter's Textbook of Small Animal Surgery, 2nd ed. Philadelphia: WB Saunders, 1991, pp. 2276–2278.

Martin DD: Trauma patients. In Thurmon JC, Tranquilli WJ, Benson JG (eds): Veterinary Anesthesia. Baltimore: Williams & Wilkins, 1996, pp. 829–843.

McLeskey CH: Anesthesia for the geriatric patient. In Barash PG, Cullen BF, Stoelting RK (eds): Clinical Anesthesia. Philadelphia: JB Lippincott, 1989, pp. 1301–1337.

Olivier NB: Pathophysiology of cardiac failure. In Slatter D (ed): Textbook of Small Animal Surgery, 2nd ed. Philadelphia: WB Saunders, 1993, pp. 709–723.

Osborn I: Choice of neuroanesthetic technique. Anesthesiology Clin North Am 5:531–540, 1987.

Paddleford RR: Anesthesia for cesarean section in the dog. Opinions in small animal anesthesia. In Haskins SC, Klide AM (eds): Veterinary Clinics: Small Animal Practice Series, Philadelphia: WB Saunders, 1992, pp. 481–484.

Paddleford RR: Anesthesia. In Goldston RT, Hoskins JD (eds): Geriatrics and Gerontology of the Dog and Cat. Philadelphia: WB Saunders, 1995, pp. 363–378.

Peterson ME: Pathophysiological changes in the endocrine system. In Short CE (ed): Principles and Practice of Veterinary Anesthesia. Baltimore: Williams & Wilkins, 1987, pp. 251–260.

Quandt JF, Raffe MR: Anesthesia for upper airway and thoracic surgery. In Slatter D (ed): Textbook of Small Animal Surgery, 2nd ed. Philadelphia: WB Saunders, 1993, pp. 2278–2283

Raffe M: Anesthetic management of the unstable trauma patient. Proceedings of 4th International Veterinary Emergency and Critical Care Symposium, San Antonio, Texas, 1994, pp. 281–287.

Robinson EP: Anesthesia of pediatric patients. Compend Cont Educ Pract Vet 5:1004, 1983.

Schatzmann URS: Clinical considerations of complications of the pulmonary system. In Short CE (ed): Principles and Practice of Veterinary Anesthesia. Baltimore: Williams & Wilkins, 1987, pp. 208–221.

Stoelting RK: Pharmacology and Physiology in Anesthetic Practice. Philadelphia: JB Lippincott, 1987.

Tranquilli WJ: Anesthesia for cesarean section in the cat. Opinions in small animal anesthesia. In Haskins SC, Klide AM (eds): Veterinary Clinics: Small Animal Practice Series. Philadelphia: WB Saunders, 1992, pp. 484–486.

Trim CM: Anesthesia and the liver. In Slatter DH (ed): Textbook of Small Animal Surgery. Philadelphia: WB Saunders, 1985.

Trim CM: Anesthesia and the endocrine system. In Slatter D (ed): Textbook of Small Animal Surgery, 2nd ed. Philadelphia: WB Saunders, 1993, pp. 2290–2294.

Tuker A: Pathophysiology of the respiratory system. In Slatter D (ed): Textbook of Small Animal Surgery, 2nd ed. Philadelphia: WB Saunders, 1993, pp. 709–723.

VanPoznak A: Special consideration for veterinary neuroanesthesia. In Short CE (ed): Principles and Practice of Veterinary Anesthesia. Baltimore: Williams & Wilkins, 1987.

Chapter 13

Anesthesia for Small to Medium Sized Exotic Mammals, Birds, and Reptiles

Charles J. Sedgwick

Many zoologic veterinarians would agree that more than 95% of the general anesthetics given in large North American zoos serve subjects, of less than 350 kg body size, well. Animal subjects addressed in this chapter include mammals, birds, and reptiles weighing from 0.02 kg (20 g) to 350 kg in body size. The machine in Figure 13–1 can maintain general inhalant anesthesia for animals weighing from a few grams to 500 kg with assisted ventilation. The specific requirements for various exotic animals, however, challenge the most resourceful and innovative of technologists. We can never be finished accumulating, modifying, and adapting the instruments and machines for anesthesia to service diverse zoologic species.

Metric notation is best for *all* calculations, because it gives a better perspective of the continuity of the range of body sizes encountered in zoologic anesthesiology and makes it clearer how *body size* and *metabolic size* affect dosage and dose rate. That is, metric notation facilitates treatment extrapolations from one subject to the next, from the very small to the very large animals. Some guidelines follow:

1. Express all body sizes in kilograms (kg).
2. Avoid wasting time struggling with mixed metric and avoirdupois conversions when faced with demands for precision and speed.
3. Anesthesias described herein employ potent injectable and inhalant chemical agents that profoundly alter consciousness and physiologic function. Anesthetics potentially impose profound alteration to essential cardiopulmonary homeostasis.
4. *Etorphine* and *carfentanil*, two extremely potent opioid anesthetics used in veterinary anesthesia for the very large zoologic species and for immobilization of adult wild horses, will not be addressed in this chapter because those most potent opioids require highly regulated care. (See pages 354 and 355.)

CAUTIONARY NOTE

Direct human contact with alpha$_2$-adrenergic agonists (xylazine, medetomidine, detomidine) and dissociative anesthetics, the arylcycloalkylamines (ketamine, tiletamine, phencyclidine) mentioned in this discussion, should be avoided, especially by technicians who have heart, lung, or neurologic disease. Skin and mucous membrane contact is not always easily avoided when syringe darts are shot from blow pipes or guns or when drugs are accidentally spilled or splashed. Use rubber gloves to assemble and load dart syringes, use great caution pressurizing dart syringes, and be prepared to flush any splashed drug from the skin or mucous membranes using running water.

Anesthesiology should be logical as well as practical, regardless of the type of

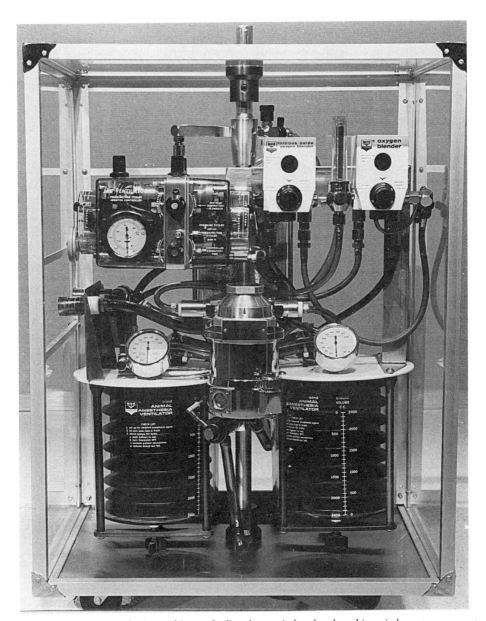

Figure 13–1. This anesthesia machine embodies the semi-closed, rebreathing circle system concept employed by most contemporary medical and veterinary systems. Instead of exchanging breaths with a rebreathing bag, the patient exchanges breaths with bellows. The inherent compliance resistance of the bellows is overcome and balanced precisely by a technician against any ventilatory compliance needs of the subject. Thus, the patient is servomechanized, i.e., "servoed." A pressure limited respirator (Bird Ventilator) having the capability to perform continuous positive airway pressure (CPAP) lung ventilation as well as intermittent demand ventilation (IDV) or intermittent mandatory ventilation (IMV) is used. The respirator is set up at a nominal 4 cm of water CPAP and 24 cm of water IDV (sigh). With this setting, any animal (amphibian, reptile, bird, or mammal), from those weighing a few grams to those weighing 500 kilograms, can be carried for indeterminate periods of stimulus-responsive general anesthesia.

Specifications

Tidal volumes (ml)	to	4800
Minute volumes	to	48,000

patient to be anesthetized. It is the goal of this chapter on exotic animal anesthesia to show logic and mathematical continuity in the principles and methods suggested and to assist those who must medically handle diverse types of wild animals, many of which cannot be handled without prior chemical restraint or anesthesia. Zoologic species (wildlife) should not be considered physiologically unique as compared against domesticated animals or even human beings. Wild animals are, after all, the major constituency of the physiologic continuum that includes domestic animals and mankind. Consider the anesthetic chemicals used herein in terms of their physiologic effects and not merely as ingredients for a cookbook approach, that is, "doses to knock down wild animals."

The use of wildlife *anesthesia and chemical immobilization methods* for various zoologic species tends to be highly speculative among the zoo and field veterinarians who routinely employ them. They are not decisively standardized by any one discipline of practitioners, institutions, or venues.

I. *Veterinary injectable anesthetic methods are known by various expressions.*

    A. Chemical immobilization

    B. Chemical knock-down or take-down

    C. Chemical restraint or remote immobilization

    D. Intramuscular or injectable anesthesia

II. The groups of wild animals for which anesthesia is applied in various zoologic veterinary fields are diverse and should be viewed from several aspects that influence anesthetic pharmacokinetics.

    A. *Body size*

        One of the factors that determines rates of anesthetic uptake, distribution, and elimination—that is, pharmacokinetics—is *body size* (kg).

        1. Body size diversity. *Zoologic veterinarians anesthetize animals of great diversity* in size:

            a. In 20 g deer mouse, uptake, distribution, and elimination of anesthetic are very rapid, with a nominal circulation time of but a few seconds (see Table 13–3).

            b. In a 5000 kg elephant, uptake, distribution, and elimination are relatively slow, lasting several minutes (see Table 13–3).

            c. Birds ranging in size from 0.004 kg (4 g) for a hummingbird to 150 kg for an ostrich have been anesthetized.

            d. Reptiles ranging in size from 0.004 kg for a lizard to 300 kg for a tortoise have been anesthetized.

    B. *Surface-area-to-mass ratios* (consideration of diversity of morphology). Like body size, surface-area-to-mass ratios influence the pharmacokinetics of anesthetics. Examples of vast diversity in *body surface area to mass* (see Table 13–2) ratios influenced by morphology include the following:

        1. Multi-appendaged arthropods (see Fig. 13–18), legless animals (see Fig. 13–8), both cold-blooded (see Fig. 13–7) and warm-blooded quadrupeds

        2. Animals with winglike appendages, which have *increased* ratios

        3. Marine animals with "torpedo-shaped" bodies, which have *decreased* ratios compared with most domesticated animals

    C. *There are five discrete energy taxa in nature* (Table 13–1).

        The five energy groups (taxa) in biology position themselves (metabolically) on straight logarithmic regression lines, with slopes of approximately 0.75. These taxa represent individuals with discrete species-specific core body temperatures, that is, optimal core body temperature set points that influence anesthetic pharmacokinetics (see suggested readings at end of chapter).

Table 13–1. Scaling Dosages Using Metabolic Energy Equations

Energy Taxa	Energy Constants (K)	Core Body Temperature Set Points
Passerine birds	129	42°C
Nonpasserine birds	78	40°C
Placental mammals	70	37°C
Marsupial mammals	49	36°C
Reptiles (at optimal body temperature)	10	37°C

K is the minimum energy cost (MEC) *or* specific minimum energy cost (SMEC) of a 1 kg
individual of each energy taxon.

Metabolic energy equations as the modality for calculating MEC and SMEC used in extrapolating
treatment regimens:

$$MEC = K(W_{kg}^{0.75})$$
$$SMEC = [K(W_{kg}^{0.75})] \div W_{kg}$$
$$= K(W_{kg}^{-0.25})$$

Using the metabolic energy equation as the allometric scaling modality: An empirical ketamine dose
rate for a 20 g white-footed mouse ($W_{kg} = 0.020$) was found to be 1.5 mg ($1.5 \div 0.020 = 76$
mg/kg). Based on the mouse's empirical data, what follows is an allometrically extrapolated
ketamine dose rate for another rodent, a large 50 kg capybara:

$$Mouse\ SMEC = 70(0.02_{kg}^{-0.25})$$
$$= 186$$
$$SMEC\ Dose = 75 \div 186$$
$$= 0.4$$
$$Capybara\ SMEC = 70\ (50_{kg}^{-0.25})$$
$$= 26.3$$
$$26.3 \times 0.4 = 10.5\ mg/kg$$
$$= 526\ mg$$

Table 13–2. Body Surface Area

Body surface area (Meeh's constants and formulas) as the modality for extrapolating treatment
regimens:

$$\text{Body surface area in square meters (m}^2) = [K(W_g^{0.66})] \div 10^4$$
$$= [K(W_{kg}^{0.66})] \div 10^2$$

Surface area constants (K)

Bat	57.5	Man	10
Cat	10	Mouse	11
Cattle	10	Opossum	11.3
Dog	10	Rabbit	10
Elephant	10	Sheep	10
Goat	10	Shrew	7
Guinea pig	10	Swine	10
Horse	10	Whale (fin)	8.3
Lion	12.3		

Using body surface area (body surface area in squared meters) as the allometric scaling modality
for dosage and dose rate treatment extrapolations:

Medetomidine hydrochloride (Domitor), an alpha$_2$-adrenergic agonist, has the dose rate of *1000
mcg per m²*.

Example: You wish to treat a 1.5 kg kit fox and a 125 kg bear with medetomidine. Compare the
dose rates, mcg/kg for the two zoo animals thus:

Body surface area for a 1.5 kg fox:
$$[10(1.5^{0.66})] \div 10^2 = 0.13\ m^2$$
$$0.13\ m^2 \times 1000\ mcg\ medetomidine = 130\ mcg \div 1.5\ kg$$
$$= 86\ mcg/kg$$

Body surface area for a 125 kg bear:
$$[10(100^{0.66})] \div 10^2 = 2.42\ m^2$$
$$2.42\ m^2 \times 1000\ mcg\ medetomidine = 2420\ mcg \div 100\ kg$$
$$= 24.2\ mcg/kg.$$

Notice that the *dose rate* of medetomidine for the very small fox is more than three times that
for the larger bear. This example illustrates the essence of the allometric principle.

III. Professional experience and expertise in wildlife anesthesia technology are highly individualized among practitioners and for the many categories of veterinary species. But principles of anesthesia technology vary little. Before anesthetizing any animal, a profile of physiologic variables useful for monitoring anesthesia may be estimated as demonstrated in Table 13–3.

A. *Birds* (Tables 13–4 and 13–5)

1. Currently veterinarians can successfully perform *long-term* inhalation anesthesia for birds with the inhalant anesthetic isoflurane, using anesthesia machines with the ability to support avian ventilation (see Fig. 13–17).

2. Avian respiration is physiologically served through their unidirectional-flow air sacs and parabronchial lungs instead of the less efficient to-and-fro-flow alveolar lungs of mammals and other animals.

3. Many species of injured, free-ranging birds are treated by veterinarians working in wildlife rehabilitation.

   a. Birds with fractured bones may require isoflurane anesthesia and support from an anesthesia-ventilator in order to tolerate surgeries lasting hours.

   b. It is now routine to hold wild birds under general anesthesia for hours in varying planes of anesthesia. Previously, injectable anes-

---

Table 13–3. Scaling Biologic Values and Metabolic and Anatomic Sizes

Formulas:

a. Energy groups	K
Passerines	129
Nonpasserines	78
Placental mammals	70
Marsupials	49
Reptiles (37°C)	10

b. $MEC = K(W_{kg}^{0.75})$
d. *Tidal volume* (V_T)
   Birds 13.2 $(W_{kg}^{1.08})$
   Mammals 6.2 $(W_{kg}^{1.01})$
g. *Minute vol* (V_T, V_D)
   $V_T \times RR$
   $V_D \times RR$

c. $SMEC = K(W_{kg}^{-0.25})$
e. *Anatomic dead space* (V_D)
   Mammals 2.2 $(W_{kg}^{1.01})$
f. *Respiratory rate (RR)*
   Birds 17.2 $(W_{kg}^{-0.31})$
   Mammals 53.5 $(W_{kg}^{-0.26})$

h. *Oxygen consumption* (V_{oxygen}): passerine birds = 18 $(W_{kg}^{0.75})$; nonpasserine birds = 11 $(W_{kg}^{0.75})$; placental mammals = 10 $(W_{kg}^{0.75})$; marsupial mammals = 7 $(W_{kg}^{0.75})$; reptiles and amphibians (37°C) = 1.4 $(W_{kg}^{0.75})$

i. *Blood volume*
   Mammals 65 $(W_{kg}^{1.02})$
l. *Heart size*
   Birds 8.2 $(W_{kg}^{0.91})$
   Mammals 5.8 $(W_{kg}^{0.99})$

j. *Heartbeat frequency (hbf)*
   Birds 155.8 $(W_{kg}^{-0.23})$
   Mammals 241 $(W_{kg}^{-0.25})$
   Marsupials 106 $(W_{kg}^{-0.27})$
   Reptiles 33.4 $(W_{kg}^{-0.25})$

k. *Cardiac output (Q)*
   Mammals 187 $(W_{kg}^{0.81})$
m. $t_{circ} = 17.4 (W_{kg}^{0.25})$
n. $t_{500\ hb} = 500/hbf$

Example species	Koala	Squirrel	Wolf
Weight (kg)	4	0.1	50.0
a. Energy (K) group	49	70	70
b. Minimum energy cost (MEC)	139	12	1316
c. Specific minimum energy cost (SMEC)	35	124	26
d. Tidal volume (ml)	25	0.6	298
e. Anatomic dead-space volume (ml)	9	0.2	91
f. Respiratory rate (R/min)	28	97	20
g. Minute volume (ml/min)	364	58	5140
h. Oxygen consumption (ml/min)	16	1.7	159
i. Blood volume (ml)	199	6.2	2799
j. Heartbeat frequency (bpm)	128	429	96
k. Cardiac output (ml/min)	319	29	3711
l. Heart size (g)	12	0.6	223
m. t_{circ} (seconds)	16	10	44
n. $t_{500\ heartbeats}$ (minutes)	4	1	5

Source: WA Calder: Size, Function, and Life History (Cambridge, MA: Harvard University Press, 1984); FR Hainsworth: Animal Physiology: Adaptations in Function (Reading, PA: Addison-Wesley, 1981); RH Peters: The Ecological Implications of Body Size (New York: Cambridge University Press, 1983); K Schmidt-Nielsen: Scaling: Why Is Animal Size So Important (New York: Cambridge University Press, 1984).

Table 13–4. Ketamine (Ketaset)

Ketamine (Ketaset) is an arylcycloalkylamine dissociative anesthetic. It has a wide range of safe dosages but may not be suitable for certain investigations involving long-term brain wave pattern studies. Renarcotization may occur but is not a clinical problem except in animals that may climb and then fall. Ketamine is available for veterinary use as a 10% solution (100 mg/ml). A 10% ketamine concentration can be inconvenient for administration to small subjects because of the required minuscule volume. Make a tenfold dilution by adding one part ketamine to nine parts water, thus moving the decimal point one place to the right and converting the 10% to a 1% solution (10 mg/ml instead of 100 mg/ml).

Directions

1. Make a best estimate of subject weight (kg). If possible, weigh the subject with a scale.
2. Based on the subject's health assessment and considerations for handler safety, decide whether a low, medium, or high dosage (in milliliters) is indicated. In the table below, dosages are given in the three bold-type columns for animals weighing 0.02–350 kg. If a subject's weight does not fit a table category precisely, make an extrapolation. If a low dosage does not provide for suitable handler safety or adequate chemical immobilization of a subject, and it is not feasible to use a face mask to administer isoflurane or inject a second "low" dosage (ml), an additional *low* dosage may be added.
3. Wherever possible, augment injectable anesthetics with isoflurane given by face mask.
4. For prolonged procedures, endotracheally intubate the subject, use isoflurane to increase depth of anesthesia, and support ventilation with effective mechanical ventilation.

Weight (kg)	Dosage (ml)			Dosage (mg)			Dose Rate (mg/kg)		
	Low	*Med*	*High*	*Low*	*Med*	*High*	*Low*	*Med*	*High*
0.02	0.0074	0.015	0.022	0.74	1.5	2.2	37	75	110
0.25	0.045	0.1	0.15	4.5	10	15	18	40	60
0.5	0.08	0.17	0.25	8	17	25	16	34	50
1.5	0.19	0.38	0.57	19	38	57	12.6	25	38
4	0.4	0.8	1.2	40	80	119	10	20	30
12	0.9	1.80	2.7	90	180	270	7.5	15	22.5
25	1.6	3.13	4.7	156	313	470	6.25	12.5	19
50	2.63	5.26	7.9	263	526	790	5.26	10.5	16
125	5.23	10.5	15.7	523	1046	1570	4.2	8.4	12.5
250	8.8	17.6	26.4	880	1760	2641	3.5	7	10.5
350	11.3	22.65	34	1133	2265	3399	3.2	6.4	9.7

thetics and ventilatory machine support were such that surgery for birds was limited to relatively short procedures, subjecting them to high mortality rates.

B. *Reptiles* (see Table 13–4)
   1. Handling reptiles (ectotherms) poses challenges.
      a. Many reptiles are quick, powerful, aggressive, and able to focus on handlers as potential adversaries.
      b. They are strong, have sharp claws and teeth, and can inflict injury on handlers (see Fig. 13–7).
      c. Some are venomous (see Fig. 13–8).
      d. Many are delicate and vulnerable to the injurious effects of improper anesthesia.
   2. Working with reptiles requires a special interest in reptilian physiology and biology
      a. Interest and training, plus the ability to provide isoflurane anesthesia and ventilatory support for diverse reptile species, are now the practice standard.
      b. Reptiles are animals with reticulated, saclike lungs that are amenable to isoflurane anesthesia and mechanically assisted ventilation.
C. *Very small mammals* (see Tables 13–4 and 13–5)
   1. Laboratory mammals, the "pocket pets," may be successfully intubated

Table 13–5. Ket-xyl: Ketamine (Ketaset) 10% Plus Xylazine (Rompun)
2% or 10%

Combination injectable (intramuscular) anesthetic. Ketamine (Ketaset) and xylazine (Rompun) can be mixed using either of two concentrations available for xylazine, 2% (20 mg/ml) or 10% (100 mg/ml) solutions. Using xylazine (2%), *#1,* ketamine and xylazine are *mixed in equal parts* (V:V 1:1). Using xylazine (10%), *#2,* ketamine and xylazine are *mixed five parts ketamine to one part xylazine* (V:V 5:1). Reverse xylazine with yohimbine or atipamezole (Table 13–10). When very minute volume dosages are indicated, make tenfold dilutions (one part ket-xyl, nine parts water) to move the decimal points one place to the right, thus making syringe measurement more precise.

Directions

1. Weigh, or make a best estimate of weight, for an anesthesia subject and express that weight in kilograms (kg).
2. Based on a health assessment, select a dosage (ml) from column #1 or #2 (if the patient is not healthy, consider using *only* ketamine and go to Table 13–3 for dosages). If dosage volumes are impracticably too minute, make a tenfold dilution of either mixture #1 or #2 by taking one part of a #1 or #2 mixture and diluting it with nine parts of water, thus moving the decimal point one place to the right and providing a practical volume to measure out and inject.
3. In large animals, if projected dosage volumes become impracticably too large (even using 10% xylazine in the #2 column), consider using a mixture of ketamine plus medetomidine or tiletamine-zolazepam (Telazol) plus medetomidine (Table 13–5).
4. Use isoflurane via mask or endotracheal tube to augment or prolong general anesthesia, and be prepared to provide ventilatory support through an endotracheal tube.

Weight (kg)	Dosage Volumes (ml)		Dosage (mg)		Dose Rate (mg/kg)	
	#1	*#2*	*Ketamine*	*Xylazine*	*Ketamine*	*Xylazine*
0.1	0.05	0.03	2.5	0.5	25	5
0.25	0.1	0.06	5	1	20	4
0.5	0.2	0.12	10	2	20	4
1.5	0.5	0.3	25	5	16.5	3
4	1	0.6	50	10	12.5	2.5
12	2	1.2	100	20	8	1.5
25	3.5	2.1	175	35	7	1.4
50	6	3.6	300	60	6	1.2
125	13.5	7.1	675	135	5	1.1
250	20	12	1000	200	4	0.8
350	25	15	1250	250	3.6	0.7

for inhalation anesthesia with isoflurane and supported with mechanical ventilation (see Figs. 13–4, 13–5, 13–6, and Table 13–3).

2. Small mammals include the following:

   a. The rodents (see Figs. 13–5 and 13–6), lagomorphs, mustelids, marmosets and tamarins, bats, and insectivores can all be anesthetized.

   b. In laboratory animal practice with rodents, retrograde transcutaneous penetration into the trachea has been demonstrated. A large hypodermic needle was directed rostrad from the trachea through the larynx and into the pharynx in order to "find" the laryngeal orifice for intubation. This technique is not survivable by the subject and is not called for.

   c. Intubation can be accomplished orally in the small mammals (see Figs. 13–4, 13–5, and 13–6).

D. *Primates* (Tables 13–5 and 13–6, and Table 13–11)

   1. Includes the smallest primates, that is, the marmosets, tamarins, and tarsiers (see Fig. 13–9).

   2. Also includes the largest primates, that is, the great apes (Figs. 13–2, 13–10, and 13–11).

Text continued on page 329

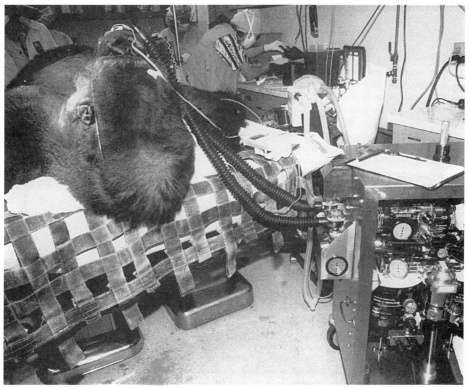

Figure 13–2. This robust, healthy 285 kg male gorilla was taken down with a syringe dart. Options for chemical take-down include chemicals from Tables 13–4 through 13–6, 13–8. Ket-xyl was selected to immobilize this gorilla (Table 13–5). He was endotracheally intubated and placed on the anesthesia ventilator (Fig. 13–1) for 3 hours of delicate surgery involving an invasive tumor of a parotid salivary gland. Postsurgically, he aspirated gastric reflux and had to be returned to the anesthesia ventilator for an additional 14 hours of pulmonary therapy.

Physiologic variables (see Table 13–3)	
Tidal volume (ml)	1869.7
Respiratory rate	12
Minute volume	22,436
Heart beat frequency (resting)	58
Bradycardia frequency	46

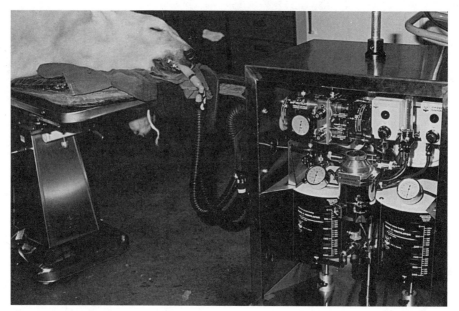

Figure 13–3. This healthy, young 350 kg polar bear was taken down with a syringe dart (see Tables 13–5 through 13–7). Ketamine alone would not be a good selection for the bear. Instead, ket-xyl (Table 13–5) was selected from the available chemicals for intramuscular injection. For a robust North American bear living in a zoo on full ration, full time, we must assume that up to 20% of the body size is subcutaneous fat. Thus, we should calculate physiologic variables (Table 13–3) and injectable anesthetics (Tables 13–5 through 13–8) based on lean body size (350 × 0.2 = 70), i.e., 280 kg. Further, we should endeavor to place the syringe dart for induction in a muscle mass, avoiding fat. This animal was endotracheally intubated (see Fig. 13–5) and placed on the anesthesia ventilator (Fig. 13–1) for 2 hours of surgery on a broken canine tooth.

Physiologic variables (see Table 13–3)	
Tidal volume (ml)	1836.6
Respiratory rate	12
Minute volume	22,039
Heart beat frequency (resting)	59
Bradycardia frequency	47

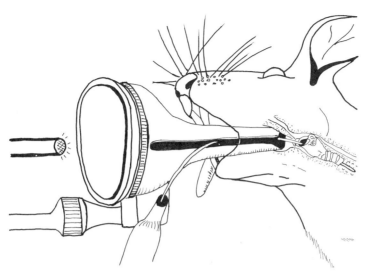

Figure 13–4. A modified canine otoscope can be used as a laryngoscope for a very small mammal such as a rodent. A narrow tom-cat urinary catheter (stylus) can be passed into the animal's laryngeal orifice and a Cole endotracheal tube passed over the stylus and directed into the larynx. (Lynn LB: Techniques for endotracheal intubation and inhalation anesthesia for laboratory animals. Calif Vet, March 1980, 32–33.)

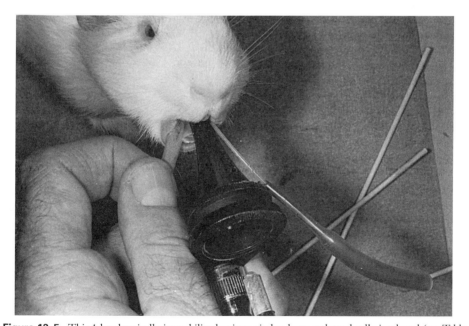

Figure 13–5. This 1 kg chemically immobilized guinea pig has been endotracheally intubated (see Table 13–4). The guinea pig's laryngeal orifice was visualized using a modified canine otoscope as the laryngoscope. A tom-cat urinary catheter was passed into the larynx, and a Cole infant endotracheal tube was then passed over the tom-cat catheter into the larynx.

Physiologic variables (see Table 13–3)

Tidal volume	6.2
Respiratory rate	53.5
Minute volume	332
Heart beat frequency	241
Bradycardia frequency	193

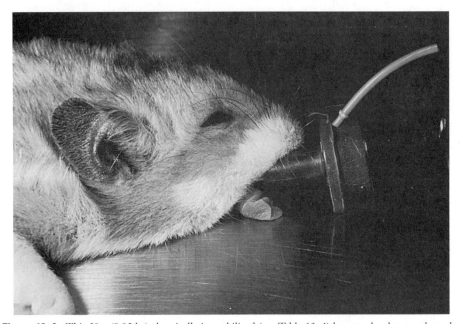

Figure 13–6. This 50 g (0.05 kg) chemically immobilized (see Table 13–4) hamster has been endotracheally intubated. A modified canine otoscope was used as a laryngoscope (see Fig. 13–12).

Physiologic variables (see Table 13–3)	
Tidal volume	0.3
Respiratory rate (resting)	116
Minute volume	35
Heart beat frequency (resting)	509
Bradycardia frequency	407

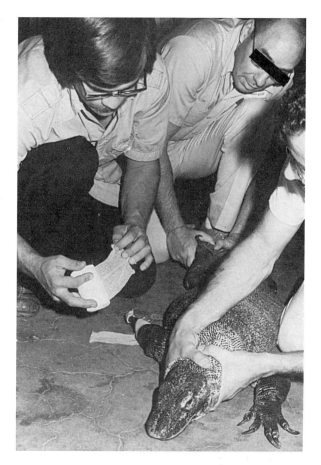

Figure 13–7. This large monitor lizard (Komodo dragon) is a formidable antagonist. It is quick, very strong, armed with sharp claws, and possesses flint-sharp cutting edges on its mouth. It is an animal that is potentially aggressive toward anything. General anesthesia is performed on this animal by first restraining it as shown. The mouth is gagged open with looped towels, and an endotracheal tube is inserted into its laryngeal orifice. With the tube connected to the anesthesia ventilator, the patient is forced to breathe 3% isoflurane and is thus anesthetized.

E. *Large mammalian Carnivora* (see Tables 13–4 through 13–7, and Table 13–11)

   1. Anesthetizing of the medium to large Carnivora is a regular part of veterinary practices that have access to zoos, performing zoo animals, or field projects with zoologic Carnivora.

      a. Included in the Carnivora are cats, bears, wolves, coyotes, jackals, hyenas, and foxes. They all can be chemically immobilized by injection.

      b. For all long-term anesthesia, the large mammalian carnivores should routinely be intubated endotracheally, given inhalation anesthesia with isoflurane, and supported with assisted mechanical ventilation once they are immobilized by injectable agents (see Figs. 13–12 through 13–14).

F. *Marine mammals* (see Tables 13–4 and 13–5)

   1. Anesthesia for marine mammals requires a demanding technology dealing with animals prone to CO_2 tolerance and to apnea (because of their diving adaptation) when under general anesthesia.

      a. Seals, sea lions, walruses, and cetaceans often hold their breath when anesthetized.

      b. Isoflurane inhalation anesthesia with assisted mechanical ventilation is routinely indicated for marine mammals following chemical immobilization with the injectable agents shown in Table 13–8. Diving

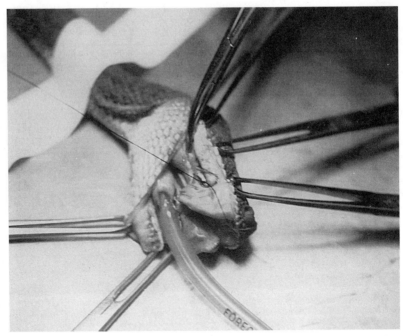

Figure 13–8. A venomous reptile can be head-pinned with a snake hook, gagged with a role of cotton gauze, and intubated, as shown. General anesthesia is induced by connecting the animal to the anesthesia ventilator and forcing it to breathe 3% isoflurane.

mammals are often apneic under general anesthesia and require ventilatory support.

G. *Medium to large ungulates* (hooved mammals)

1. These animals constitute a highly challenging group for the veterinarian to anesthetize because they possess explosive physical power and speed and are often self-destructive as well as aggressive while being handled.

2. Because such animals are difficult to handle, they may require specialized chuting and holding facilities and may need to be chemically immobilized (see Tables 13–5 through 13–7).

3. They should be endotracheally intubated and ventilated during isoflurane anesthesia (ruminating species easily regurgitate and aspirate rumen contents when anesthetized or when they become hypoxemic). Included are the following:

a. Antelope

b. Large bovids

c. Wild sheep and mountain goats

d. Camelids (ruminating nonruminants)

e. Cervids (see Fig. 13–15)

H. *Huge mammals*, elephants (see Fig. 13–16), rhinoceroses, hippopotamuses, giraffes, etc.—and *horses*

1. Anesthesia should not be undertaken for such species by most practitioners before those practitioners have served a significant internship with an experienced technologist. Practitioners must understand the principles of hands-on versus protected-contact practices plus the use of restraint machines that have been developed to better handle such wild species. The Equidae (horses) usually require the potent opioids

Table 13–6. Ket-med: Ketamine (Ketaset) 10% Plus Medetomidine (Domitor) 0.1%

Be prepared to reverse medetomidine (Domitor) with atipamezole (Antisedan) (see Table 13–10). Be concerned for animals potentially suffering preexisting respiratory or cardiac disease. Medetomidine causes bradycardia and hypotension.

Mix one part 10% ketamine with two parts 0.1% medetomidine (V:V 1:2). If dosage volume is too small, make a tenfold dilution by adding one part ket-med with nine parts water, thus moving the dosage (ml) decimal point one place to the right. Medetomidine is also available for experimental purposes in a 0.5% solution (5 mg/ml). Avoid using ket-med on diving animals or others that are potentially CO_2 tolerant and might experience apnea when anesthetized unless you are prepared to support pulmonary ventilation with a mechanical respirator.

Directions

1. Weigh, or make best estimate of weight, as precisely as possible and avoid treating ill or aged animals or animals with possible heart or respiratory disease with this powerful field anesthetic mixture. Administer atropine intravenously (Table 13–9).
2. To accomplish endotracheal intubation, mask the subject with isoflurane, intubate quickly, and start ventilatory support. Monitor EKG, oxygen saturation, and end-tidal CO_2. Insert an intravenous line and start a physiologic saline drip.
3. Reverse medetomidine with intravenous atipamezole (Table 13–10), and ventilate the subject until it is substantially recovered from anesthesia.

Weight (kg)	Dosage (ml)	Dosage (mg)		Dose Rate (mg/kg)	
		Ketamine	*Medetomidine*	*Ketamine*	*Medetomidine*
0.1	0.036	1.2	0.024	12	0.24
0.25	0.068	2.25	0.045	9	0.18
0.5	0.12	4	0.08	8	0.16
1.5	0.27	9	0.18	6	0.12
4	0.56	18.8	0.37	5	0.09
12	1.27	43	0.86	3.5	0.07
25	2.25	75	1.5	3	0.06
50	3.75	125	2.5	2.5	0.05
125	7.5	250	5	2	0.04
250	12	400	8	1.6	0.03
350	15	500	10	1.5	0.03

(etorphine or carfentanil) for field take-down. These agents are not discussed in this chapter.

IV. Specialized applications exist for various kinds of anesthetic equipment. Special ways of combining drugs are possible to achieve effective field take-down and general anesthesia. Unique methods also exist for administering drugs to capture free-ranging animals. Special techniques are used to monitor anesthesia for wild animals once chemical immobilization has been achieved.

A. The alpha$_2$-adrenergic agonists (xylazine, medetomidine, detomidine) are used only in veterinary medicine as adjuncts to anesthetics; they are not used as such in medical practice. They have profound physiologic effects that beg familiarity with subjects' potentially defective cardiovascular status. They require careful monitoring of subjects' resting-state physiologic variables (see Table 13–3), including blood pressure, blood pH, oxygen saturation, and end-tidal CO_2.

1. Veterinarians need to know how to measure indirect blood pressure using the sphygmomanometer with an ultrasonic Doppler pulse detector (Fig. 13–9).
2. Unfamiliarity with monitoring instruments can result in the inability to respond to developing emergencies involving hypotension and bradycardia caused by the alpha$_2$-adrenergic agonists.
3. The inability to use ventilators to support a subject invariably results in

Table 13–7. Tel-med: Tiletamine Combined with Zolazepam (Telazol) Plus Medetomidine (Domitor)

Add 5 ml of medetomidine (0.1% solution) *to 500 mg of crystalline Telazol* (contains 250 mg tiletamine and 250 mg zolazepam). This combination could be dangerous for animals suffering respiratory or cardiac disease. Each milliliter of tel-med contains Telazol 100 mg/ml (50 mg tiletamine and 50 mg zolazepam), *plus* 1 mg *medetomidine*. Tel-med may cause profound bradycardia and hypotension. Estimate a nominal heart rate for a subject in order to monitor for bradycardia. Avoid using this combination on diving mammals or others that are potentially CO_2 tolerant and prone to apnea unless there is a pulmonary ventilator available. Make a tenfold dilution by adding one part tel-med to nine parts water, thus moving the dosage (ml) decimal point one place to the right and making administration more convenient.

Directions

1. Determine body weight as precisely as possible and avoid treating ill or aged animals or animals with heart or respiratory disease with this potent field anesthetic combination. Establish an intravenous line. Administer atropine intravenously (Table 13–9).
2. If more anesthetic is needed to accomplish endotracheal intubation, mask the subject with isoflurane, intubate quickly, and start ventilatory support. *Monitor EKG, oxygen saturation, and end-tidal CO_2.*
3. *Reverse medetomidine with intravenous atipamezole* (Table 13–10).

Weight (kg)	Dosage (ml)	Dosage (mg)		Dose Rate (mg/kg)	
		Telazol	**Medetomidine**	**Telazol**	**Medetomidine**
0.1	0.007	0.7	0.007	7	0.07
0.25	0.015	1.5	0.015	6	0.06
0.5	0.025	2.5	0.025	5	0.05
1.5	0.05	5	0.05	3.3	0.03
4	0.12	12	0.12	3	0.03
12	0.27	27	0.27	2.25	0.02
25	0.47	47	0.47	1.9	0.02
50	0.79	79	0.79	1.6	0.01
125	1.6	160	1.6	1.28	0.01
250	2.6	260	2.6	1	0.01
350	3.4	340	3.4	0.9	0.01

low oxygen saturation in ill subjects that are obese, aged, cardiovascular or respiratory compromised.

B. The arylcycloalkylamine dissociative anesthetics (ketamine, tiletamine, and cyclohexylamine) produce good analgesia but cause side effects that are troubling to a clinician.

1. With the arylcycloalkylamines, subjects can sometimes be roused by too rough shaking and bumping (see Fig. 13–14).
2. Arylcycloalkylamines can cause clonic seizure-like activity and breath holding.
3. They can cause changes in a subject's electroencephalograph, indicating chemical CNS disruption of some order. Also, renarcotization can occur hours after apparent recovery.

C. Veterinarians and technologists who immobilize wildlife must understand the following:

1. Dart syringe mechanisms and syringe firing devices
2. The effects of anesthetic chemicals and combinations of chemicals on normal physiology
3. Endotracheal instruments and intubation techniques
4. Inhalation anesthesia machines with ventilatory support (see Figs. 13–1 through 13–3, 13–15, and 13–17)

D. Remember that chemical immobilization of wild, potentially dangerous animals presents daunting challenges to veterinarians (experienced or not). To cause the death or injury of a subject for lack of the appropriate instruments, machines, or experience is a price any veterinarian or technologist should be unwilling to pay.

V. Some field challenges in wild-animal anesthesia practices follow:

   A. Knowledge of anesthetic chemicals or combinations of chemicals is necessary because of the following reasons:

     1. They must be administered rapidly, usually remotely, and *intramuscularly.*

     2. They must be injected without the opportunity to test the injection site for underlying structures.

   B. Practitioners must try to determine an animal's preexisting health status in order to safely have it undergo general anesthesia. Making this determination is an art, a technology, and sometimes a guess.

     1. Note whether an animal has suffered lung disease, is obese (Figs. 13–10 and 13–11), or has other visible impediments to adequate respiratory ventilation or cardiovascular function.

     2. Skillful observation should alert the veterinarian to any possibility of previously developed respiratory compromise such as pneumonia, lung granuloma, or trauma.

     3. Obese animals should always be endotracheally intubated, provided ventilatory support, and monitored for *blood pressure, EKG, oxygen satura-*

Table 13–8. Ket-diaz or ket-midaz: Ketamine (Vetalar) 10% with (#1) Diazepam (Valium) 0.5% or (#2) Midazolam (Versed) 0.5%

Either diazepam or midazolam dosages may be given separately from a ketamine component, and either may be given orally.

When combined in the same syringe:
For #1 (ket-diaz), mix one part ketamine with one and a quarter parts diazepam.
For #2 (ket-midaz), mix eight parts ketamine with one part midazolam.

Directions

1. Weigh, or make a best estimate of weight, for the subject, and express the weight in kilograms (kg). Match the subject to the closest weight on the chart and, based on the most convenient volume, decide whether you will mix (#1) diazepam or (#2) midazolam with ketamine. Volumes using midazolam with ketamine will be lower than those using diazepam with ketamine.
2. Use isoflurane via mask or endotracheal tube to augment or prolong general anesthesia. Be prepared to provide ventilatory support via an endotracheal tube. Wear surgical gloves when intubating marine mammals.
3. Monitor EKG, oxygen tension, end-tidal CO_2, and blood pressure. Use a pulmonary ventilator to support respiration.

Weight (kg)	Dosage (ml)		Dosage (mg)			Dose Rate (mg/kg)		
	#1 Ketamine with Diazepam	#2 Ketamine with Midazolam	Ketamine	#1 Diazepam	#2 Midazolam	Ketamine	#1 Diazepam	#2 Midazolam
0.1	0.055	0.028	2.5	0.15	0.015	25	1.5	0.15
0.25	0.11	0.056	5	0.3	0.03	20	1.2	0.12
0.5	0.18	0.09	8	0.5	0.05	16	1	0.1
1.5	0.38	0.18	16	1.1	0.11	10.6	0.73	0.073
4	0.86	0.45	40	2.3	0.23	10	0.57	0.057
12	1.8	0.9	80	5.4	0.54	6.6	0.45	0.045
25	3.44	1.7	156	9.4	0.94	6.24	0.38	0.038
50	5.8	2.93	263	15.8	1.58	5.26	0.32	0.032
125	11.5	5.86	523	31.4	3.14	4.2	0.25	0.025
250	19.3	9.85	880	52.8	5.28	3.5	0.2	0.021
350	24.8	12.5	1120	68	6.8	3.2	0.19	0.019

Table 13–9. Atropine and Glycopyrrolate

Atropine (500 mcg/ml) or glycopyrrolate (200 mcg/ml) can be injected intramuscularly or intravenously. Either can cause bradycardia.

Weight (kg)	Dosage (mcg)		Dose Rate (mcg/kg)	
	Atropine	*Glycopyrrolate*	*Atropine*	*Glycopyrrolate*
0.25	10	6.5	40	26
0.5	16	10	32	20
1.5	38	25	25	16.5
4	79	51	20	10
12	180	117	15	9.75
25	313	203	12.5	8
50	526	342	10.5	7
125	1000	680	8	5
250	1760	1144	7	4.5
350	2265	1472	6.5	4

tion, and end-tidal CO_2 during prolonged anesthetic procedures (see Fig. 13–10).

4. It is necessary to be equipped with an effective mechanical ventilator to provide ventilatory assistance, "sighing," oxygen enrichment, and varying respiratory patterns when effective spontaneous ventilation is in question (see Figs. 13–1 through 13–3, 13–15 through 13–17).

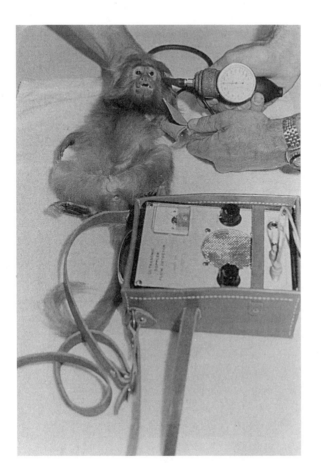

Figure 13–9. For the smallest primates, ketamine (by itself) works very well for chemical immobilization (Table 13–4) during diagnostic procedures or minor surgery.

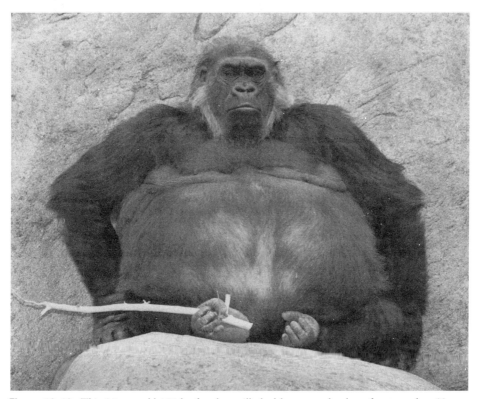

Figure 13–10. This 36-year-old 196 kg female gorilla had been grossly obese for more than 20 years and was thought to be pickwickian. She presented with difficulty moving; in fact, she staggered. The subject was chemically immobilized with the low-dosage ketamine alone (Table 13–4) for diagnostic procedures. She immediately became apneic. She was endotracheally intubated and was placed on the anesthesia ventilator. On the ventilator, her oxygen saturation was above 98%. When she was removed from assisted ventilation, her saturation immediately dropped below 18%. Even after ketamine effects had ceased (the subject could reach about and grasp), she did not breathe normally without the ventilator.

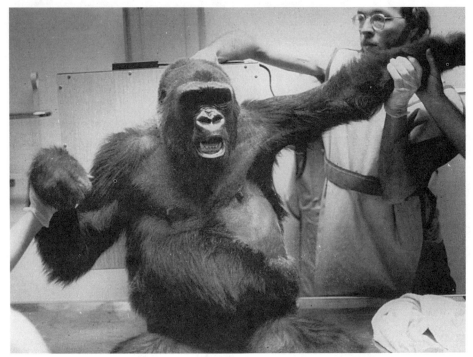

Figure 13–11. This 15-year-old, 80 kg female gorilla presented with severe dyspnea caused by a *Coccidioides immitis* lung granuloma, a fluid-filled left chest, and a collapsed lung. The subject was chemically immobilized with low-dosage ketamine alone (Table 13–4) for diagnostic procedures. Arterial pH was normal, but CO_2 was elevated. Following general anesthesia, the subject died.

5. Postural (pulmonary) ventilatory compromise
   a. Some species that cannot tolerate certain postures during anesthesia take-down might not ventilate effectively as a result.
   b. Animals should have end-tidal CO_2 monitored when it is necessary to position them in a compromising surgical posture that could impede adequate ventilation. *For example:*
      (1) Adult elephants should not be anesthetized prone (in sternal recumbency) because the weight of displaced abdominal viscera impairs effective ventilatory action of the diaphragm. Adult elephants can better tolerate lateral recumbency (see Fig. 13–16) than sternal recumbency, although that, too, compromises optimal ventilation in this species. Infant and juvenile elephants do not suffer the same problem. Adult elephants normally spend substantial sleep time standing (as do adult giraffes and others).
6. Animals that develop reduced sensitivity to the regular central respiratory drive of increased arterial CO_2 may unexpectedly become apneic while under general anesthesia.
   a. Veterinarians accustomed to the usual respiratory responses of terrestrial mammals to elevated arterial CO_2 levels ($\geq$30–50 mm Hg) expect to see regular ventilation stimulated, not apnea occurring, when the patient is placed under a moderate level of general anesthesia.
   b. Tolerance to hypercarbia while under light to moderate general anesthesia is a condition seen in animals with chronic respiratory disease and is a normal phenomenon in birds and diving mammals.

    c. Usually hypercapnea decreases cerebral spinal pH, which increases pulmonary ventilation. Animals subjected to long-term chronic hypercapnea develop compensatory mechanisms to stabilize lowered cerebral spinal fluid pH; thus, increased arterial CO_2 no longer functions to effectively drive pulmonary ventilation (see Figs. 13–12 and 13–13).

C. Special techniques are needed to endotracheally intubate a subject for application of assisted pulmonary ventilatory support (see Figs. 13–2, through 13–6, 13–8, 13–12, 13–13, 13–15 through 13–17).

    1. Many larger animals are endotracheally intubated by passing a handheld endotracheal tube into the pharynx and guiding the tip into the larynx with the fingers (see Figs. 13–12 and 13–13).

    2. Smaller animals can be intubated by visually placing a narrow stylus into the larynx and passing the endotracheal tube over the stylus (see Fig. 13–4).

    3. Tracheostomy and tracheal trocarization may be last resorts. These are traumatic methods for intubation and may condemn a subject to ultimate euthanasia as a result of irreparable injury.

D. A dart syringe anesthetic delivery system must be selected that accommodates the required volume of anesthetic for successful immobilization yet constitutes a projectile weight that will not cause excessive pain or serious injury to the subject. Making the correct selection is the art of remote anesthesia induction.

    1. Heavy dart syringes propelled at high velocity have sometimes pierced a small subject's body.

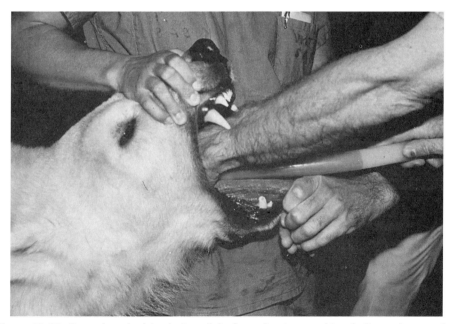

Figure 13–12. For endotracheal intubation of the large *Carnivora*, nothing facilitates the procedure better than the hand to introduce the tube into the laryngeal orifice. This manual procedure is the least traumatic for the animal and the quickest way to intubate. The anesthetist spreads open the laryngeal orifice with the fingers, and gently introduces the tube to the airway. This 350 kg subject was taken down with ket-xyl (Table 13–5) and placed on the anesthesia ventilator for 2 hours of surgery on a fistulated canine tooth. See Table 13–1 for the physiologic variables calculated from Table 13–3.

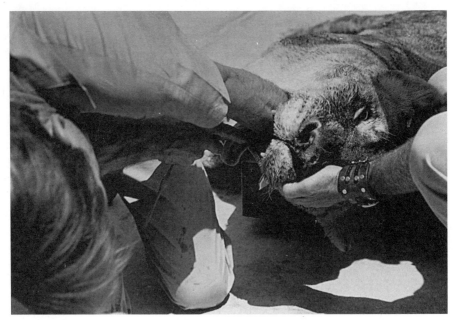

Figure 13–13. An African lioness is being endotracheally intubated. The great (roaring) cats offer a unique experience in intubation and inhalation anesthesia for the veterinarian. Because of very loose laryngeal suspensory structures, the laryngeal orifice falls away toward the thoracic inlet in an adult anesthetized lion or tiger. Consequently, the veterinarian must introduce the endotracheal tube by hand. In addition, tracheal diameters are much greater than one would expect. This 125 kg lioness easily accommodates a 36 mm diameter endotracheal tube, whereas an elk with the same body size would have taken a tube not greater than 28 mm. Perhaps this large tracheal diameter, in such predators who stalk their prey and then charge with a short rush, represents an adaptation to facilitate the exchange of very large volumes of air over a short time period. Because of this large diameter, the anesthetist must fit the endotracheal tube snugly in the great cats. Otherwise, it is possible for air to pass around the outside of the tube. Then the mechanical ventilator will set up a Venturi effect that imbibes air into the trachea and dilutes anesthetic gas. The cat will start to wake, the anesthetist will increase anesthetic concentration, and a false impression of gas concentration requirement will result.

2. The options include the following:
   a. Using a handheld syringe to be injected by the clinician through a fence or other barrier with the traditional veterinary "quick-shot" technique or with a pole syringe (common practice)
   b. Using one of the lightweight, pressurized dart syringes (Telinject) employing a sliding cuff and a side-ejecting needle port to be shot into the subject's muscle by means of a dart gun or a blow pipe (common practice)
   c. Using blow pipe dart syringes that are pressurized prior to being fired (these are reliable with smaller volumes but not so reliable with large volumes)
   d. Using one of the heavier, explosive-actuated dart syringe systems (Cap-Chur) in which syringe function depends on substantial dart velocity coupled with an inertial mechanism that fires the syringe plunger as the dart-syringe strikes the animal
3. Substantial trauma can result from certain dart syringes, and there is potential for failure of the syringe to function.
4. Inertia triggers an explosive charge inside the dart syringe, pushing the piston forward in Palmer systems.
5. An explosive syringe system accommodates large volumes, and injection is both instantaneous and reliable but often injurious.

6. Remember that one of the main families of chemicals used in syringe darts, the arylcycloalkylamines (ketamine, tiletamine, phencyclidine), are painful upon intramuscular injection.

7. The challenge in field anesthesia is to accomplish endotracheal intubation and inhalation anesthesia without the clinician being injured by the patient or the patient without being injured, frightened, or killed.

No dart syringe system has all the advantages with none of the disadvantages: Each syringe dart delivery system has both advantages and disadvantages. The anesthetist may sometimes need the advantage of range and high syringe capacity but then must accept the disadvantage of increased potential trauma from projectile increased weight and velocity. Lightweight (blow dart) syringes are not so traumatic, but cannot hold large volumes and are less reliable when ejecting an entire load.

VI. It is well to understand the importance that variations in *body sizes* versus *metabolic sizes* impose when extrapolating anesthetic treatment regimens between animals of widely disparate body sizes.

   A. Variations of *body sizes*—weight expressed in kilograms (kg)—encountered in wildlife practice can be on the order of thousands when extrapolating treatment regimens between certain categories of wild animals.

      1. For example, various subgroups of the Rodentia mammals or the Passeriformes birds can exhibit such variations in size as follows:

         a. The 20 g mouse versus the 50 kg capybara

         b. The 16 g finch (Passeriformes) versus the 1.5 kg raven (Passeriformes)

         c. The 60 kg infant elephant versus the 6000 kg adult elephant

   B. Variations in *metabolic sizes*—expressed as minimum kilocalorie (kcal) expenditures—are among the basic considerations in dose rates when ex-

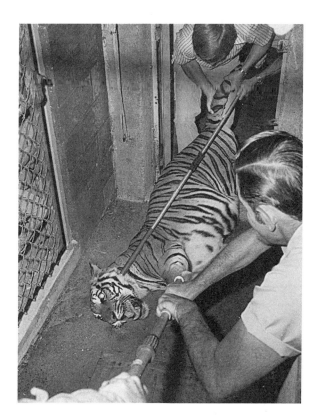

Figure 13-14. This adult tiger was chemically immobilized solely with ketamine (Table 13–4). Removing the animal from a very cramped holding area resulted in an inordinate amount of pushing and prodding, bumping and bending of the animal. It was probably a little too noisy in this environment as well. As a result, the anesthetic effect of ketamine was reduced, and the animal actively resisted treatment. The anesthetic effects of the arylcycloalkylamine dissociative anesthetics (ketamine, tiletamine, phencyclidine) can be reduced by too much stimulation and should not be relied upon (solely) for the large, dangerous zoo animals when clatter and body manipulation cannot be well controlled. I once "bounced" a tiger to her feet that was presumed to be overly depressed by phencyclidine.

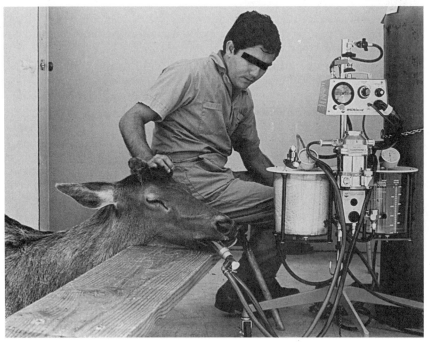

Figure 13–15. This 100 kg elk was chemically immobilized (Tables 13–5 through 13–7), endotracheally intubated, and connected to the anesthesia ventilator.

Physiologic variables (Table 13–3)	
Tidal volume (ml)	649
Respiratory rate	16
Minute volume	10,384
Heart beat frequency	76
Bradycardia frequency	61

trapolating treatment regimens between subjects of widely divergent body sizes, as is commonly required for wildlife anesthesia.

1. With *body surface area*—expressed in square meters per unit of mass (kg)—we have one facet of *metabolic size* that helps answer the questions of anesthetic treatment extrapolations from one subject to the next.

   a. Relative body sizes and metabolic sizes are problematic in comparing drug dose rates.

   b. The elephant and the mouse have the same *mean core body temperature set points.* They are both placentals, with a core body temperature of 37°C. Most of the mouse's mass is within 1 cm of its body surface, whereas very little of the elephant's mass is within that 1 cm of its body surface.

   c. The problem for the mouse is how to keep metabolic machinery working at a high enough rate to compensate for rapid loss of body heat. The problem for the elephant is how to keep metabolic machinery operating without creating more body heat than can be radiated effectively and thus prevent hyperthermia.

   d. *The preceding principles account for the relatively high metabolic rates, translatable into high dose rates for anesthetics (and other drugs), for small animals compared against the low metabolic rates, translatable to low dose rates, for large animals.*

   e. Although the body size of the elephant is many thousand times that of the mouse, the elephant's *metabolic size* is many times less than that of the mouse.

f. *Metabolic size* (kcal/kg) relates to *dose rate* (mg/kg). *Body size* (kg) relates to *treatment dosage* (mg).

Example: The ketamine dose rate for a small, 20 g rodent (mouse) is 75 mg/kg, or 1.5 mg, while the clinically equivalent dose rate for a very large, 50 kg rodent (capybara) is 10.5 mg/kg, or 75 mg (body size) (see Table 13–4).

g. Considering the foregoing, one must recognize the fallacy of saying, "The range of ketamine dose rates for rodents is 10.5 to 75 mg/kg," because the dose rate for a 0.020 kg rodent is 75 mg/kg whereas the dose rate for 50 kg rodent is 10.5 mg/kg. It needs to be recognized that such errors sometimes occur in the literature. There is a range of dose rates for 20 g mice, but, there is *another range* of dose rates for 50 kg capybaras. These differences must be heeded to avoid underdosing mice and overdosing capybaras. The two animal sizes have very different ranges for their respective dose rates.

h. Any dose rate to be doubled must be the one that is allometrically scaled for the subject's body size with its attendant *metabolic size* and its discrete energy class. Do not use a dose rate that "fits" another subject from a different energy or weight class. For example, double

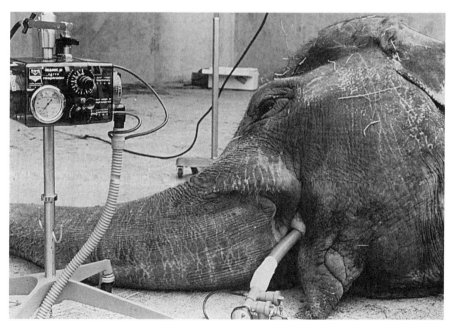

Figure 13–16. This 4000 kg elephant was anesthetized with etorphine HCl (M99). The subject was endotracheally intubated and placed on a Bird Corporation Mk 9 respirator. The Mk 9, with its minute volume capacity of 270 liters, is capable of ventilating the 4000 kg animal. A peak positive transpulmonic pressure from the ventilator of 24 cm of water will ventilate an elephant as effectively as a mouse. It is of interest that a 20% reduction of the elephant's resting-state heart beat frequency, 6 beats per minute, constitutes bradycardia.

Physiologic variables (see Table 13–3)	
Tidal volume (ml)	27,000
Respiratory rate	6
Minute volume	162,000
Heart beat frequency	30
Bradycardia frequency	24

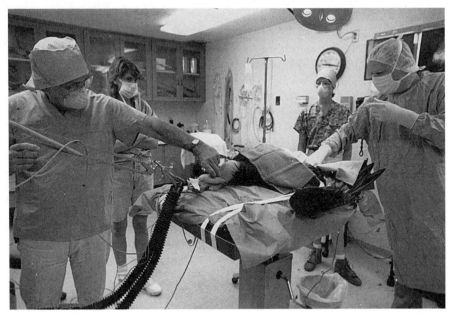

Figure 13–17. This California condor was manually restrained and had isoflurane anesthesia induced by mask. When relaxed, the subject was endotracheally intubated and attached to the anesthesia ventilator for surgery involving an oviduct.

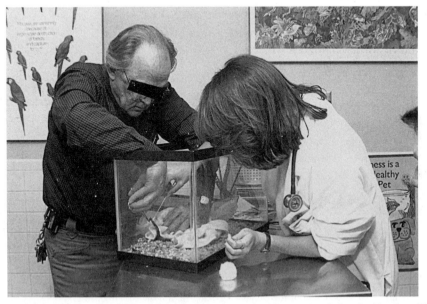

Figure 13–18. This very large African giant scorpion, a pet for 18 years, was infested with mites. When the subject was placed in an induction box with 3% isoflurane, it became anesthetized, as did the mites. All mites fell off the scorpion after a few moments in the isoflurane. The scorpion was removed from the box and recovered from the anesthetic minus its mites.

the ketamine dose rate for the 20 g mouse would be 150 mg/kg, and double the dose rate for the 50 kg capybara would be 21 mg/kg.

2. Species-specific core body temperature set points (there are five discrete energy taxa) are aspects of metabolic size. Extrapolating dose rates among individuals from different energy taxa (e.g., from placental mammals to marsupial mammals) must mathematically factor in the different energy constants (*K value*) for each *energy taxon* into the equation used in making a dosage extrapolation (see Table 13–1).

3. Injectable anesthetic *dose rates* from empirical treatment data gathered during clinical experience with one subject or a group of subjects may be used to estimate (allometrically) dose rates for another patient or group using body surface area or using metabolic formulas (something that does not work for linear extrapolations). This is *the* critical concept in *allometric scaling of drug doses.*

ALLOMETRIC SCALING AND SURFACE AREA, METERS SQUARED: A HISTORICAL NOTE

Widespread application of *allometric scaling* for dosage extrapolations among different species followed a landmark paper by Freireich and coworkers.* The flaw with using surface area as the modality for treatment extrapolations in all veterinary species lies in the fact that this approach ignores the large variations in surface-area-to-mass ratios that exist among hundreds of veterinary species. This is obviously not the case in human medical extrapolations dealing with a single species (*Homo sapiens*) with one morphology. Also, differences exist in species-specific core body temperature set points of animals other than the placental mammals (see Table 13–1). Energy formulas that describe the similarities that exist for metabolic chemistry and fluidics common to all species seem to work well for the veterinary extrapolations.

VII. Using allometric scaling to extrapolate dose rates, the clinician recognizes that the largest body sizes of any given energy taxon take the *highest* treatment dosages but the *lowest* dose rates, whereas the smallest body sizes of any energy group take the *highest* dose rates but the *lowest* treatment dosages.

EXTRAPOLATION OF DOSAGES AND DOSE RATES

In Table 13–4, note that 1.5 mg (75 mg/kg) of ketamine is one of the anesthetic treatments for a 20 g mouse, whereas 526 mg (10.5 mg/kg) of ketamine is the treatment for a 50 kg capybara. The 50 kg capybara weighs 2500 times the 0.02 kg mouse. The clinically equivalent dosage and dose rate of each subject obviously *cannot be the same.* The mouse ketamine dosage (1.5 mg) would not anesthetize the capybara and the capybara ketamine dosage (526 mg) would kill the mouse.

VIII. It is important to consider that the injectable combination anesthetics currently used in many wildlife immobilizations center around arylcycloalkylamine *dissociative agents* (ketamine, tiletamine, phencyclidine) combined with *alpha*$_2$-adrenoceptor agonists (xylazine, medetomidine, detomidine).

A. Assessment of strengths and weaknesses of injectable anesthetics and combinations.

---

*EJ Freireich, EA Gehen, DP Rall, et al.: Quantitative comparison of toxicity of anticancer agents in mouse, rat, hamster, dog, monkey and man. Cancer Chemother Rep 50(4): 74–76, 219–229, 1966.

IMMOBILIZATION PRINCIPLE #1:

Larger subjects, such as adult great cats or apes, immobilized solely with ketamine, tiletamine, or the older phencyclidine (arylcycloalkylamines) may stretch out, hold their breath, and undergo clonic seizures. While under the effect of the arylcycloalkylamine, they may sometimes be "roused," bounced, shaken, or clattered into a plane of consciousness and potential aggressiveness that is dangerous for handlers (see Fig. 3–14). The combination of (1) a dissociative arylcycloalkylamine anesthetic (ketamine, tiletamine, phencyclidine) with (2) an alpha$_2$-adrenoceptor agonist *is more effective* and requires smaller dart volumes for remote induction of anesthesia for wild animals than either of the two classes of chemical agents alone. But the alpha$_2$-adrenoceptor agonists bring bradycardia and hypotension to the mix of clinical problems faced by the veterinarian.

1. Dissociative anesthetics provide good analgesia. They do not, by themselves, offer good muscular relaxation for highly invasive or meticulous surgery.

2. Having a large carnivore jerking and twitching each time the surgeon makes an incision or places a suture has led to unnecessary repeated dosing, then overdosing (with the cyclohexylamine). The subject's muscular tension and movement that lead to operator distraction can be alleviated by administering the alpha$_2$-adrenergic agonist.

   a. The addition of an *alpha$_2$-adrenergic agonist* enhances arylcycloalkylamine (ketamine, tiletamine) anesthesia, but alpha$_2$-adrenergic agonists *reduce blood pressure* and *cause bradycardia* by activating alpha$_2$-adrenergic receptors in the cardiovascular control centers of the CNS. Such activation suppresses the outflow of the sympathetic nervous system from the lower brain stem. That is, *the preponderant clinical effects of alpha$_2$ adrenergic agonists* are centrally mediated hypotension and bradycardia.

   b. Alpha$_2$-adrenergic agonists decrease and "smooth" take-down; however, "smooth" means cause a *reduction in vital function* (something to consider during the preanesthetic health assessment).

   c. Alpha$_2$-adrenergic agonists alleviate some musculoskeletal movement associated with arylcycloalkylamine anesthetics.

   d. Alpha$_2$-adrenergic agonist components are reversible with alpha$_2$-adrenergic antagonists such as *yohimbine* and *atipamezole* (Table 13–10).

3. Alpha$_2$-adrenoceptor agonists *will not* by themselves always render animals immobile until high dosage or great potency renders a subject severely hypotensive.

   a. A wolf lying quietly and apparently anesthetized with xylazine (as the sole agent) has been observed to suddenly snap "awake" and menace a handler.

   b. An "excitement stage" has been observed in camels apparently anesthetized with xylazine. In this excitement stage, they suddenly jumped up and kicked and bit at a handler holding the halter rope.

   c. Zebras not taken down by heavy dosages of intramuscular xylazine have been observed to finally go down and succumb from very high dosages of this alpha$_2$-adrenergic agonist.

4. When using alpha$_2$-adrenergic agonists (see Tables 13–5 and 13–6), administer anticholinergics (see Table 13–9) for bradycardia. *Nominal bradycardiac rates can be predicted for animals* (see Table 13–3, item j).

5. Monitor blood pressure and blood oxygen saturation, especially if tran-

Table 13–10. Yohimbine (Antagonil) and Atipamezole (Antisedan)

Yohimbine (Antagonil) and atipamezole (Antisedan) are competitive antagonists that are selective for reversing the effect of alpha$_2$-adrenergic agonists. Both can be administered intravenously to subjects in which *xylazine* or *medetomidine* has been used when it is desired to reverse the agonist drug effects.

If subjects anesthetized by combinations of ketamine and xylazine or medetomidine are to receive an antagonist (yohimbine or atipamezole), some time should have elapsed before antagonist administration in order to allow ketamine to have had time to be substantially eliminated.

Both yohimbine and atipamezole are available in 0.5% solutions (concentrations of 5 mg/ml). In the following table, select the appropriate weight, and look along its data line for the most convenient agent (yohimbine or atipamezole) to use in antagonizing whichever alpha$_2$-adrenergic agonist (xylazine or medetomidine) is to be reversed.

Weight (kg)	Dosage Volumes (ml)		Dosages (mg)		Dose Rates (mg/kg)	
	Yohimbine	*Atipamezole*	*Yohimbine*	*Atipamezole*	*Yohimbine*	*Atipamezole*
0.1	0.03	0.004	0.15	0.02	1.5	0.2
0.25	0.06	0.008	0.3	0.04	1.2	0.16
0.5	0.1	0.01	0.5	0.05	1.1	0.1
1.5	0.2	0.03	1	0.15	0.66	0.1
4	0.55	0.05	2.75	0.25	0.68	0.06
12	1.26	0.1	6.3	0.5	0.52	0.04
25	2	0.2	10	1	0.4	0.04
50	3.7	0.3	18.5	1.5	0.37	0.03
125	7	0.5	35	2.5	0.3	0.02
250	12	0.8	60	3	0.24	0.016
350	15.8	0.9	80	3.5	0.22	0.01

Yohimbine or atipamezole can be given intramuscularly, although the intravenous route better serves their value as alpha$_2$-adrenergic antagonists in emergencies.

quilizers are to be included with injectable anesthetic cocktails like that of tiletamine and zolazepam (Telazol).

6. Combinations of dissociative anesthetic plus alpha$_2$-adrenoceptor agonist provide better anesthesia but they are not always safe for subjects with subtle or hidden disabilities.

7. Be prepared to endotracheally intubate, provide assisted pulmonary ventilation, and inject every anesthesia patient on xylazine, medetomidine, or detomidine with an alpha$_2$-adrenergic antagonist if indicated (see Table 13–10).

   a. Calculate a physiologic variables database for each anesthesia patient (Table 13–3).

   b. Calculate a nominal bradycardiac heartbeat rate (Table 13–3).

B. Consideration of dart syringe volume is critical in selecting which injectable agents will be used for remote application.

1. Select the combination anesthetics that give the most convenient dart volume (Table 13–11; see also Tables 13–4 through 13–8) and that work best for the species.

IMMOBILIZATION PRINCIPLE #2:

The best combination of available arylcycloalkylamine dissociative anesthetics (ketamine, tiletamine, phencyclidine) with an alpha$_2$-adrenoceptor agonist (xylazine, medetomidine, detomidine) depends on critical *volumes* imposed by available dart or handheld syringe capacities. Remember that alpha$_2$-adrenergic agonists are not anesthetics per se but rather agents that seem to "smooth" the effects of anesthetics by centrally blocking sympathetic outflow from the cardiovascular control center of

Table 13–11. Ket-tel: Ketamine (Ketaset) Plus Tiletamine Combined with Zolazepam (Telazol)

Ket-tel is an emergency field anesthetic for quick take-down.

Directions for constitution (ket-tel): Mix 5 ml of 10% ketamine solution (100 mg/ml) to reconstitute one vial of crystalline Telazol. When thus reconstituted, each milliliter of active ingredients will consist of ketamine (100 mg/ml) and Telazol solution (100 mg/ml).

Injections must go intramuscularly.

Weight (kg)	Dosage (ml)	Dosage (mg)		Dose Rate (mg/kg)	
		Ketamine	*Telazol*	*Ketamine*	*Telazol*
0.25	0.02	2	2	8	8
0.5	0.03	3	3	6	6
1.5	0.07	7	7	4.6	4.6
4	0.15	15	15	3.7	3.6
12	0.34	34	34	2.8	2.8
25	0.6	60	60	2.4	2.4
50	1.0	100	100	2	2
125	2.0	200	200	1.6	1.6
250	3.3	330	330	1.3	1.3
350	4.3	430	430	1.2	1.2

Advantages

1. Requires relatively small volumes for use in low-volume (blow) dart syringes.
2. Short induction time is useful for rapid take-downs of escaped animals.
3. Reconstitution is quick and simple: merely *add 5 ml of ketamine solution to a vial of Telazol.*

Disadvantages

1. Be prepared to endotracheally intubate and assist ventilation in subjects as with all other general anesthetic agents.
2. Renarcotization has been reported with tiletamine in tigers. Animals under anesthesia should be assiduously monitored for 24–48 hours or longer for renarcotization while confined.
3. Apparently no drugs act as antagonists to the cyclohexylamine anesthetics. Overdosage with them causes respiratory depression, and assisted mechanical ventilation will likely be needed.
4. Anticholenergics—atropine (short acting) or glycopyrrolate (longer acting)—are sometimes indicated.

---

the CNS. That is, these agents cause hypotension. Be concerned and careful if a subject might have preexisting cardiovascular, respiratory, or miscellaneous degenerative diseases that compromise vital function as a sequel to designer combination chemicals for anesthesia.

    2. Small volumes are sometimes an advantage.

    3. With the potent anesthetic agents, volumes may be too small to be practical.

       a. Less than 1–2 ml volumes work well in blow dart syringe systems (Telinject) but not so well in the heavier, explosive-charged syringe (Cap-Chur) darts.

       b. To increase a volume, make tenfold dilutions of the drug by adding nine parts water to one part drug (move the decimal point one place to the right).

  C. The ultimate goal of anesthesia applied for indeterminate periods should be to place a subject in a position for readily adjustable anesthesia levels or planes with optimal physiologic support using an anesthesia-ventilator machine.

IMMOBILIZATION PRINCIPLE #3:

The ultimate goal for extended, *stimulus-responsive anesthesia* is to have the subject endotracheally intubated and converted to an inhalant anesthetic (isoflurane) supported by a machine that is capable of providing effective *ventilatory assistance*. Field immobilization with injectable agents is to be employed for capture, transport, and short diagnostic or simple surgical procedures. Inhalation anesthesia with ventilatory support is required for long-term, stimulus-responsive general anesthesia. Otherwise, if an emergency requires long-term ventilatory support, the practitioner could be sitting for hours blowing on a gorilla's or tiger's endotracheal tube with his or her mouth, trusting someone to titrate appropriate alliquots of injectable anesthetic agent intramuscularly or intravenously.

1. Most veterinarians experienced with anesthesia for some group of animals have mastered how to intubate endotracheally and ventilate that group.

2. The unfortunate occasional alternative (not to intubate and support ventilation) is to helplessly watch an anesthetized animal expire unnecessarily while casting frantically about for the necessary intubation endotracheal tube and ventilatory support equipment.

D. Tables 13–4 through 13–8, and 13–10 can be used to estimate rational anesthetic treatments for diverse species and for animals of great variation in body size. The tables also illustrate the clinical aspects of allometric scaling.

1. The choice of (a) ketamine as an exclusive anesthetic agent, (b) ketamine plus xylazine (20–100 mg/ml), (c) ketamine plus medetomidine (1–5 mg/ml), (d) tiletamine-zolazepam (Telazol) plus medetomidine to be used with ketamine (100 mg/ml), or (e) tiletamine-zolazepam (100 mg/ml) will depend on the practicality of the volumes that are needed for their use in a dart syringe or other field delivery system.

2. Remember that as animal size increases, dosage increases (direct relationship), but dose rate decreases (indirect relationship). Conversely, as animal size decreases, dosage decreases, but dose rate increases. A nominal *bradycardiac heart rate* may be estimated allometrically for establishing a database for a patient (see Table 13–3).

Clinical definition of bradycardia: Bradycardia can be characterized as a 15–20% reduction in heart rate *below* that of the resting heart rate (see Table 13–3, item j), beats per minute (bpm). An allometric *estimate of resting heart rate* can be made for mammals using the following calculation:

$$\text{Resting Heart Rate in Mammals (bpm)} = 241 \ (W_{kg}^{-0.25})$$

a. *Example:* A healthy 125 kg zoo mountain lion with a resting heart rate of about $241(125^{-0.25}) = 72$ has bradycardia when the heart rate falls 15–20% below 72; i.e., $72 - (72 \times 0.20) = 57$ bpm is bradycardia in the 125 kg mountain lion.

b. Thus, if a 125 kg lion were anesthetized with either a xylazine or medetomidine combination anesthetic, the animal might be presumed to have *bradycardia* when its heart rate falls to a nominal 57–72 beats per minute. Atropine or glycopyrrolate treatment should then be administered (see Tables 13–7 and 13–9) in the following dosages: atropine 1000 mcg (8 mcg/kg) or glycopyrrolate 680 mcg (5 mcg/kg).

E. Benzodiazepines (diazepam, midazolam, zolazepam) used in conjunction with the arylcycloalkylamine dissociative anesthetics are CNS-active drugs.

Their effects are very useful in combination with ketamine (diazepam, midazolam) and tiletamine (zolazepam) (see Tables 13–7 and 13–8). Desirable benzodiazepine effects when used with anesthesia are as follows:

1. Sedation and hypnosis
2. Decreased anxiety
3. Anticonvulsive and muscle-relaxant effects
4. Amnesia

Because of their effect of decreased anxiety, the benzodiazepines are sometimes used for nonanesthetic treatments of animals that have been introduced to a new environment or in some other way have become frightened or aversively conditioned and need to increase locomotor activity, appetite, and willingness to drink.

IX. Birds

    A. Use of injectable anesthetics for birds has been unnecessary in most cases since isoflurane was placed in the veterinarian's armamentarium. Even the ostrich can usually be restrained by experienced handlers and "masked down" with isoflurane. One exception is the cassowary. Most experienced handlers would prefer to syringe dart an adult cassowary rather than have this very dangerous ratite try to eviscerate them with its lethal and persistent kicking.

        1. The dose rates of injectable anesthetics for birds vary according to body size (kg) *and* metabolic size (kcal) and approximate those of mammals (see Table 13–4).

            a. Body sizes vary from 5 g hummingbirds to 150 kg ostriches.

            b. *Two* metabolic sizes exist for birds (see Table 13–3):

                (1) *Song birds* (so-called passerines) have core body temperatures of 42°C.

                (2) *All other birds* (nonpasserines) have core body temperatures of 40°C.

        2. Passerines have a considerably higher metabolic rate for each weight class than do nonpasserines because of a higher core body temperature set point, controlled by the hypothalamus.

            a. Two different dose rates should be used for injectable anesthetics, one for nonpasserines and the other for passerines. But isoflurane is a far superior option to injectable anesthetics for both passerines and nonpasserines. (see Table 13–4).

        4. Muscular relaxation is poor with ketamine anesthesia in birds (as in other animals).

            a. Recoveries from injectable anesthesia are stormy, with the sometimes disastrous result of broken feathers.

            b. Usually an excitement stage occurs during recovery from ketamine in birds, and it may last for a long time in larger birds.

        5. Small birds recover more rapidly than larger ones from clinically equivalent levels or planes of ketamine anesthesia.

        6. If isoflurane anesthesia cannot be employed in an avian subject and anesthesia must be extended by repeated injectable anesthetic renarcotization, expect a concomitant high risk of mortality.

IMPORTANT BIRD RESPIRATION CONCERNS

Sedated or anesthetized birds do not effectively ventilate spontaneously. Their ventilation is apparently less dependent on arterial CO_2 drive than is the ventilation of mammals. Birds should usually be endotracheally intubated and receive intermittent mandatory ventilation (IMV) to assure extraction of CO_2 from the blood in any prolonged anesthesia procedure. Oxygen and IMV should be available regardless of the anesthetic agent used or the period of anesthesia.

    B. Inhalation anesthetics (see Fig. 13–6)

        1. Inhalation anesthesia with isoflurane is the preferred method for general anesthesia in birds, even for short-term applications.

            a. Isoflurane offers rapid induction, good analgesia, good muscular relaxation, and rapid recovery with little struggling.

            b. Even in large birds (condors, ostriches), general anesthesia can be induced effectively using isoflurane.

        2. Induction can be achieved by head cone with 3% isoflurane, and a bird can then be endotracheally intubated with a noncuffed or Cole style endotracheal tube to receive IMV.

            a. A pulse oximeter (VET/OX 4402) can be used to monitor oxygen saturation.

            b. An ultrasonic Doppler blood flow detector (Parks Model 811) is an ideal monitor for cardiovascular monitoring.

            c. A special challenge to the exotic animal clinician is the trained falcon because owners will not tolerate damage to the bird's feathers. A feline induction box can be set up vertically, the hooded falcon placed (standing) in the chamber by its owner, and anesthesia induced with isoflurane. No excitement will occur, and no aversive "manning" restraint will be needed. The falcon can be removed smoothly from the box and quickly intubated for IMV inhalation anesthesia.

            d. Endotracheal tubes without cuffs are recommended for birds because they have complete tracheal rings with less circumferential elasticity than mammals have.

    C. The allometric formula for avian resting heartbeat frequency is as follows:

Resting Heart Rate in Birds $= 155.8 \, (W_{kg}^{-0.23})$ (Table 13–3, item j)

    1 *Examples:*

        a. A 12 kg California condor:

$$155.8 \, (12^{-0.23}) = 88 \text{ bpm}$$

        b. A 0.02 kg (20 g) house finch:

$$155.8 \, (0.02^{-0.23}) = 383 \text{ bpm}$$

X. Reptiles

    A. Core body temperature and body size are important considerations in anesthetizing ectotherms with injectable agents (Table 13–12).

    It is essential to understand two principles when anesthetizing reptiles:

        1. In treating reptilian ectotherms with any therapeutic agent, there is little hope for consistent results from subject to subject without understanding the dependence of dosage, uptake, distribution, and excretion on a variable (ectothermic) body temperature that is, in turn, dependent on environmental temperatures.

        2. In order to maintain effective blood levels, drug dose rates (mg/kg) will be greater and will need to be administered more frequently for small specimens than for large specimens (just as with mammals and birds).

Table 13–12. Heart Rate Ranges for Reptiles

The heartbeat rate ranges of reptiles at preferred body temperature by body size follow:

Body Weights	Heart Beat (per min.)
≤50 g	70–90
>50 g–1 kg	35–70
>1–5 kg	23–35
>5–10 kg	19–23
>10–20 kg	16–19
>20–50 kg	12–16
>50–100 kg	10–12

An indication that a specimen is at its preferred optimal core body temperature is when it has achieved its predicted heartbeat rate. Heartbeat rate in reptiles depends on core body temperature, not subjective alarm or excitement.

B. The importance of core body temperature
1. Metabolism in the ectothermic reptiles presumably functions most efficiently when core body temperature of most species reaches a temperature of around 37°C, a (physiologic) preferred body temperature (PBT).
2. Any reptile may survive varying periods of time with a core body temperature that is reduced and with the animal in a state of torpor or hibernation.
3. Trying to bring reptile patients close to their PBT is, therefore, essential when treating such animals with injectable therapeutic agents.
4. Even though reptiles are ectothermic—meaning their core body temperatures fluctuate with that of the environment—some reptiles function in cool native environments with body temperatures higher than ambient.
5. Whether or not a reptile is at its metabolic optimal state may be determined by taking the *cloacal temperature* and *determining the animal's heart rate.*
   a. Any reptile with a cloacal temperature of 27–30°C is probably close to its optimal core body temperature.
   b. When at its PBT, the reptile should exhibit its resting heart rate.
   c. Pulse may be determined with a Doppler ultrasonic blood flow detector. An *allometric formula for calculating resting pulse rate squamata and terrestrial chelonia,* (assuming PBT) follows:

   $$\text{Resting Heart Rate in Reptiles} = 34\ (W_{kg}{}^{-0.25})$$

   (1) Examples
      (i) A 500 g python:

      $$34\ (0.5^{-0.25}) = 40\ \text{bpm}$$

      (ii) A 32 kg python:

      $$34\ (32^{-0.25}) = 14\ \text{bpm}$$

D. The following injectable anesthetics are used in reptiles:
1. Ketamine (see Table 13–4)
   a. Ketamine is a readily available, rather ineffective agent for anesthesia

in reptiles. It only slows them down, but it sometimes facilitates endotracheal intubation and inhalant anesthesia with isoflurane.

   b. It provides poor muscle relaxation and, as with any anesthetic, *should never be relied upon to render venomous reptiles incapable of biting.*

   c. Overdosage with ketamine can result in death in reptiles via respiratory depression just as it does in other animals.

   d. The injectable anesthetics should be used to facilitate endotracheal intubation and inhalation anesthesia.

   e. Subjects should be accurately weighed before administration of injectable anesthetics.

   f. All injections should be placed deep within the muscle.

2. Ketamine plus xylazine (see Table 13–5)

   a. Ketamine (100 mg/ml) in combination with xylazine (20 mg/ml) is mixed in equal volumes.

   b. The combination is a dubious improvement over ketamine used by itself. It is, however, useful in extricating the head of a recalcitrant tortoise from its shell in order to endotracheally intubate the animal for inhalant (isoflurane) anesthesia.

3. The volatile liquid anesthetic, *isoflurane*, is highly recommended for prolonged anesthesia procedures in reptiles, as it is for other animals (see Figs. 13–7 and 13–8).

   a. Cuffed endotracheal tubes are not recommended for reptiles because excessive inflation of the cuff can easily damage their tracheal rings.

   b. As planes of general anesthesia with isoflurane deepen, muscular relaxation progresses from the head to the tail. Induction with isoflurane (4–5%) in oxygen is rapid in the intubated subject when supported by intermittent mandatory ventilation (IMV) of the lungs. Prior acclimation of reptiles to preferred body temperature is not necessary with inhalation anesthesia supported by IMV.

4. Although long periods of apnea caused by torpor or breath holding may be commonplace in normal reptiles, anesthetized subjects in which apnea occurs should be endotracheally intubated and mechanically ventilated.

5. An ultrasonic Doppler blood flow detector (Parks Electronics) is a very useful heart monitoring instrument for anesthesia in reptiles (as it is in birds and mammals).

XI. Amphibia and Anura

  A. Amphibia may be intubated *laryngeally* for inhalation anesthesia with isoflurane.

  B. Bifurcation of the bronchi occurs immediately caudad to the larynx in the Anura (frogs and toads), and bronchial attachments to the larynx are very delicate. Be careful not to tear them off trying to force the tube too far.

PHARMACEUTICALS

1. ANTAGONIL, Wildlife Laboratories (yohimbine HCl)
Sterile injection: 5 mg/ml. For intravenous use
Xylazine reversing agent
Wildlife Laboratories, Inc., 1401 Duff Drive, Suite 600, Fort Collins, CO 80524
2. ANTISEDAN, Orion Corporation (atipamezole HCl)
Sterile injectable solution: 5 mg/ml. For intramuscular use in dogs only
Medetomidine reversing agent

Distributed by Animal Health, Exton, PA 19341
Division of Pfizer Inc., New York, NY 10017
3. VALIUM, Roche Laboratories (diazepam solution)
Sterile injection: 5 mg/ml. For intramuscular and intravenous use. Insoluble in water
Benzodiazepine derivative tranquilizer for relief of anxiety and for muscle relaxation
Mfd. by Steris Labs, Inc., Phoenix, AZ 85043
4. DOMITOR, Orion Corporation (medetomidine HCl)
Sterile injectable solution: 1 mg/ml. For intramuscular and intravenous use in dogs only
Sedative and analgesic
Distributed by Pfizer Animal Health, Pfizer Inc., West Chester, PA 19380
5. DORMOSEDAN, Orion Corporation (detomidine HCl)
Sterile solution: 10 mg/ml. For intramuscular and intravenous use in horses only
Sedative and analgesic
Dist. by Pfizer Animal Health, Pfizer Inc., West Chester, PA 19380
6. TELAZOL, Elkins-Sinn, Inc. (Cherry Hill, NJ 08003) (tiletamine HCl and zolazepam HCl)
To each vial, add 5 ml of sterile water. For intramuscular use in dogs and cats only
Anesthetic agent
Distributed by Fort Dodge Laboratories, Inc., Fort Dodge, IA 50501
7. ROMPUN, Bayer Corp. (xylazine HCl)
Solutions of 2% or 10%. For intravenous and intramuscular use in cats, dogs (2%), and horses (10%)
Sedative and analgesic
Bayer Corporation, Agriculture Division of Animal Health, Shawnee Mission, KS 66201
8. VERSED, Roche Laboratories (midazolam HCl)
Solution of 0.5%. For intramuscular and intravenous use
Benzodiazepine derivative tranquilizer and muscle relaxant
Hoffmann-La Roche Inc., 340 Kingsland Street, Nutley, NJ 07110-1199
9. KETASET, (ketamine HCl)
Solution of 10%. For intramuscular and intravenous use
Fort Dodge Laboratories, Inc., Fort Dodge, IA 50501

SYRINGE DART SYSTEMS

1. TELINJECT, USA, Inc., 23655 San Femando Rd., Newhall, CA 91321; 805-255-0617
2. CAP-CHUR EQUIPMENT, Palmer Chemical & Equipment Co., Inc., Palmer Village, Box 867, Douglasville, GA 30133
3. PNEU DART Inc., P. O. Box 1415, Williamsport, PA 17703

INSTRUMENTS FOR MONITORING ANESTHESIA

1. SENSOR DEVICES, INC., VET/OX 4402
Veterinary Specific Pulse Oximeter.
SpO_2 and pulse rate
2. VET/CAP 7000
End-Tidal CO_2 Monitor.
SDI Sensor Device Inc., 407 Pilot Court, #400 A, Waukesha, WI 53188, 800-246-8300

3. ULTRASONIC DOPPLER BLOOD FLOW DETECTOR, Model 811-B, Parks Medical Electronics, Inc., Aloha, OR

Suggested Readings

Abrams JT: Fundamental approach to the nutrition of captive wild animals. In Crawford A (ed): Symposia of the Zoological Society of London. New York: Academic Press, 1968, pp. 41–62.

Brody S: Bioenergetics and Growth. New York: Reingold, 1945.

Freireich, EJ, Gehan, EA, Rall, DP, et al.: Quantitative comparison of toxicity of anticancer agents in mouse, rat, hamster, dog, monkey and man. Cancer Chemother Rep 50(4): 219–229, 1966.

Ginsberg N, Tager I: Practical Guide to Antimicrobial Agents. Baltimore: Williams and Wilkins, 1981, pp. 74–76, 82–84.

Hainsworth FR: Animal Physiology Adaptations in Function. Reading, PA: Addison-Wesley, 1981, pp. 160–163.

Hardman JG (ed): Goodman & Gilman's The Pharmacological Basis of Therapeutics, 9th ed. New York: McGraw-Hill Co., 1996, pp. 217, 227.

Mordenti J: Dosage regimen design for pharmaceutical studies conducted in animals. J Pharm Sci 75(9): 852–856, 1986.

Mordenti J: Man versus beast. J Pharm Sci 75(1): 1028–1040, 1986.

Mordenti J, Chappell W: The use of interspecies scaling in toxicokinetics. In Yacobi JS, Batra V (eds): Toxicokinetics and New Drug Development. New York: Pergamon Press, 1989, pp. 42–96.

Ogilvie GK, et al.: Efficacy of mitoxantrone against various neoplasms in dogs. JAVMA 198(9): 1618–1621, 1991.

Peters RH: The Ecological Implications of Body Size. Cambridge, MA: Cambridge University Press, 1987, pp. 45–53.

Riviere JE, Craigmill, AL, Sundlof, SF: Handbook of Comparative Pharmacokinetics and Residues of Veterinary Antimicrobials. Boca Raton, FL: CRC Press Inc, 1991, pp. 22–23.

Schmidt-Nielsen K: Scaling—Why Is Animal Size So Important? Cambridge, MA: Cambridge University Press, 1984, pp. 90–98.

Sedgwick C: Scaling emergency treatments allometrically: The importance of body size. In Fowler ME (ed): Zoo and Wild Animal Medicine, 3rd ed. Philadelphia: WB Saunders Co, in press.

Sedgwick C: Extrapolating Rational Drug Doses and Treatment Periods by Allometric Scaling. Scientific Proceedings of the American Animal Hospital Association, 55th annual meeting, Denver: American Animal Hospital Association, 1988, pp. 156–161.

Sedgwick CJ, Kaufman G: Metabolic scaling: Using estimated energy costs to extrapolate drug doses between different species and different individuals of diverse body sizes. Proceedings American Association of Zoo Veterinarians, annual meeting, pp. 249–254.

Shapiro BA, et al.: Clinical Application of Respiratory Care. Chicago, IL: Year Book Medical Publishers, Inc., 1975, pp. 299–301.

Etorphine or Carfentanil

Doses for Chemical Immobilization of Very Large Mammals

Multiply an animal's MEC by the MEC/SMEC dose to obtain a takedown dose in micrograms (μg); or, multiply by its SMEC to obtain the comparative dose rate as micrograms per kilogram (μg/kg), i.e., MEC = 70 ($W_{kg}^{0.75}$); SMEC = [70 ($W_{kg}^{0.75}$)]/W_{kg} = 70 ($W_{kg}^{-0.25}$). Low doses may be given intravenously at moderate rates and intramuscularly if the patients are calm. High doses of etorphine or carfentanil are usually necessary for intramuscular administrations and for animals that are agitated. The antagonist MEC/SMEC doses for **diprenorphine** are used to calculate reversal doses for etorphine and carfentanil.

MEC/SMEC Doses
(Dimensionless Numbers)

Agonists (Antagonist)	Etorphine			Carfentanil		
	Low	High	Diprenorphine	Low	High	Diprenorphine
Subject category A						
1 rhinoceroses, tapirs	0.09	0.2	0.5	0.067	0.15	0.5
2 elephants	0.15	0.25	0.4	0.11	0.2	0.4
Subject category B						
3 giraffids	0.2	0.75	1.2	0.15	0.56	1.2
4 zoo bovids	0.22	1.1	1.4	0.16	0.82	1.4
5 large cervids (>150 kg)	0.37	1.2	1.6	0.27	0.9	1.6
6 small cervids (<150 kg)	0.65	1.5	1.8	0.5	1.1	1.8
7 large antelopes (>150 kg)	0.6	1.8	3.0	0.5	1.3	3.0
8 small antelopes (<150 kg)	0.75	1.5	3.0	0.56	1.1	2.0
9 zoo ovids	0.75	1.5	3.0	0.56	1.1	2.0
10 zoo caprids, antelocaprids	0.75	1.5	3.0	0.56	1.2	2.0
11 zoo equids (zebras)	0.75	1.5	5.0	0.64	1.2	3.0
12 suids, tayassuids	0.85	2.5	3.5	0.63	1.5	3.5
Subject category C						
13 bears	0.25	0.45	0.75	0.18	0.33	0.75

Etorphine or Carfentanil in combination with xylazine or medetomidine for Takedown

Multiply the animal's MEC by the MEC/SMEC dose of etorphine or carfentanil plus xylazine or medetomidine to obtain a takedown dose in micrograms (μg), i.e., MEC = 70 ($W_{kg}^{0.75}$); SMEC = [70 ($W_{kg}^{0.75}$)]/W_{kg} = 70 ($W_{kg}^{-0.25}$); or, multiply by the animal's SMEC to obtain the dose rates as micrograms per kilogram (μg/kg). The MEC/SMEC doses for the opioid antagonist **diprenorphine** and the alpha$_2$-adrenergic antagonist **yohimbine** are given under Antagonists (IV). Antagonists are administered intravenously.

MEC/SMEC Doses
(Dimensionless Numbers)

Agonists (IM)	Etorphine with xylazine or medetomide			Carfentanil with xylazine or medetomidine		
Subject category A						
1 elephants	0.08–0.15	3.0	0.03	0.06–0.11	3.0	0.03
Subject category B						
2 giraffids	0.15–0.5	3.3	0.03	0.11–0.37	3.3	0.03
3 zoo bovids	0.15–0.75	3.3	0.05	0.11–0.56	3.3	0.05
4 lg cervids (>150 kg)	0.25–0.8	30.0	0.3	0.18–0.6	30.0	0.3
5 small cervids	0.45–1.0	40.0	0.4	0.33–0.75	40.0	0.4
6 lg antelopes (>150 kg)	0.45–1.0	40.0	0.4	0.33–0.75	40.0	0.4
7 small antelopes	0.5 –1.5	40.0	0.4	0.37–1.1	40.0	0.4
Antagonists (IV)	Diprenorphine 0.16–3	Yohimbine 15–35		Diprenorphine 0.12–3	Yohimbine 15–35	

Opioid-Opiate Analgesic Dose Rates for Mammals Postsurgery

Each analgesic in the following list is arranged according to potency; the most potent is carfentanil, the least is codeine. For example, for a 70-kg animal: Analgesic regimens would be #1 carfentanil, 0.12 μg/kg q10h, or #10 meperidine, 0.7 mg/kg q3h. A clinician would use regimens in the following list to provide analgesia, to make a patient more comfortable postsurgically, or after trauma.

Directions for Scaling Opioid-Opiate Analgesic Treatment Regimens from SMEC

Multiply a patient's SMEC by the SMEC dose (dimensionless number) to obtain a dose rate of mg/kg, i.e., $SMEC = [70(W_{kg}^{0.75})]/W_{kg} = 70(W_{kg}^{-0.25})$. Multiply the patient's SMEC by the SMEC frequency (dimensionless number) to obtain the frequency of treatments per day (24 hr). Divide 24 by treatments per day to estimate the time between treatments. *Dose rates may be doubled (except for felids and equids) based on the judgment of a clinician.*

		Dimensionless Numbers	
Opioid Analgesics	Route	SMEC Dose	SMEC Frequency
Carfentanil	IM	5.0×10^{-6}	1.0×10^{-1}
Etorphine	IM	6.0×10^{-6}	1.0×10^{-1}
Fentanyl	IM, SC	6.0×10^{-5}	1.0×10^{-1}
Buprenorphine	IM	2.4×10^{-4}	2.5×10^{-1}
Oxymorphone	IM, SC	6.0×10^{-4}	2.5×10^{-1}
Butorphanol	IM	1.2×10^{-3}	2.5×10^{-1}
Morphine	IM, SC	6.0×10^{-3}	2.5×10^{-1}
Nalbuphine	IM	6.0×10^{-3}	2.5×10^{-1}
Pentazocine	IM, SC	2.0×10^{-2}	2.5×10^{-1}
Meperidine	IM, SC	4.4×10^{-2}	3.3×10^{-1}
Codeine	IM	7.7×10^{-2}	3.3×10^{-1}
Felids			
Oxymorphone	IM, SC	3.0×10^{-4}	2.5×10^{-1}
Morphine	IM, SC	3.0×10^{-3}	2.5×10^{-1}
Meperidine	IM, SC	1.5×10^{-3}	3.3×10^{-1}
Equids			
Oxymorphone	IM, SC	2.0×10^{-4}	2.5×10^{-1}
Morphine	IM, SC	2.0×10^{-4}	2.5×10^{-1}
Meperidine	IM, SC	1.0×10^{-3}	3.3×10^{-1}

Index

Note: Page numbers in *italics* refer to illustrations; page numbers followed by (t) refer to tables.

357

Breathing *(Continued)*
  irregular, 165–166
  Kussmaul, 166
  labored, 166–167
    during recovery from anesthesia, 205–211
      causes of, 206–207, 208(t)
    rates of, 129
    vs. agonal gasps, 130
Breathing system(s), 97–101
  Bain, 100–101, *101*
  circle, *93*, 97–100
  noncircle, 100
  pediatric, 100
  vaporizer-inside-circuit, 95, 96
  vaporizer-outside-circuit, 93
Breath sounds, 131–132
Breed predispositions, of dogs, in responding to
    anesthesia, 1–2, 314–316
Bronchospasm, 160, 162
  treatment of, 162
    drugs used in, 148, 149(t), 162
Bronchovesicular breath sounds, 131
"Bubbling" sounds, on auscultation, 132
Bulldogs, intubation of, obstacles to, 149–150
Bupivacaine, for pain, 199, 233, 234
Buprenorphine, 28
  action of, duration of, 13(t)
  postoperative pain control with, 198(t), 241(t)
    dose scaling for, in large mammals, 355(t)
  premedication with, dosage for, 13(t)
Butorphanol, 28
  action of, duration of, 13(t)
  combined with ketamine, dosage of, 44(t)
  combined with Telazol, to sedate fractious ani-
      mal, 51
  combined with tranquilizer, in neuroleptanalge-
      sia, 30(t)
    for geriatric patient, 277(t)
    for patient with systemic dysfunction, 286,
      313
    for pediatric patient, 270
  control of ketamine-induced behavioral distur-
      bances with, in cat, 213
  enhancement of anesthetic depth with, dosage
      for, 155, 186
  limiting of muscle activity with, in hyperther-
      mic cat, 217
  postoperative pain control with, 198(t), 241(t),
      242(t)
    dose scaling for, in large mammals, 355(t)
  premedication with, 13(t)
    in pediatric patient, 270
Butyrophenone-derived preanesthetic agents, 17
  dosages of, for dog or cat, 13(t)

Cachexia, anesthetic considerations in presence of,
    2, 4
Cage, oxygen, 203
California condor. See also *Birds.*
  anesthesia in, *342*
Carbicarb, for metabolic acidosis, 259
Carbon dioxide, partial pressure of, in arterial
    blood, 132
Carbon dioxide absorber, rapid heat build-up in,
    significance of, 173
Cardiac arrest, 176–180
  air embolism and, 174
  EKG findings associated with, 177, *177*

Cardiac arrest *(Continued)*
  management approach based on, 178–179
  respiratory arrest preceding, 177
Cardiac dysrhythmias, complicating anesthesia,
    179–183
Cardiac massage, external, in cardiopulmonary
    resuscitation, 178, 179, 180
  in treatment of sinus bradycardia, 176
  internal, in cardiopulmonary resuscitation, 178,
    180
Cardiomyopathy, 280
Cardiopulmonary resuscitation, 178–180
Cardiovascular function, adverse effects of
    anesthesia on, 174–190
  impaired, 278–282
    anesthesia in presence of, 280–281
Cardiovascular monitoring, 135–143
Cardioversion, 180
Carfentanil, effects of, diprenorphine dosages for
    reversal of, 354(t)
  scaling of dosage of, for large mammal, 354(t),
    355(t)
Carnivores, large mammalian. See also *Large
    mammals.*
  anesthesia in, 329
    wearing off of, and resistance to handling,
      339
  intubation of, *337, 338*
Carprofen, for pain, 235–236, 236(t)
Cat(s), aged. See *Geriatric patient(s).*
  blood pressure in, 186
    abnormal. See *Hypertension; Hypotension.*
  blood volume in, 184
  hyperthermia in, muscle activity and, treatment
    of, 217
  ketamine-induced behavioral disturbances in,
    211
    butorphanol for, 213
  ketamine-preanesthetic combinations used in,
    dosages of, 44(t)
  muscle relaxant dosage for, 82, 83, 84, 85
  neuroleptanalgesic dosages for, preanesthetic,
    30(t), 277(t)
  neuromuscular blocking agents used in, dosages
    of, 82, 83, 84, 85
  NSAIDs used in, dosages of, 236(t)
    ulcer risk associated with, management of,
      238(t)
  opioid dosages for, 241(t), 242(t)
  preanesthetic dosages for, 13(t)
    combined narcotic and non-narcotic, 30(t),
      277(t)
  preanesthetic-ketamine combinations used in,
    dosages of, 44(t)
  six to 12 weeks old. See *Pediatric patient(s).*
  urethral obstruction in, 297
  wild. See also *Large mammals.*
    intubation of, *338*
    opioid dosages for, calculation of, 355(t)
    resistance of, to handling, despite anesthetiza-
      tion, *339*
Catheter(s), nasal, oxygen delivery via, 203–204
Catheterization, urethral, anesthesia for, 297
Central nervous system. See also *Brain.*
  adverse effects of anesthesia on, 152, 220–221
  organic disease of, anesthesia in presence of,
    298
Central sensitization, and pain sensation, 229
Central venous pressure (CVP), 138–140

Morphine *(Continued)*
  premedication with, 26
    dosage for, 13(t)
  sedation with, in treatment of pulmonary
    edema, 224
Mouth specula, 107
Mucous membranes, assessment of, for cyanotic
  discoloration, 131. See also *Cyanosis.*
Murphy-style endotracheal tube, 105, *106*
Muscle relaxants, 78–88
  adverse side effects of, 79
  antagonists to, 86–87
  depolarizing, 79–80
    effects of, 82–83
  dosage of, for cats, 82, 83, 84, 85
    for dogs, 82, 83, 84, 85
  nondepolarizing, 80
    antagonists to, 86–87
    effects of, 83, 84, 85, 86
  persistence of effects of, 200–201
    management approach to, 210
    tests for, 87
      in animal slow to recover from anesthesia,
        222
Myelography, candidate for, anesthesia in, 300
  complications of, 299, 300

Nalbuphine, postoperative pain control with,
  241(t)
  dose scaling for, in large mammals, 355(t)
Nalorphine, reversal of opioid effects with, 20(t),
  29
Naloxone, reversal of opioid effects with, 20(t),
  29, 149(t), 153, 209
  in newborn, 306
Narcotics. See *Opioid* entries.
Nasal catheter, oxygen delivery via, 203–204
Neostigmine, 86–87
  use of, as antagonist to neuromuscular blocking
    agents, 86–87
    atropine administration preceding, 87
    dosage for, 87
Nerve blocks, for pain, 233–234
Nerve end plates, acetylcholinesterase in. See
  Acetylcholinesterase.
Neuroleptanalgesic(s), 29, 30(t)
  for geriatric patient, 277, 277(t)
  for patient with systemic dysfunction, 286, 313
  for pediatric patient, 270
  use of lidocaine with, in patient undergoing ce-
    sarean section, 303
Neurologic dysfunction. See *Brain; Central
  nervous system.*
Neuromuscular blocking agents, 78–88
  adverse side effects of, 79
  antagonists to, 86–87
  depolarizing, 79–80
    effects of, 82–83
  dosage of, for cats, 82, 83, 84, 85
    for dogs, 82, 83, 84, 85
  nondepolarizing, 80
    antagonists to, 86–87
    effects of, 83, 84, 85, 86
  persistence of effects of, 200–201
    management approach to, 210
    tests for, 87
      in animal slow to recover from anesthesia,
        222

Newborn. See also *Pediatric patient(s).*
  management of, after cesarean delivery, 305–
    306
  response of, to anesthesia, 2
Nitrous oxide, 71–73
  advantages of, 72
  disadvantages of, 73, 165, 168
    in cases of gastrointestinal dysfunction, 312,
      313
  effects of, 71–72
  expanded pneumothorax due to, 168
  human exposure to, dosimetry of, 76
  minimum alveolar concentration of, 59(t)
  physical properties of, 58(t), 71
  solubility of, 71
    partition coefficients for, 59(t)
Nociceptors, stimulation of, and pain, 227, 228
Noncircle breathing systems, 100
Nondepolarizing muscle relaxants, 80
  antagonists to, 86–87
  effects of, 83, 84, 85, 86
Nonrebreathing systems, 100
Nonsteroidal anti-inflammatory drugs (NSAIDs),
  for pain, 234–239, 236(t)
  ulcer risk associated with, management of,
    238(t), 238–239

Obesity, anesthesia in presence of, 2, 4, 40, 316
Obstetric anesthesia. See *Cesarean section;
  Pregnancy.*
Ohio #8 vaporizer (drawover vaporizer), 94, 96
Oliguria, 218–219. See also *Renal function,
  impaired.*
Omeprazole, for NSAID-induced ulcers, 238(t),
  239
Opioid(s), 239–240
  antagonists to. See *Opioid antagonists* and spe-
    cific agents, e.g., *Naloxone.*
  biotransformation of, in liver, 289
  effects of, on respiration, 25, 283
  for geriatric patient, 277
  for large mammal, dose scaling of, 354(t),
    355(t)
  for patient with systemic dysfunction, 280
  for pediatric patient, 270
  pain control with, 198–199, 240–246
    postoperative, 198(t), 198–199, 240–246
      dose scaling for, in large mammals, 355(t)
      oral route of administration for, 242
        dosages used in, 242(t)
      parenteral route of administration for,
        241–242
        dosages used in, 241(t)
  panting due to, 172–173
  premedication with, 24–28
  receptors for, 24, 240
  sinus bradycardia due to, prophylaxis against, in
    pediatric patient, 270
  tranquilizers used with. See *Neuroleptanalgesic(s).*
Opioid agonist-antagonists, 26
  for pain, 241
Opioid antagonists, 20(t), 26, 29. See also specific
  agents, e.g., *Naloxone.*
Oscillation, high-frequency, 121
Osmolality, 248–249
Overdose, 152–153
  atropine, signs of, 14
  causes of, 152–153

Vomiting *(Continued)*
  as indication for cimetidine or metoclopramide, 312
  complicating induction of anesthesia, 151–152

Warming, of hypothermic animal, 144–145, 194
Waste gases, hazards associated with, 73–76, 101–102
  methods of avoiding exposure to, 103
  scavenging systems for, 102, *102*
Weaning, from ventilatory support, 119–121
Weight. See also *Size differentials.*
  and response to anesthesia, 2, 4, 40, 316
Wheezes, 131
Whole blood, transfusion of. See *Blood transfusion.*
Wildlife anesthesia, 318–355. See also *Birds; Large mammals; Reptiles.*
  benzodiazepines as aid to, 348
  body size differentials in, 320, 339
    metabolic values correlated with, 322(t)
  body surface area differentials in, 320, 321(t), 340
  dissociative agents used in. See *Large mammals, dissociative anesthetics for.*
  dose scaling in, 321(t), 340, 341, 343, 354(t), 355(t)
  energy differentials in, 320, 321(t), 343

Wildlife anesthesia *(Continued)*
    metabolic values correlated with, 322(t)
  heart rate estimation in candidate for, 347
  mechanical ventilator in, 334
  "metabolic size" in, 341
  principles of, 344–348
  syringe darts in, 337–339, 345, 346
    handling of, precautions in, 318
    suppliers of, 352
Wolf, compared biostatistically with koala and squirrel, 322(t)

Xylazine, 20–22
  action of, duration of, 13(t)
  combined with ketamine, dosage of, 44(t)
    for large animal, 324(t)
    in anesthetization of reptile, 350
  overdose of, treatment of, 153
  premedication with, 22
    dosage for, 13(t)

Yohimbine, as alpha$_2$-adrenergic antagonist, 20(t), 23, 345(t)

Zolazepam, combined with tiletamine. See *Telazol.*